T0257695

Chinese Medicine and Healing

Chinese Medicine and Healing

Edited by **Patrick Lampard**

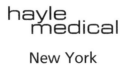

New York

Published by Hayle Medical,
30 West, 37th Street, Suite 612,
New York, NY 10018, USA
www.haylemedical.com

Chinese Medicine and Healing
Edited by Patrick Lampard

© 2015 Hayle Medical

International Standard Book Number: 978-1-63241-080-1 (Hardback)

This book contains information obtained from authentic and highly regarded sources. Copyright for all individual chapters remain with the respective authors as indicated. A wide variety of references are listed. Permission and sources are indicated; for detailed attributions, please refer to the permissions page. Reasonable efforts have been made to publish reliable data and information, but the authors, editors and publisher cannot assume any responsibility for the validity of all materials or the consequences of their use.

The publisher's policy is to use permanent paper from mills that operate a sustainable forestry policy. Furthermore, the publisher ensures that the text paper and cover boards used have met acceptable environmental accreditation standards.

Trademark Notice: Registered trademark of products or corporate names are used only for explanation and identification without intent to infringe.

Printed in the United States of America.

Contents

Preface

In the past few years, traditional Chinese medicine (TCM) has drawn the attention of researchers from all over the world. This book introduces the readers to the vast field of Chinese medicine with the help of comprehensive details and information. TCM is gradually evolving as a subject area with high potential and a possibility for original innovation. The book gives understanding of the TCM researches by discussing diagnostic approach and current clinical applications under two sections: pharmacological experimental research and pharmacodynamic material base research. This book includes contributions of eminent researchers who possess clinical knowledge and have years of experience in this field. It serves the objective of providing deep understanding of the distinct characteristics of Chinese medicine.

Significant researches are present in this book. Intensive efforts have been employed by authors to make this book an outstanding discourse. This book contains the enlightening chapters which have been written on the basis of significant researches done by the experts.

Finally, I would also like to thank all the members involved in this book for being a team and meeting all the deadlines for the submission of their respective works. I would also like to thank my friends and family for being supportive in my efforts.

Editor

Part 1

Pharmacological Experimental Research

Traditional Chinese Herbal Medicine – East Meets West in Validation and Therapeutic Application

John W.M. Yuen, Sonny H.M. Tse
and Jolene Y.K. Yung
*School of Nursing, The Hong Kong Polytechnic University, Hong Kong SAR,
China*

1. Introduction

Chinese herbal medicine has been practiced for thousands of years, and is used increasingly in western countries in conjunction with or in place of allopathic medicine. The earliest extant book of material medica, known as *Shen Nong Bencaojing* (The divine farmer's material medica), appeared in the third century AD. At that time, the Father of Chinese herbal medicine Shen Nong, had classified 365 entities of herbs and drugs (Yang, 2005). The herbal tradition reached its peak some thousand years later, in 1552-1578 AD, of when Li Shi-zhen compiled his Great Herbal *Bencao Gangmu* (Compendium of Materia Medica) of 52 volumes which described 1,892 herbal entities in details (Li, 2003). The World health Organization (WHO) estimates that at least 75% of the world's population utilizes traditional medicines for healing and curing diseases (Robinson & Zhang, 2011). However, the holistic concepts of traditional Chinese medicine (TCM) are far removed from the reductionist principles of the modern day Western approach, and are difficult to express and comprehend in western terms. Western medicine is evidence-based and disease-focused, and relies on the double blinded, randomized, controlled clinical trial as the gold standard to assess clinical utility and safety of treatment, which is usually a pure chemical with a defined pharmacological action. Conversely, TCM is based on history, experience, culture and belief, and most herbal medicines are complex mixtures of largely unknown chemical composition. In western terms, the health benefits of most herbal remedies remain unsubstantiated by scientific evidence in well-designed human studies, and this limits their acceptance by western trained health professionals. In addition to efficacy, the issues of toxicity and of herb-herb and herb-drug interaction that might be additive, synergistic or antagonistic need comprehensive scientific study. In this chapter, we overview the divergence and convergence between the two systems, and explore into nowadays methods used in herbal case-studies representing different stages of herbal use and evaluation. More importantly, the need for and feasibility of performing controlled trials for scientific validation of herbal medicine are discussed, thus repositioning the herbal research, and helping to decide the most favorable direction for East meets West.

2. The conceptual divergence between Western and Eastern perspectives

Looking into the world history, modern medicine is known to be originated from the ancient Egyptian medicine, and largely influenced by the Greek medical ideas about anatomy, physiology and practical medicine. Different cultures, from their very beginning, have established their own special ways in the care of the sick (Longrigg, 1997). The earliest written evidences (10,000-2000 BC) have mentioned the practice of Chinese medicine and imhotep in Egypt, which both commonly used medicinal herbs as the treatment modality (Bynum, 2008). Such ancient medical approaches, were largely influence by the cultural and religious beliefs, have later on transformed into scientific disciplines to its own effective and safe practice. The beginnings of true medical science in the West were laid when the reliance on superstition that underpinned tribal medicine was replaced by civilized and rational curiosity about the cause of illness. Modern medicine, at first glance, especially in the past century, is moving from triumph to triumph with the growing number of survivors, it has gained the prevailing acceptance. However, Chinese medicine, holding the key traditional beliefs of healing – holism, is divided into special disciplines e.g. herbalism and acupuncture in the alternative and complementary medicine. Scientific and alternative medical approaches have followed different paths at different speeds. Rational treatment ultimately depends upon properly understanding the true nature of disease. Orthodox and unorthodox practitioners have relied for centuries on 'tried-and-tested' methods to ensure the efficacy of empirical remedies. Empiricism has become the general principle to explain the purpose and rationale of therapy (Tong, 2010). The conundrum of east meets west - let's first look into the theory and thinking of the two perspectives.

2.1 The Western perspective

During the last two centuries, western medicine has developed and been practiced both generally and officially in those industrial nations that are collectively known as 'the West'. The modernization of medicine begun with the taxonomy and classification by grouping of signs and symptoms into disease entities (Bliss, 2011). The anatomic concept has formed the basis of disease identification, explaining and visualizing the cause of illness in the patient's internal anatomical organs (Duffin, 2010). Later on, disease and environment were bonded upon the discovery of small living organisms, i.e. microorganisms like bacteria and fungi, using microscope (Duffin, 2010). Thus, illnesses are diagnosed based on something so called the "demonstrable pathology". For cures, chemical drugs and surgery are the main therapeutic lines used to remove specifically the notable causes of the illness (e.g. antibiotics killing pathogenic bacteria, tumor removal in malignant diseases) or at least alleviation of symptoms and distress (Lock, 1997). In simple words, western medicine has a single-minded, materialistic approach that, basically, reduces all bodily function and dysfunction to material causes, mechanical mechanisms and structural flaws that can be thought of and studied in isolation from those who suffer from them – the so called 'science', which relies on objective, demonstrable, measurable, and self-evident observations. Western practitioners, at least many of them, are in fact treating the diseases rather than the patients. Empirical beliefs and tried remedies often persist beyond the actual needs of the patients and consequently affect quality-of-life, for example life-term hormone supplementation (with possible side-effects) is needed after the surgical removal of thyroid. Scientific medicine rejects all concepts of 'vitalism', the belief on immaterial spiritual or vital forces to explain natural phenomena (Lock, 1997). It has no place for 'life forces' or vital principles distinct from physical and chemical processes, and thus differs from the Eastern medical systems, particularly TCM.

2.2 The Eastern perspective

Traditional Chinese Medicine is originated from the culture and lives of the ancient orient, who considered life and death as the meaning of life forces. The underlying philosophy was established based on methods non-differentiable from the western one, namely objective observation, clinical practice, comparison, categorization, production, analysis, integration, and advancement. In other words, TCM is a subject of science specialty. The main difference between Chinese medicine and other medicine lies on "The sages in ancient times who knew the *Dao* (the tenets for cultivating health) who followed the rules of *yin* and *yang* and adjusted *Shushu* (the way to cultivate health)". According to the earliest text of Chinese medicine (206 BC-220 AD) *Huangdi neijing* (Yellow Emperor's Inner Canon), the doctrine of *Dao* is drawn from speculations of the two central theories, the creation of the universe (cosmology) and from direct observation of the natural world (Beinfield & Korngold, 2003). It postulated that all states of being, characteristics and physical phenomena could be categorized as either Yang, which was formless and existed conceptually in an association with heaven, light, heat and masculinity, or Yin, which corresponded to earth, darkness, cold and femininity. The principals of yin-yang suggest that each of these opposites produce the other, however, these verses draw lines of correspondence or association between sets of opposing states (Kaptchuk, 2000; van Wijk et al., 2010). The production of yin from yang and yang from yin occurs cyclically and constantly, so that no one principle continually dominates the other or determines the other (Mann, 2001; Unschuld, 2003). The *Tai Chi* (infinite void) symbol of yin yang (Figure 1) is emblematic of the continual change and renewal (Kaptchuk, 2000). Chinese people believe what the existence of human being is an organic whole which is integrated with the external environment. This idea is known as holism, dispute from the demonstrable anatomy in western medicine, concerning the functional rather than the physical body (Kaptchuk, 2000). Thus, the visceral organs in Chinese anatomy are actually groups of closely related physiological functions, which composed of *jing* (body essence), *qi* (energy), *shen* (spirit) – collectively known as the *San Bao* or 'three gems' and allowed the transportation of qi within the meridians for health maintenance (Kaptchuk, 2000; Unschuld, 2003). The essential qi of the five viscera, further divided into *Zang* (yin organs) and *Fu* (yang organs) are supplied by five corresponding tastes of foods, of each has its corresponding phase (known as five phases theory) (Table 1). The ingestion and storage of the five tastes nourish the five kinds of *qi* (*visceral qi*), however, the harmony of qi is essential for the production of jing and shen in the healthy body (Unschuld, 2003). The concept of five tastes of medicinal foods, derived from the long history of living and clinical experiences, has the direct linkage to the basic theories of yin-yang, five phases, viscera, meridian and collateral, in order to explain the cause of disease and therapeutic principle in TCM. Therefore, medicinal foods including large entities of herbs are commonly used for life nurturing and healing.

Disease diagnose in TCM is based on the pattern identification and syndrome differentiation. Rooting from the doctrine of yin and yang, the 'eight principles' were developed as the guiding principle to categorize illnesses into yin and yang, exterior and interior, cold and heat, deficiency and excess (Shiang & Li, 1971; Unschuld, 2003). Signs and symptoms of illness were comprehensively analyzed through the four examinations known as inspection, listening and smelling, inquiry, and palpation. With then, Chinese practitioners can determine the cause, nature and location of the pathogens, consider the disharmony between the disease and healthy qi, and conclude to identify the pattern of a certain nature following the rules of the eight principles. Upon identifying the disease pattern, a treatment plan, normally using herbal medicine and/or acupuncture, can be determined to rebalance the patient's inner yin and yang energy, and thus treating the root of the illness. Herbs may be prescribed individually or as part of a formula, of which formula are polyherbals including four typical components (Table 2) that promote the effective use of herbs (Covington, 2001). The ultimate aim of Chinese healing is to preserve or restore the healthy equilibrium of the body to adapt to the living environment. Chinese also believed that changing states either of body or of mind could affect the healthy balanced state, and therefore, an excessive emotion might cause a bodily illness or vice versa. Asian healers and practitioners treat consciousness as an organ of the body rather than a separate entity residing within it.

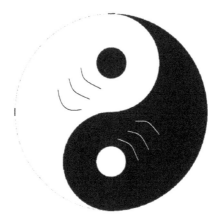

Fig. 1. Taijitu in motion. The forces of yin and yang are expressed in dark and white, respectively, are interdependent and interact constantly to form the integrated whole. Furthermore, the small circles of opposite shading illustrate that within the yin there is yang and vice versa, whereas the dynamic curve dividing them indicates that yin and yang are continuously merging, overall representing yin and yang's ability to create, control, and transform into each other (Yuen & Gohel, 2008).

Phases (Elements)	Tastes	Zang (yin organs)	Fu (yang organs)	Tissues	Sense organs
Wood	Sour	Liver	Gallbladder	Tendons	Eye
Fire	Bitter	Heart	Small intestine	Vessels	Tongue
Earth	Sweet	Spleen	Stomach	Muscles	Mouth
Metal	Pungent	Lung	Large intestine	Skin/hair	Nose
Water	Salty	Kidney	Bladder	Bones	Ear

Table 1. The Five phase theory. The five elements control the corresponding tissues and organs that are also correspondent with the five tastes of foods.

Components	Purpose
Principal	Use to treat the principal pattern of disease.
Associate	Use to assist the principal ingredient(s) in treating the major syndrome or serve as the main ingredient against a coexisting syndrome.
Adjutant	To enhance the effect of the principal ingredient, moderate or eliminate the toxicity of the principal or associate ingredients, or can have the opposite function of the principal ingredient(s) to produce supplementing effects.
Guide	To focus the actions of the formula on a certain meridian or area of the body or harmolize and integrate the actions of the other ingredients.

Table 2. The composition of typical herbal formula in TCM. Each component may consist of more than one herb, and a formula may not consist of all four components.

3. Junctions between the two systems of medicine – The dynamic equilibrium of the body as yin-yang interplay

While the maintenance of health and the treatment of disease are expressed in very different terms in the two cultures, the physiological processes and pathological changes that define human health are common in many aspects on each side of the East-West divide. Yet despite how difficult it is being illustrated in the language of modern medicine, the yin-yang theory governs the underlying principle of occurrence and development of diseases in TCM (Kaptchuk, 2000). An algorithmic scoring system is now available to group human subjects quantitatively into broad categories of yin and yang, in accordance to their health conditions expressed in the western terms (Langevin et al., 2004). More recently, a mathematical reasoning model using steady multilateral systems was successfully applied to guide the treatment of diseases based on the "*yin yang wu xing*" principle of TCM (Zhang, 2011). This is an important milestone, in East meets West, expressing the yin and yang entities numerically, which permits the mathematical manipulation and provides quantitative parameters for statistical analysis, which eventually make acceptance of TCM diagnosis to modern medicine with a standardized method and scientific validity. Maintaining yin and yang in harmony is akin to attaining the homeostatic state in modern medicine. However, the logic of yin-yang is often misunderstood as a matter of two complementary opposite qualities only, whereas the compensatory, synthetic and dialectical natures are entirely omitted. On the other hand, researchers have attempted to align the yin-yang concept with different physiological mechanisms of the body.

3.1 Oxidation and antioxidation

Reactive oxygen species (ROS), by-products of mitochondrial combustion, are generated alongside the adenosine triphosphate (ATP) during the process of oxidative phosphorylation in metabolism (Halliwell, 2009). ROS are known to be detrimental leading to oxidative damage of DNA, protein and lipid molecules, while the accumulation of such damage has been regarded as an endogenous cause of ageing as well as age-related disorders inclduing cancers (Finkel & Holbrook, 2000; Halliwell, 2009). Fortunately, our body has an antioxidant defense mechanism, in forms of endogenous enzymatic and dietary non-enzymatic molecules, to counteract the harmful activities of ROS *in vivo* (Gutteridge, 1994). Therefore, the balance between antioxidation and oxidation play an important role in health maintenance. The analogy of yin-yang balance with that of antioxidation-oxidation has been suggested by different researchers (Ko et al., 2004, 2006; Ou et al., 2003; Szeto & Benzie, 2006), who come up with a general agreement that yin corresponds to antioxidation and Yang corresponds to oxidation involved in energy metabolism. Researchers (Ou et al., 2003) proposed that, inside the body, yang represents the driving force for energy-generating oxidation processes, while yin exhibits the protective role of antioxidation. Pharmacologically, the 'yang-invigorating' herbs were found to promote ATP-generation capacity through stimulating the mitochondrial electron transport, in rat heart homogenates *ex vivo* (Ko et al., 2004, 2006) and cultured cardiomyocytes *in vitro* (Wong et al., 2011). In TCM, the heart plays a pivotal role in fueling the vital activities in all organs, hence promoting the body function in terms of 'Qi' (Kaptchuk, 2000;Ko et al., 2004). Experimental analysis has demonstrated that yang-herbs processed protective effects on DNA *ex vivo* from hydrogen peroxide challenge (Szeto & Benzie, 2006). Authors of the work then argued that the antioxidation-oxidation relationships are not necessarily obeyed to the opposite nature of yin and yang. In fact, apart from the antioxidant activities derived from the phytochemicals, ROS such as superoxides and nitric oxide, are also present in herbs (Achike & Kwan, 2003; Lin et al., 1995). In general, yin-herbs were found to have higher free-radical scavenging activities than yang-herbs (Ko & Leung, 2007; Szeto & Benzie, 2006). Herbs by themselves are not explicitly absolutely antioxidant or oxidant in nature. Antioxidant and ATP generation (oxidation) actions could be coexisted amongst yang-promoting herbs, while the ATP generation capacity was absence in yin-tonic herbs (Ko et al., 2004). Therefore, it is not surprising that yang-invigorating herbs are able to enhance the antioxidant status of human red cells after ingestion (Mak et al., 2004) and simultaneously protect DNA (Szeto & Benzie, 2006), further supporting the important role of the yin nature of yang-herbs being played in safeguarding the ATP generation process with ROS production. According to the Chinese Materia Medica (Bensky et al., 2004), some single herbs such as *Ganoderma lucidum* (Lingzi), are neutral in nature as they presumably contain complex chemical constituents and so have both yin and yang properties. The differential biochemical analysis of Lingzhi indicated that the water-soluble extract containing higher antioxidant capacities than its ethanol counterpart, were designated as the yin and yang, respectively (Yuen & Gohel, 2008). Functionally, in this study, the former (yin) reduced the carcinogen-induced oxidative DNA damage, while the later (yang) induced the formation of ROS and oxidative DNA damage resulting in apoptosis, in a pre-cancerous cell line (Yuen & Gohel, 2008). The authors anticipated that, even in a single herb, phytochemicals are interacting as yin and yang interplay that may be responsible for its multiple functions-bearing characteristic.

3.2 Immune balance

Given that many antioxidants are immunomodulating. The herb Cordyceps (*Cordyceps sinensis*) enhanced the concanavalin A (Con A)-stimulated splenocytes proliferation and the myocardial ATP generation capacity, which were disseminated in terms of TCM as 'yin-nourishment' and 'yang-invigoration', respectively (Siu et al., 2004). This is consistent with the notion of Ko and Leung (Ko & Leung, 2007) that yin-herbs, in addition to their significant antioxidant capcities, also possess immunomodulatory properties, including mitogen-stimulated proliferation of mouse splenocytes, cytokines secretion, leukocyte migration, and antibody production. In TCM, "Fu-zheng" therapy is one of the basic principles, literally equivalent to the promotion of the natural host defense mechanism, following the immunological balance of yin and yang (Macek, 1984). The Chinese believe that the herbal regimens may not only stimulate host defense but also enhance the vitality of their patients, hence the immune system resembles the yin aspect to support such vital yang aspects as the heart force and energy generation (Ko & Leung, 2007). The immunological yin-yang is considered as the cross-talk between the innate and adaptive arms of the immune system: the former serving to initiate a response of the latter, and the latter amplifying the former, defending the body from pathogens but sometimes exaggerating it certain immunological disorders (Lafaille & Mathis, 2002). The intricate immune network is composed of uncountable pairs of cells with activating/suppressive activities and stimulatory/inhibitory molecules, analogous regulatory interplay (Lafaille & Mathis, 2002; Macek, 1984). No doubt, T-suppressor and T-helper cells are in opposition but are totally interdependent, and an imbalance of either cell population can result in disease (Macek, 1984). Proinflammatory and antiinflammatory processes formed another interplaying pair that must be balanced to maintain health (Mann, 2001; Mills & Bhatt, 2004; Zhang, 2007). The interplay of interferon-gamma (IFN-γ) with other immune components was crucial to the development of autoimmune disease (Zhang, 2007). Hence, the inside views of yin-yang in the system denoted inflammatory process as yang, while its regulation as yin. Once an inflammatory process (yang) is initiated, IFN-γ is produced to promote inflammation until reaching the peak level, the inflammation then intensifies and compresses its opposite to activate a regulatory process (yin), and finally resulting in the reduction of inflammation. The differential immunological study of Lingzhi demonstrated that the ethanol extract in yang nature induced the secretion of proinflammatory interleukins (IL)-2, -6, and -8 via nuclear factor-kappaB (NF-κB) pathway in the apoptotic pre-cancer cells, but such effects were not exhibited by the water extract in yin nature (Yuen et al., 2011). This is explained that "yang initiates the expression of yin. Yang controls the origination and enjoys the completion of a process while yin follows the effects produced by yang and completes the work of yang" (Chan, 1969). In viral myocarditis, interleukin 6 (IL-6) played the paradoxical roles in promoting and suppressing the inflammation, to avert deleterious viral effects and to increase tissue destruction, respectively (Mann, 2001). Given that C-reactive protein (CRP) plays critical roles in atherosclerosis central to plaque progression and plaque rupture, the interplay of proinflammation and antiinflammation, that affecting the CRP levels is considered as a determinant for vascular health or illness (Mills & Bhatt, 2004). Such arterial inflammatory process is closely regulated by the local T-helper 1 (Th1)-type and Th2-type responses, with the principal inducers IL-12 and IL-10, respectively (Yang et al., 2010). Previous researches have demonstrated the presence of both IL-12 and IL-10 in atherosclerotic lesions, and the increase of IL-10 secretion led to the reduction in lesion size, that suggesting IL-10 is a counterbalancing factor that exerts its effect on Th1-Th2 cooperation by downregulating IL-12 and IL-18 production and inhibiting the Th1-based immune response, altogether to fully illustrate the yin-yang picture (Yang et al., 2010). The Th1/Th2 imbalance, an expression of yin-yang disharmony, causing the dichotomy between the humoral and cellular arms is related to pathological changes, such that cancerous tumor with Th2 dominant (Witz, 2008) and spontaneous abortion when Th1 reaction is in excess during pregnancy (Wilczynski, 2005).

3.3 Hormonal harmony

The biochemical meaning of yin-yang is extendable to the interaction between the immune system and other systems, involving a variety of hormones as key mediators. The endocrine system is known as one of the regulatory machineries to the immune response. Established literatures have documented that high levels of stress elevate the concentration of hormones such as glucocorticoids (cortisol or corticosterone) and catecholamines (epinephrine or norepinephrine), which exert immunosuppressive activities by binding the receptors on lymphocytes and impairing the immune defense, so that overall health will be altered (Kaye & Lightman, 2005; Vegiopoulos & Herzig, 2007). Consequently, certain soluble factors of the immune system, i.e. cytokines and interleukins, are altered to act on the brain and variety of endocrine pathways, to trigger feedback reactions in the Hypothalamic-pituitary-adrenal (HPA) axis (Dunn, 1996). The bidirectional interaction between the immune and the endocrine system is also reflected by its influence on the reproductive system, probably via the hypothamus-gonadal axis. Gonadal hormone like estrogen involves in the development of the thymus (an important lymphoid organ for lymphocyte differentiation), while the removal of thymus can induce pathologies in ovaries, testes and thyroid endocrine tissues, hence changes in one system will likely influence the other (Ahmed, 2000). The gender differences in brain development and immune response, possibly also in other non-gonadal organs, were explained as the compensatory yin-yang effects between sex chromosome and sex hormone status (Palaszynski et al., 2005). Furthermore, the functions of endocrine glands are explicitly controlled by the antagonizing sympathetic and parasympathetic activities of the autonomic nervous system in response to stimulation. In a recent human psychophysiological study, the decreases of parasympathetic and sympathetic activity were associated with the deficiency of yin and yang, respectively (Taitano et al., 2003). This is exemplified by the cardiac autonomic control that the activation of parasympathetic and sympathetic inputs to the heart in tandem results in greater cardiac output, demonstrating the synergistic and complementary properties of yin-yang interplay (Paton et al., 2005). In patients with hypothyroidism they are classified as having a deficiency of yang in terms of the TCM diagnosis, and the usage of yang tonifying herbs was shown to help in alleviating the symptoms (Kuang et al., 1988). As previously mentioned, yang-herbs actively promote the ATP-generation capacity and cardiac activity, and in hypothyroid rabbits, serum levels of thyroxine (T_3) and triiodothyronine (T_4) were elevated by intake of selected yang tonifying herbs, following the enhancement of myocardial β-adrenoceptor density and affinity (Min et al., 1998).

4. Feasibility of validating Eastern medicine by Western methods

The theory of yin-yang is explanatory to the biochemical activities of various biological phenomena, which supporting the feasibility of using western methods for TCM validation.

Regardless of what treatment principle behind, science and technology provide objective, accurate and reliable platforms for examining the effectiveness and efficacy of traditional therapeutic modalities. Herbal remedies are often marketed as dietary supplements, where they are not required to meet with the stringent clinical testing of pharmaceuticals, even though their usage may be for the same purpose, i.e. treatment of disease. Most herbal-derived medicines are complex mixtures of largely unknown chemical composition. They may be decoctions, infusions or extracts of one or many herbs, the quality and identity of which may vary widely, whose active ingredients are not well defined and whose molecular action is unknown. In light of the increasing globalization of herbal medicines, the WHO-leading authorities have put plenty of efforts to setup guidelines and regulations for the herbal identification and quality control (World Health Organization Special Programme for Research and Training in Tropical Diseases (WHO-TDR, 2005).

4.1 Authentication of herbal identity and quality control of ingredients
In TCM, herbs are traditionally authenticated by smell, taste and appearance that are totally dependent on the prescriber's experience. Even a famous herb such as ginseng, cases of misidentification have caused adverse reactions after use have been reported (Yap et al., 2008). Right herb possessing the right properties must be given to a right person for the right purpose. Therefore, reliable authentication becomes an important issue to safeguard the efficacy and safety about the usage of herbal medicine. Fingerprint analysis is accepted as the standard methodology for the assessment of natural products (WHO-TDR, 2005). Each herbal species has its unique fringerprint chemical profile containing an array of individual compounds separated and developed by chromatographic technique coupled with suitable detection methods (Schaneberg et al., 2003; Tistaert et al., 2011). There are several chromatographic techniques that can be used for the fingerprint profiling, including *Thin layer chromatography* for fast screening of samples, *High performance liquid chromatography (HPLC)* for high resolution, selectivity and sensitivity, *Ultra-High performance liquid chromatography* for superior sensitivity and resolution to HPLC, *Hydrophilic interaction chromatography* for retention and separation of hydrophilic compounds, and *Gas chromatography* for characterization and identification for volatile compounds (Tistaert et al., 2011). Additionally, there are some pattern recognition methods (some sort of statistical methods), which enable the visualization and further exploratory data analysis on information that is included in the chromatographic profile, are available for addressing the difficult differentiation of some closely related species (Lu et al., 2005; Tistaert et al., 2011; Zhao et al., 2009). The quality of herbs may vary due to the cultivation conditions, breeds and places of origin, for examples, liquid chromatographic coupled with multistage mass spectrometry (HPLC-MS) technique has revealed there to be non-stable and inconsistence of chemical constituents amongst different batches of Lingzhi samples (Chen et al., 2008a). In this regard, the research team (Chen et al., 2008b) has demonstrated the feasibility of employing multiple statistical analyses of HPLC fingerprints of Lingzhi to discriminate samples in accordance of origin of cultivation (Chen et al., 2008b). For fingerprinting the complicated decoctions, multi-herb botanical drug products, multiple chromatographic fingerprinting was suggested, in order to capture the complete picture of chemical profile (Fan et al., 2006). By employing such chromatographic technology, herbs of different species that share the identical bioactive ingredients, or at least a particular chemical fraction, can be merged and classified to facilitate the standardization of herbal products (Xie et al., 2010). In

the past decade, the rapid growth of molecular techniques has also benefited the herbal authentication. Numerous polymerase chain reaction (PCR)-based and sequencing methods using specific probes have shown to be applicable for validating the herbal identities (Chang et al., 2009; Herrero et al., 2010; Law et al., 2011). Particularly, random amplified polymorphic DNA (RAPD) profiling, a newly developed cost-effective PCR-based technique, has extensively used to differentiate large number of medicinal species from their close relatives or adulterants (Khan et al., 2011; Kiran et al., 2010). Not surprising, encouraging outcomes support the development of DNA barcoding technique, which enables the fast screen of botanical identities just like we checking out at the supermarkets (Song et al., 2009).

4.2 Extraction and fractionation of herbs – recovery of the active ingredients

For pharmaceutical preparation, the technique of HPLC-MS is still promising the characterization and isolation of chemical constituents from medicinal plants (Han et al., 2009; Yang et al., 2009). In addition to polysaccharides and flavanoids which have been commonly identified in many herbs, phytochemical analyses revealed 'marker components' that could be used for quality evaluation and standardization of specific herbs, for example, triterpenoids and β-glucans in *Ganoderma* (Wang et al., 2006), cordycepin and ergosterol in Cordyceps (Paterson, 2008), ginsenoside in *Ginseng* (Chen et al., 2009). The complexity of TCM samples, particularly multiple active constituents and low concentration levels of active compounds, poses a big challenge to analytical chemistry for active ingredients recovery (Tang et al., 2009). To solve this problem, researchers have devoted to develop and optimize a wide variety of sample preparation methods for herbs, such as shaking, ultrasonic, soxhlet, boiling, distilling, high/ultrahigh pressure, heat reflux, supercritical-fluid (CO_2), microwave, etc (Chen et al., 2009, 2007; Shouqin et al., 2004). Usually, traditional techniques for extraction are time consuming and with low efficiency in recovery and purification of active ingredients. The technique of high pressure extraction coupled with selective solvents have been suggested in providing cost-effective and time-saving methods for obtaining single components of high purity (Shouqin et al., 2004). With the ultrahigh pressure extraction, not only the yielding of ginsenosides extracted from ginseng roots was increased, but the extract was shown to have enhanced free radical scavenging activity, when compared with other extraction methods (Chen et al, 2009). However, the extraction conditions and solvents being used need to be carefully decided based on the chemical characteristics and physical natures of the target molecules. For Lingzhi as an example it was found that the fraction of polysaccharides and triterpenes, each contains more than 100 molecules, can be simply extracted by water and ethanol (Yuen & Gohel, 2005). The most abundant polysaccharides type found in Lingzhi was β-glucans (Askin et al., 2010; Yuen & Gohel, 2005). The problems with β-glucan are low extraction yielding and poor purity, although various extraction methods using organic solvents have been applied (Askin et al, 2010). Recently, Askin and co-workers (Askin et al., 2010) have used a hydrothermal extraction method with 'subcritical water', conditioned at 473 K temperature at 10 MPa atmospheric pressure, and successfully obtained the maximum total amount (57.4% yielding) of β-glucans from Lingzhi. Besides, extraction of total triterpenes with organic solvents and water have long been practiced, however, isolation of the acidic triterpenes, mainly highly oxygenated triterpenoids which responsible for the bitter taste of the Lingzhi, from the total triterpenes fraction can be achieved with 95% aqueous ethanol under reflux and evaporation under reduced pressure, followed by chloroform extraction under acidic condition (Huie & Di, 2004). Silica gel column chromatography has also been described as an additional purification procedure for such acidic triterpenes (Huie & Di, 2004). To extract the specific triterpenoid saponins from another *Ganoderma species*, microwave-assisted extraction was demonstrated to be superior over other techniques, in terms of high yielding and short extraction time (Chen et al., 2007). Because of its gentle extraction conditions of supercritical CO_2 used with relatively low viscosity, high diffusivity, low extraction temperature, rapid and minimal use of halogenated solvents, supercritical fluid extraction (SFE) is a widely accepted extraction technique, however, its application is largely limited by the non-polar nature of CO_2 (Chen et al., 2011; Tang et al., 2009). Nonetheless, the dissolving and penetrating powers of SFE were employed to aid the breaking of extremely hard and resilient sporoderm of *Ganoderma lucidum* spores, in order to obtain the spore components and easy the subsequent extraction (Fu et al., 2009; Liu et al., 2002). Furthermore, activity-guided fractionation of herbal remedies has remained a hot field in the separation science. Constituents sharing similar chemical structures or physical properties can be isolated together into fraction during the chromatographic separation. Hence, the time-specific fraction can be tested for certain desired bioactivities such as anti-tumor (Li et al. 2010), antimicrobial (Kitzberger et al., 2007), antioxidant (Chen et al., 2009; Kitzberger et al., 2007), and many other activities by using any *in vitro* platforms and animal models. Results will then guide to identify the potent fractions and the effective bioactive ingredients. For example, in the study of Wang et al (Wang et al., 2005), four fractions namely R, F1, F2 and F3 were produced by the SFE of Cordyceps sinensis with CO_2, followed by bioassays that indicated that fraction R was the most active fraction to scavenge free radicals and induce apoptosis on human colorectal and liver cancer cells, while the remaining fractions exhibited only low to moderate levels of scavenging activities but no antitumor effect.

4.3 *In vitro* experiments and animal studies

In translational research, tissue culture and animal models serve as convenient tools for drug screening and mechanistic investigation. As presented in a scientific review (Yuen & Gohel, 2005), huge numbers of cancer cell lines and tumor-bearing animal models were used to address the antitumor properties of Lingzhi, its extracts or isolated compounds. By employing a well-established tumorigenic transformation model of uroepthelial cells, a series of chemopreventive properties were demonstrated by the ethanol extract of *Ganoderma lucidum* (GLe) to inhibit the carcinogen-induced tumorigenesis of bladder cancer through the inhibition of growth and cell migration (Lu et al., 2004; Yuen et al., 2008), telomerase-associated apoptosis (Yuen et al., 2008), oxidative DNA damage (Yuen & Gohel, 2008), and stimulation of selected cytokines and neutrophilic migration (Yuen et al., 2011). Meanwhile, an *ex vivo* orthotopic organ culture model is being used to establish the synergistic effects between GLe and other conventional chemotherapeutics. Anticancer effects of Lingzhi were also supported by the induction of cell cycle arrest and apoptosis amongst human and rodent tumor cells of various origins through signaling pathway controlling cell death, inhibition of cell adhesion, invasion and migration in foci formation assays, and stimulation of anti-angiogenesis, anti-metastasis and tumor regression in tumor-bearing rat/mice models (Wachtel-Galor et al., 2011). To delineate the cause-and-effect mechanism of particular genes and/or proteins, sometimes techniques of cell transfection and transgenic mice will be applied to create overexpression or suppression of certain gene(s), and used to test the herbal products. These experimental models are excellent to study the mechanism of action under the well-controlled microenvironments; however, they also limit on a focused pathway, ignoring the holism, and might not reflect the actual response inside the human bodies, especially issues about bioavailability and drug distribution. On the other hand, animal studies allow the determination of therapeutic and toxic dosage ranges, which are crucial before human trials can be admitted. Furthermore, animal models enable the whole body physiological examination and individual organ tissues can be isolated to study the drug effects as well as toxicities. Some pathological conditions, for example diabetic rats can be induced by intraperitoneal injection of streptozotocin, and was used to establish the mechanism underlying the antioxidant enzyme activity of Lingzhi polysaccharides to diminish pancreatic damage through the bax/bcl-2 modulation (Yang et al., 2010). In another experiment conducted by Tam et al. (Tam et al., 2011), a two-herb formula (with Radix Astragali and Radix Rehmanniae) was designed according to the classical theory of Chinese medicine, that was shown to elicit the actions of fibroblast proliferation, angiogenesis and anti-inflammation which favored the wound healing, in a chemically induced diabetic foot ulcer rat model. Nowadays, advanced molecular technology such as DNA micro-arrays also allowed the rapid high-throughput gene expression screening to conclude the outcomes of herbal remedies when tested on animal and cell culture studies (Hudson & Altamirano, 2006).

4.4 Safety and efficacy issues

For anything being applied inside the human body, regardless it is for treatment or health maintenance purpose, safety and efficacy are the first concerned. Despite the general public perceived herbal products as low risk because of the long history of usage, the current body of scientific evidence is seldom conveyed. In fact, herbal medicines may carry potential harms due to contamination, adulteration, misidentification, as well as unknown interactions with other herbal products, pharmaceutical drugs or even diets (Jordan et al., 2010). Unlike conventional drugs which are single chemical compounds, the complex composition of whole herbs or their extracts contain a myriad of phytochemicals, making the toxicological evaluation difficult, especially the therapeutic effects are also possibly based on the interaction of these different components could hardly be separated (Jordan et al., 2010). In terms of quality control, it is suggested that markers used for Chinese herbal medicine should be strongly correlated with their safety and efficacy, and thus 'marker components' of specific herb should be the 'effective components' which consisting both the active (bioactivity for therapeutic effects) and relative (no specific action but affect the therapeutic effects of active components) components, rather than just the most abundant chemical constituents mentioned in 4.1 as convenient (Li et al., 2011). One more challenge is that, the *in vivo* target sites for herbal remedies are usually unknown because of their complicated natures, and thus antidotes are unavailable in case of adverse reactions occur (Li et al., 2011). Therefore, scientifically, not so much can be done regarding the safety and efficacy concerns of traditional herbal medicine, but only taking the passive role in waiting for the case reports of adverse reaction are inadequate, demanding proper designed randomized controlled trails to conduct.

4.5 *In vivo* human trails – randomized controlled trails

Human controlled trails that use randomized allocation are the gold standard to restrain bias and confounding in trials evaluating pharmaceuticals. So as for TCM, randomized controlled trials (RCTs) of herbal medicine were not uncommon, at least in China. During 1999-2004, a total of 7,422 RCTs has been identified from 13 randomly selected journals published in Mainland China, and the number is kept increasing (Wang et al., 2007). However, by reviewing these RCTs, outcomes were discouraging, not because of the treatment outcomes themselves, but the poor qualities as assessed by using international standards, i.e. the Jadad score scare and the Consolidated Standards of Reporting Trials (CONSORT) checklist, more than 90% of these studies were poorly designed or reported with poor scientific rigor (Gagnier et al., 2011; Wang et al., 2007; Wolsko et al., 2005; Zhong et al., 2010). Some essential RCT components, such as sample size calculation, randomization sequence, allocation concealment, implementation of the random-allocation sequence, analysis of intention-to-treat (ITT), lacking syndrome differentiation of TCM, and the use of placebo was not justified and was ethically contradictory, were not sufficiently described in the methodologies of the studies (Gagnier et al., 2011; Wang et al., 2007; Zhong et al., 2010). Even limiting to the RCTs published in English, many investigators have failed to provide proper characterization to the study herbs such as identity, purity, quality, strength, and composition in their articles (Wolsko et al., 2005). A systemic review has conducted to assess 49 trials which included 3992 cancer patients who have given Chinese medicinal herbs concurrently with conventional cancer treatments (Molassiotis et al., 2009). Majority of the studies has shown positive herbal drug effects in terms of treatment toxicity, quality of life, survival, and tumor regression, however, no clinical recommendation could be concluded because of the poor intervention qualities (Molassiotis et al., 2009). Up to 2005, there were at least 127 Chinese RCTs identified of studying a single compound β-Elemene isolated from the Chinese herb *Curcuma wenyujin*, in order to characterize its efficacy on antitumorgenecity (Peng et al., 2006). Since the middle 1990s, although this chemical component has already been widely used in clinical practice for cancer treatment in China, there were less than two percents of trials performed with the double-blinding in the subject allocation, just four percents have carried out statistical analysis on baseline data, and none have used the intention-to-treat analysis (Peng et al., 2006). On the other hand, an international research team has conducted a series of well-designed RCTs (at phase I/II) on advanced cancer patients, which supported the efficacy of use of Lingzhi as an adjunct cancer therapy where it enhanced the conventional treatment outcome, by improving the immune response, increasing quality of life and survival, and decreasing side effects from conventional treatments (Gao et al., 2002, 2003a, 2003b, 2005). More recently, a perspective, multiple-center, randomized, double-blind, placebo-controlled trial was conducted to study the efficacy and safety of Antiwei granule (with ma huang and Baimaogen as the principals) on infected adults of influenza (Wang et al., 2010). The report provided sufficient evidence to recommend antiwei as an effective influenza treatment based on the positive outcomes, of which increased the patients' recovery by 17% and reduced the severity of illness by 50%. The study was considered as perfectly designed since there was a well characterized herbal prescription, the use of visually indistinguishable starch coupled with a bitter agent as a placebo, fulfillment of all items listed in the CONSORT checklist as an objective outcome measurement using median symptom scores was used, and objective side effects monitored using ECG and vital signs.

5. The spectrum of East meets West: The transition from traditional cure to conventional drug really necessary?

Many folk remedies have maintained their reputation for effectiveness, to be handed on from generation to generation, on the word of the village elders. Faith in the efficacy of a treatment plays a large part in feeling better. Confidence in a remedy is reinforced by word-of-mouth repetition, when everyone tells everyone else in everyday conversation that they simply know it works. Their over-the-counter availability and reputation as natural, 'safe' and effective alternatives to drug treatment makes herbal products attractive to consumers. The great increase in consumption of herbal products is a cause for concern, however, because, in addition to their efficacy, the issues of toxicity and of herb-herb and herb-drug interactions that might be additive, synergistic or antagonistic will require comprehensive scientific study. Scientists all over the world consider herbal species as a rich source for new chemical entities and used them successfully to isolate compounds, such as ephedrine, digoxin, morphine, taxol, atropine and vinblastine, are nowadays conventional drugs in allopathic medicine (Tistaert et al., 2011). To develop a new drug from herbs, the WHO has setup guidelines related on chemical drug development and traditional experience of using herbs. The paradigm of chemical drug development: drug discovery, drug design, pre-clinical studies, and clinical studies. A chemical drug always requires 10-12 years for optimization and evaluation to allow in prescription. Herbal medicine starts with human use and finally become an isolated purified form of chemical(s) for approval to be marketed. Considering the unique features of herbal products are multiple component mixtures and that substantial prior human use precedes their formal investigation, the WHO has issued a set of clear and concise recommendations for preparing well supported clinical trials to evaluate the actual benefits and risks of traditional herbal products being used for clinical purpose (WHO-TDR, 2005). Such operational guidance was built according to the principles of modern clinical sciences with four sets of issues: chemical manufacturing-control (CMC) issues, non-clinical issues, clinical issues, and ethical issues, and considerations have to translate into terms appropriate to support the justification for a clinical trial of a traditional herbal remedy, as summarized in a flowchart (Figure 2). Looking into the recommendations, the WHO has acted supportively in preserving the traditions of herbal medicine, i.e. candidate herbal substance or product should be prepared in accordance with the traditionally-used formulation, where purified chemicals are not required WHO-TDR, 2005).

6. The current positioning: Right or wrong direction of research in traditional Chinese herbal medicine

In western terms, the health benefits of most herbal remedies remain unsubstantiated by scientific evidence in well-designed human studies, and this limits their acceptance by western trained health professionals. Nonetheless, herbal medicine offers an enormous potential for health promotion and treatment of disease, and several commonly used western drugs have their origins in herbal medicine. On the other hands, the traditional essence of TCM is reconsidered by other investigators, who have used western criteria to validate scientifically the traditional theories and their usage. Based on what are the personal beliefs, the applications of herbal medicine are splitting into either one of the two paths: transition into pure chemicals or holding the traditional way of practice. Right or wrong is always up your decision, or actually there is no answer. However, whatever it is decided will lead the future research direction of herbal medicine very differently.

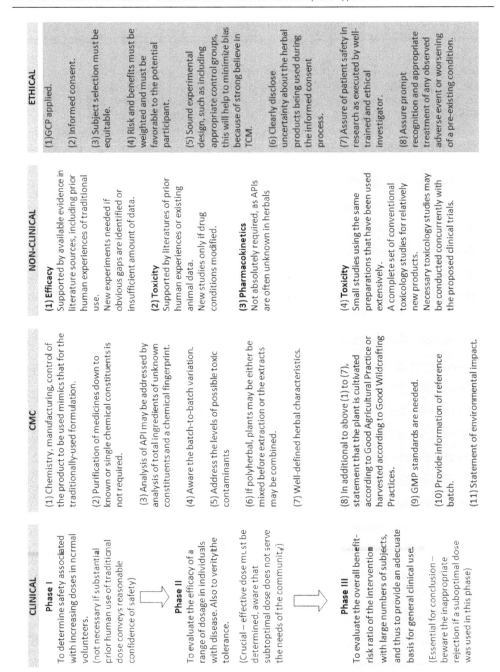

Fig. 2. Recommended information needed to support a clinical trial for an herbal medicine (WHO-TDR, 2005). CMC: chemical-manufacturing-control; API: Active pharmaceutical ingredient; GMP: Good Manufacturing Practices; GCP: Good Clinical Practice.

6.1 The transition of herbs into pure chemicals

Referring to the development of plant-derived medicines, the Western approach with clinically effective plant extracts was to ask "what is the active principle?", and then to isolate, purify, determine its structure and produce a standardized dosage form. Herbal medicine has made many contributions to commercial drug preparations manufactured today including ephedrine from ma huang (*Ephedra sinica*) (Gaddum & Kwiatkowski, 1938). Ephedra, which is being used for weight loss, antiasthmatic, or as stimulant for athletic performance, and clinical trials recognized common side effects as increased risk of psychiatric, autonomic or gastrointestinal symptoms, and heart palpitations (Schaneberg et al., 2003; Shekelle et al., 2003). Serious adverse reactions, including death, have occurred; in most cases, the people were abusingly taking two or four times the recommended dose (Samenuk et al., 2002). In this relation, one should realize the fact that definite phytopharmaceuticals are highly concentrated that no longer represent the whole herb. In many cases they are vast more effective than the whole herb, but some effects of the herb may be lost and the potential for adverse effects and herb/drug interactions may increase.

In the last 30 years, no plant compounds discovered have generated as much public interest and excitement as has taxol (paclitaxel). Pure taxol, a complex polyoxygenated diterpene, was isolated in 1969 in 0.01% yield from the bark of *Taxus brevifolia Nutt*, following a series of screening experiments for anticancer activity (Kingston, 2007). Later on, taxol was known to be extractable from other *Taxus* species of Yew trees including the Chinese yew Hong Dou Shan (*Taxus chinensis*) grows in china (Siow et al., 2005). Upon the selection of taxol as a development candidate in 1977 and the approval as anticancer drug by U.S. Food and Drug Administration in 1992, efforts were non-stopped to explore methods to enhance its production and synthesis, although the current yielding has achieved over 90% of pure paclitaxel (Khosroushahi et al., 2006; Pyo et al., 2007). The drug is nowadays the first-line treatment for advanced ovarian and breast cancer, the second-line treatment for AIDS-related Kaposi's sarcoma, and used in combination with cisplatin for treating nonsmall-cell lung carcinoma (Siow et al., 2005), however, intensive studies are still underway for its anti-cancer mechanisms (Varbiro et al., 2001) as well as its toxic side effects (Atas et al., 2006; Rabah, 2010). Nonetheless, according to the *Dongbei Yaozhi zhi* (Records of Plant Herb in Northeast China), TCM used *Hong Dou Shan* to detoxify the body and releases cough (Siow et al., 2005) Perhaps, the traditional use of *Hong Dou Shan* has long been forgotten which attract no more attention at the rear of the successful toxal (Figure 3). Of course, taxol is not the only TCM-derived anticancer drug, but many others such as homoharringtonine from *Cephalotaxus species*, camptothecin from *Camptotheca acuminate*, and vincristine from *Catharanthus roseus*, are all used for cancer chemotherapy in Western medicine (Efferth et al., 2007). This is not East-meets-West, by just turning herbal species into conventional chemical drugs, which contradict the theory and application of traditional medicine.

At edge, Lingzhi is standing at the middle point waiting for you to decide which way to go. Not mentioning it is named to be a superior tonic in the very first pharmacopeia - The divine farmer's material medica, Lingzhi has been used over two thousand years for the promotion of health and longevity. Thousands of studies have been performed with large proportion was focused on its anticancer effects, ranging from experiments *in vitro* and animals to humans' *in vivo*, merely supported its applicability for cancer treatment and prevention (Yuen & Gohel, 2005). Effective and toxic dosages have long been established by animal studies (Kim et al., 1986) in addition to the substantial prior human use. Toxicities were rarely reported, and the safe usage has been convinced by scientific evidence and history (Mizuno et al., 1995). Several Lingzhi products have already been well characterized by fingerprinting and genotyping techniques for authentication and quality control (Chen et al., 2008a, 2008b). The above conditions explicitly supported the clinical trials at phase I and II. In fact, A New Zealand-based research team (Gao et al., 2002, 2003a, 2003b, 2005) has conducted several phase II trials with advanced cancer patients as mentioned; however, the study aims were just placing Lingzhi as an adjunct therapy, where the outcome measurements were not really the valid disease endpoint. Besides, several isolated compounds, such as ganoderic acids and lucialdehydes, and their efficacy and safety have already characterized by using tissue culture and animal models (Yuen & Gohel, 2005). According to the WHO recommendations (WHO-TDR, 2005), both the crude mushrooms and isolated compounds are justified proceeding to large-scale phase III clinical trials, at least for their anticancer properties. Therefore, the choices are up to your decision, for traditional or conventional? Remember, your determination will lead the future research.

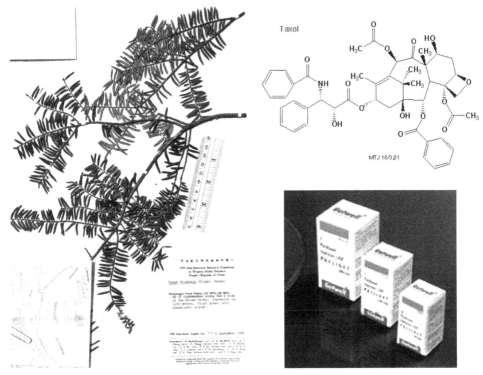

Fig. 3. The chemical structure of taxol in the package of Paclitaxel ®, reminding *Hong Dou Shan (Taxus chinensis)* available in Hubei China (diagram adopted from © The world Botanical Associates Web page) is one of the herbal sources of taxol.

6.2 The validation of holistic application of herbal formulations
We have seen for ourselves herbal medicine's ability both to heal those disorders that often fail to respond to the best of Western medicine, and treat major diseases with methods that

are more sympathetic to the human system and have fewer harmful side effects. The WHO has published a list of ailments and conditions for which treatment or alleviation with Chinese medicine is considered appropriate which include diabetes. In Western medicine, diabetes is deemed as an incurable disease that patients have persistent hyperglycemia associated with high morbidity and mortality due to complications if blood glucose levels are not controlled. In view of TCM, diabetes is referred as *Xiao Ke* which is a syndrome of "wasting and thirsting" (Duan, 2008). The disease is described as the constitutional deficiency of yin of the kidney and lung and associated with the internal heat that consumes fluids, and thus causes wasting and thirst (Covington, 2001; Duan, 2008). There were 13 traditional herbal formulations for treating Xiao Ke according to the Yellow Emperor's Inner Canon, and later on derived into hundreds of prescriptions to aim at different symptoms of diabetes (Duan, 2008; Li et al., 2004). Whilst 33 most frequently used Chinese herbs for clinical treatment of diabetes and its complications were listed (Li et al., 2004). The "Herbal drink to strengthen muscle and control swelling", which is a six-component formula using Radix Astragali (*Astragalus membranaceus*) and Radix Rehmanniae (*Rehmannia glutinosa*) as principals, have been shown to promote the healing of diabetic foot ulcers effectively (Chan et al., 2007). Experimental studies revealed that all individual components of the formula were active in modifying tissue glucose homeostasis *in vitro* but inactive to improve glycaemic control of diabetes in diabetic rats *in vivo* (Chan et al., 2007). Focusing on its mechanism for the ulcer healing effects, a chemically induced diabetic foot ulcer rat model was used to establish the *in vivo* anti-inflammatory activities of the two principal ingredients (Tam et al., 2011). This is a typical example of herbal case demonstrating the feasibility of examining the traditionally used cures using of Western approach. More of this caliber should be conducted to eventually place TCM onto the context of modern medicine, and thus East meets West.

7. Conclusion – A need for compromise and agreement – A new model for investigation

The holistic views of TCM generally have no conflicts with the western medicine, perhaps they were just expressed in different terms. Western medicine is usually more concrete in diagnosis and judgment. Treatment is often quicker, particularly in acute cases, and surgery is its strength. Its weak points are that it sees disease as something to be measured and quantified and often ignores the psychological, social and behavioral factors involved in illness. Chinese medicine, on the other hand, can be too flexible and too general where diagnosis and judgment are concerned, and sometimes relies too heavily on the individual practitioner's experiences. Its strong points are its highly flexible approach, which enabling treatments to be changed as the patient improve, and its emphasis on prevention. The Chinese way tends to treat the whole body rather than to try to isolate a particular infected area. And, finally, the herbs themselves, compared with chemically produced medicines, are relatively cheap and easy to use. They have minimal side-effects, and most have been tried and tested for over many thousand years. Western medicine focuses more on symptomatic management, whereas TCM focuses more on cause and effect. Western medicine is more useful for first-aid and surgical interventions, whereas TCM is more useful in treating internal and chronic illnesses. An ideal health care system should be established to concern people's physical and mental health, to deal with all personal problems, and to improve people's quality of life. A new model of health care should be composed by a different medical system to provide a holistic approach. TCM, today as an alternative and complementary medicine should be included into the conventional medicine to form the new modern medicine. This is in line with the aim of the WHO to promote recognition of traditional medicine and to support its integration into the mainstream health service. There is space of integration for TCM and modern medicine. A new paradigm for developing medicine is needed, and Chinese medicine could make a significant contribution in this field. To achieve such integration, modern science and technology had to be used to study the action, efficacy and toxicity of Chinese medicines. Although, there are many issues to concern, especially safe and effectiveness, some compromise and agreement are needed. Thus botanicals should be defined, authenticated and documented as to their source and conditions of cultivation using modern methodology. Manufacturing and preparation processes of Chinese medicine should be carefully monitored and standardized. Claims for Chinese medicine should be verified from rigorous controlled trials. Interaction between Western and Chinese medicines should be better studied and information obtained centralized into accessible databases. This would be an enormous undertaking requiring international collaboration and participation of governments worldwide. In fact, the feasibility of herbal validation by using Western methods is well-illustrated. In particular, concerns about identity authentication, quality control, evidences of efficacy and safety of herbal remedies, are being addressed with the modern science and technology, and ultimately allow the gathering of information necessarily to support clinical trials. Along with this route, efforts being played will return with the transition of TCM into a recognized science specialty to fill up the gaps between Eastern and Western medical approaches. In this perspective, it may not be necessary to isolate the active ingredients from herbal remedies or purity them to finally become chemical drugs. To promote the effectiveness, Chinese herbal medicine can remain in formulae but standardizations are needed. Meanwhile, both Chinese and western practitioners should come together and sort out the best treatment they can offer to patients, which very often may be the combination of the modern and Chinese medicine, instead of favoring one over the other. Conventional Western medicine and Chinese medicine should be seen as complementary to each other, rather than as alternatives. Both types of medicine have their advantages and drawbacks, which is why they need to work hand in hand for optimal results. Together, Chinese and Western medicine could form the most effective disease treatment the world has ever known.

8. Acknowledgement

The authors are grateful to be supported the research by the Hong Kong Polytechnic University Grants G-997 and G-U979.

9. References

Achike, F.I. & Kwan, C.Y. (2003). Nitric oxide, human diseases and the herbal products that affect the nitric oxide signalling pathway. *Clinical and Experimental Pharmacology and Physiology*, Vol.30, No.9, (September 2003), pp. 605-615, ISSN 0305-1870

Ahmed, S.A. (2000). The immune system as a potential target for environmental estrogens (endocrine disrupters): a new emerging field. *Toxicology*, Vol.150, No.1-3, (September 2000), pp. 191-206, ISSN 0300-483X

Askin, R., Sasaki, M., & Goto, M. (2010). Recovery of water-soluble compounds from Ganoderma lucidum by hydrothermal treatment. *Food and Bioproducts Processing*, Vol.88, No.C2-3, (July 2009), pp. 291-297, ISSN 0960-3085

Atas, A., Agca, O., Sarac, S., Poyraz, A., & Akyol, M.U. (2006). Investigation of ototoxic effects of Taxol on a mice model. *International Journal of Pediatric Otorhinolaryngology*, Vol.70, No.5, (May 2006) pp. 779-784, ISSN 0165-5876

Beinfield, H. & Korngold, E. (2003). Dao and the doctor: The thought and practice of Chinese medicine. *Seminars in Integrative medicine*, Vol.1, No.3, (September 2003), pp. 136-144, ISSN 1543-1150

Bensky, D., Clavery, S., & Stoger, E. (2004). Substances that clam the spirit, In: *Chinese Herbal Medicine: Materia Medica*, A. Gamble, (Ed.), pp. 933-935, Eastland Press, ISBN 0939616424, Seattle

Bliss, M. (2011). *The marking of modern medicine: Turning points in the treatment of disease* (1st edition), The University of Chicago Press, ISBN 9780226059013, Chicago, London

Bynum, W.F. (2008). *History of medicine* (1st edition), Oxford University Press, ISBN 9780199215430, Oxford

Chan, C.M., Chan, Y.W., Lau, C.H., Lau, T.W., Lau, K.M., Lam, F.C., Che, C.T., Leung, P.C., Fung, K.P., Lau, C.B., & Ho, Y.Y. (2007). Influence of an anti-diabetic foot ulcer formula and its component herbs on tissue and systemic glucose homeostasis. *Journal of Ethnopharmacology*, Vol.109, No.1, (January 2007), pp. 10-20, ISSN 0378-8741

Chan, W.T. (1969). *A source book in Chinese philosophy* (1st edition), Princeton University Press , ISBN 1400811228, Princeton, New Jersey

Chang, H., Huang, W., Tsao, D., Huang, K., Lee, S., Lin, S., Yang, S., & Yeh, C. (2009). Identification and Authentication of Burdock (Arctium lappa Linn) Using PCR Sequencing. *Fooyin Journal of Health Science*, Vol.1, No.1, (August 2009), pp. 28-32, ISSN 1877-8607

Chen, R.Z., Meng, F.L., Zhang, S.Q., & Liu, Z.Q. (2009). Effects of ultrahigh pressure extraction conditions on yields and antioxidant activity of ginsenoside from ginseng. *Separation and Purification Technology*, Vol.66, No.2, (April 2009), pp. 340-346, ISSN 1383-5806

Chen, T., Zhao, X., Wu, J., Yu, D., & Wu, Y. (2011). Supercritical fluid CO2 extraction, simultaneous determination of components in ultra-fine powder of Ganoderma sinense by HPLC-ESI-MS method. *Journal of the Taiwan Institute of chemical Engineers*, Vol.42, No.3., (May 2011), pp. 428-434, ISSN 1876-1070

Chen, Y., Xie, M.Y., & Gong, X.F. (2007). Microwave-assisted extraction used for the isolation of total triterpenoid saponins from Ganoderma atrum. *Journal of Food Engineering*, Vol.81, No.1, (July 2007), pp. 162-170, ISSN 0260-8774

Chen, Y., Yan, Y., Xie, M.Y., Nie, S.P., Liu, W., Gong, X.F., & Wang, Y.X. (2008a). Development of a chromatographic fingerprint for the chloroform extracts of Ganoderma lucidum by HPLC and LC-MS. *Journal of Pharmaceutical and Biomedical Analysis*,Vol.47, No.3, (July 2008), pp. 469-477, ISSN 0731-7085

Chen, Y., Zhu, S.B., Xie, M.Y., Nie, S.P., Liu, W., Li, C., Gong, X.F., & Wang, Y.X. (2008b.) Quality control and original discrimination of Ganoderma lucidum based on high-performance liquid chromatographic fingerprints and combined chemometrics methods. *Analytica Chimica Acta*, Vol.623, No.2, (August 2008), pp. 146-156, ISSN 0003-2670

Covington, M. B. (2001). Traditional Chinese medicine in the treatment of diabetes. *Diabetes Spectrum*, Vol.14, No.3, (November 2001), pp. 154-159, ISSN 1944-7353

Duan, Q.F. (2008). *Huangdi nei jing* (2nd edition), Chong wen shu ju, ISBN 9787540312350, Wuhan Shi

Duffin, J. (2010). *history of medicine: A scandalously short introduction* (2nd edition), University of Toronto Press, ISBN 9780802098252, Toronto

Dunn, A. J. (1996). Psychneuroimmunology, stress and infection, In: *Psychoneuimmunology, stress, and infection*, H.K.T.W. Friedman & A.L. Friedman (Eds.), pp. 25-78, CRC Press , ISBN 0849376386, Boca Raton, New York, London, tokyo

Efferth, T., Li, P.C., Konkimalla, V.S., & Kaina, B. (2007). From traditional Chinese medicine to rational cancer therapy. *Trends in Molecular Medicine*, Vol.13, No.8, (August 2007), pp. 353-361, ISSN 1471-4914

Fan, X.H., Cheng, Y.Y., Ye, Z.L., Lin, R.C., & Qian, Z.Z. (2006). Multiple chromatographic fingerprinting and its application to the quality control of herbal medicines. *Analytica Chimica Acta*, Vol.555, No.2, (January 2006), pp. 217-224, ISSN 0003-2670

Finkel, T. & Holbrook, N.J. (2000). Oxidants, oxidative stress and the biology of ageing. *Nature*, Vol.408, No.6809, (November 2000), pp. 239-247, ISSN 0028-0836

Fu, Y.J., Liu, W., Zu, Y.G., Shi, X.G., Liu, Z.G., Schwarz, G., & Efferth, T. (2009). Breaking the spores of the fungus Ganoderma lucidum by supercritical CO_2. *Food Chemistry*, Vol.112, No.1, (January 2009), pp. 71-76, ISSN 0308-8146

Gaddum, J.H. & Kwiatkowski, H. (1938). The action of ephedrine. *Journal of Physiology*, Vol.94, No.1, (October 1938), pp. 87-100, ISSN 0022-3751

Gagnier, J.J., Moher, D., Boon, H., Beyene, J., & Bombardier, C. (2011). Randomized controlled trials of herbal interventions underreport important details of the intervention. *Journal of Clinical Epidemiology*, Vol.64, No.7, (July 2011), pp. 760-769, ISSN 1179-1349

Gao, Y., Tang, W., Dai, X., Gao, H., Chen, G., Ye, J., Chan, E., Koh, H.L., Li, X., & Zhou, S. (2005). Effects of water-soluble Ganoderma lucidum polysaccharides on the immune functions of patients with advanced lung cancer. *Journal of Medicinal Food*, Vol.8, No.2, (Summer 2005), pp. 159-168, ISSN 1096-620X

Gao, Y., Zhou, S., Jiang, W., Huang, M., & Dai, X. (2003a). Effects of ganopoly (a Ganoderma lucidum polysaccharide extract) on the immune functions in advanced-stage cancer patients. *Immunological Investigatioms*, Vol.32, No.3, (August 2003), pp. 201-215, ISSN 1532-4311

Gao, Y. H., Dai, X. H., Chen, G. L., Ye, J. X., & Zhou, S. F. (2003b). A randomized, placebo-controlled, multicenter study of Ganoderma lucidum (W.Curt.: Fr.) Lloyd (Aphyllophoromycetideae) polysaccharides (Ganoploy (R)) in patients with advanced lung cancer. *International Journal of Medicinal Mushrooms*, Vol.5, No.4, (December 2003), pp. 369-381, ISSN 1521-9437

Gao, Y. H., Zhou, S. F., Chen, G. L., Dai, X. H., & Ye, J. X. (2002). A phaseI/II study of a Ganoderma lucidum (Curt.: Fr.) P. Karst extract (Ganopoly) in patients with advanced cancer. *International Journal of Medicinal Mushrooms*, Vol.4, No.3, (September 2002), pp. 207-214., ISSN 1521-9437

Gutteridge, J.M. (1994). Biological origin of free radicals, and mechanisms of antioxidant protection. *Chemico Biological Interactions*, Vol.91, No.2-3, (June 1994), pp. 133-140, ISSN 0009-2797

Halliwell, B. (2009). The wanderings of a free radical. *Free Radical Biolology and Medicine*, Vol.46, No.5, (March 2009), pp. 531-542, ISSN 0891-5849

Han, T., Zhang, Q.Y., Zhang, H., Wen, J., Wang, Y., Huang, B.K., Rahman, K., Zheng, H.C., & Qin, L.P. (2009). Authentication and quantitative analysis on the chemical profile of Xanthium fruit (Cang-Er-Zi) by high-performance liquid chromatography-diode-array detection tandem mass spectrometry method. *Analytica Chimica Acta*, Vol.634, No.2, (Feburary 2009), pp. 272-278, ISSN 0003-2670

Herrero, B., Madrinan, M., Vieites, J.M., & Espineira, M. (2010). Authentication of Atlantic cod (Gadus morhua) using real time PCR. *Journal of Agricultural and Food Chemistry*, Vol.58, No.8, (April 2010), pp. 4794-4799, ISSN 0021-8561

Hudson, J. & Altamirano, M. (2006). The application of DNA micro-arrays (gene arrays) to the study of herbal medicines. *Journal of Ethnopharmacology*, Vol.108, No.1, (November 2006), pp. 2-15, ISSN 0378-8741

Huie, C.W. & Di, X. (2004). Chromatographic and electrophoretic methods for Lingzhi pharmacologically active components. *Journal of Chromatography B Analytical Technologies in the Biomedical and Life Science*, Vol.812, No.1-2, (December 2004), pp. 241-257, ISSN 1570-0232

Jordan, S.A., Cunningham, D.G., & Marles, R.J. (2010). Assessment of herbal medicinal products: challenges, and opportunities to increase the knowledge base for safety assessment. *Toxicology and Applied Pharmacology*, Vol.243, No.2, (March 2010), pp. 198-216, ISSN 0041-008X

Kaptchuk, T.J. (2000). *Chinese medicine: The web that has no weaver* (1st edition), Rider, ISBN 071260281X, London, Sydney, Auckland, johannesburg

Kaye, J. M. & Lightman, S. L. (2005). Psychologucak stress and endrine axes, In: *Human psychoneuroimmunology*, K. Vedhara & M. Irwin, (Eds.), pp. 25-52, Oxford University Press , ISBN 019852840X, New York

Khan, S., Mirza, K.J., Al-Qurainy, F., & Abdin, M.Z. (2011). Authentication of the medicinal plant Senna angustifolia by RAPD profiling. *Saudi Journal of Biological Sciences*, Vol.18, No.3, (March 2011), pp. 287-292, ISSN 1319-562X

Khosroushahi, A.Y., Valizadeh, M., Ghasempour, A., Khosrowshahli, M., Naghdibadi, H., Dadpour, M.R., & Omidi, Y. (2006). Improved Taxol production by combination of inducing factors in suspension cell culture of Taxus baccata. *Cell Biology International*, Vol.30, No.3, (March 2006), pp. 262-269, ISSN 1065-6995

Kim, M. J., Kim, H. W., Lee, Y. S., Shim, M. J., Choi, E. C., & Kim, B. K. (1986). Stduies on safety of ganoderma lucidum. *Korean Journal of Mycology*, Vol.14, (March 1986), pp. 49-60, ISSN 1226-4709

Kingston, D.G. (2007). The shape of things to come: structural and synthetic studies of taxol and related compounds. *Phytochemistry*, Vol.68, No.14, (July 2007), pp. 1844-1854, ISSN 0031-9422

Kiran, U., Khan, S., Mirza, K.J., Ram, M., & Abdin, M.Z. (2010). SCAR markers: a potential tool for authentication of herbal drugs. *Fitoterapia*, Vol.81, No.8, (December 2010), pp. 969-976, ISSN 0367-326X

Kitzberger, C.S.G., Smania, A., Pedrosa, R.C., & Ferreira, S.R.S. (2007). Antioxidant and antimicrobial activities of shiitake (Lentinula edodes) extracts obtained by organic solvents and supercritical fluids. *Journal of Food Engineering*, Vol.80, No.2, (May 2007), pp. 631-638, ISSN 0260-8774

Ko, K.M., Leon, T.Y., Mak, D.H., Chiu, P.Y., Du, Y., & Poon, M.K. (2006). A characteristic pharmacological action of 'Yang-invigorating' Chinese tonifying herbs: enhancement of myocardial ATP-generation capacity. *Phytomedicine*, Vol.13, No.9-10, (November 2006), pp. 636-642, ISSN 0944-7113

Ko, K.M. & Leung, H.Y. (2007). Enhancement of ATP generation capacity, antioxidant activity and immunomodulatory activities by Chinese Yang and Yin tonifying herbs. *Chinese Medicine*, Vol.2, No.3, (March 2007), available from: http://www.cmjournal.org/content/2/1/3

Ko, K.M., Mak, D.H., Chiu, P.Y., & Poon, M.K. (2004). Pharmacological basis of 'Yang-invigoration' in Chinese medicine. *Trends in Pharmacoogical Science*, Vol. 25, No.1, (January 2004), pp. 3-6, ISSN 0165-6147

Kuang, A. K., Ding, T., Chen, G. L., Xu, M. Y., Zhang, D. Q., Chi, Y. S., Lo, S. Z., Chen, M. Y., Wang, X. L., & Wang, Q. Q. (1988). Study on clinical effect of treatment of myxedema with TCM alone and TCM supplemented with thyroid tablets. *Chinese Journal of Integrated Traditional and Western Medicine*, Vol.8, No.2, (Feburary 1988), pp. 74-76, ISSN 1003-5370

Lafaille, J.J. & Mathis, D. (2002). Immunological Yin-Yang. *Current Opinion in Immunology*, Vol.14, No.6, (December 2002), pp. 741-743, ISSN 0952-7915

Langevin, H.M., Badger, G.J., Povolny, B.K., Davis, R.T., Johnston, A.C., Sherman, K.J., Kahn, J.R., & Kaptchuk, T.J. (2004). Yin scores and yang scores: A new method for quantitative diagnostic evaluation in traditional Chinese medicine research. *Journal of Alternative and Complementary Medicine*, Vol.10, No.2, (April 2004), pp. 389-395, ISSN 1075-5535

Law, S.K., Simmons, M.P., Techen, N., Khan, I.A., He, M.F., Shaw, P.C., & But, P.P. (2011). Molecular analyses of the Chinese herb Leigongteng (Tripterygium wilfordii Hook.f.). *Phytochemistry*, Vol.72, No.1, (January 2011), pp. 21-26, ISSN 0031-9422

Li, M., Jiang, R.W., Hon, P.M., Cheng, L., Li, L.L., Zhou, J.R., Shaw, P.C., & But, P.P.H. (2010). Authentication of the anti-tumor herb Baihuasheshecao with bioactive mark0r compounds and molecular sequences. *Food Chemistry*, Vol.119, No.3, (April 2010), pp. 1239-1245, ISSN 0308-8146

Li, S.P., Zhao, J., & Yang, B. (2011). Strategies for quality control of Chinese medicines. *Journal of Pharmacutical and Biomedical Analysis.*, Vol.55, No.4, (June 2011), pp. 802-809, ISSN 0731-7085

Li, S.Z. (2003). *Compendium of materia medica (Bencao Gangmu)* (1st edition), Foreign Language Press, ISBN 9787119032603, Beijing

Li, W.L., Zheng, H.C., Bukuru, J., & De, K.N. (2004). Natural medicines used in the traditional Chinese medical system for therapy of diabetes mellitus. *Journal of Ethnopharmacology*, Vol.92, No.1, (May 2004), pp. 1-21, ISSN 0378-8741

Lin, W.S., Chan, W.C., & Hew, C.S. (1995). Superoxide and traditional Chinese medicines. *Journal of Ethnopharmacology*, Vol.48, No.3, (November 1995), pp. 165-171, ISSN 0378-8741

Liu, X., Yuan, J.P., Chung, C.K., & Chen, X.J. (2002). Antitumor activity of the sporoderm-broken germinating spores of Ganoderma lucidum. *Cancer Letters*, Vol.182, No.2, (Auguet 2002), pp. 155-161, ISSN 0304-3835

Lock, S. (1997). Medicine in the second half of the twentieth century, In: *Western Medicine: An Illustrated History*, I. Loudon, (Ed.), pp. 123-146, Oxford University Press, ISBN 0198205090, Oxford, New York

Longrigg, J. (1997). Medicine in the classical world, In: *Western Medicine: An Illustrated History*, I. Loudon, (Ed.), pp. 25-39, Oxford University Press, ISBN 0198205090, Oxford, New York

Lu, G.H., Chan, K., Liang, Y.Z., Leung, K., Chan, C.L., Jiang, Z.H., & Zhao, Z.Z. (2005). Development of high-performance liquid chromatographic fingerprints for distinguishing Chinese Angelica from related umbelliferae herbs. *Journal of Chromatography A*, Vol.1073, No.1-2, pp. 383-392, ISSN 0021-9673

Lu, Q.Y., Jin, Y.S., Zhang, Q., Zhang, Z., Heber, D., Go, V.L., Li, F.P., & Rao, J.Y. (2004). Ganoderma lucidum extracts inhibit growth and induce actin polymerization in bladder cancer cells in vitro. *Cancer Letters*, Vol.216, No.1, (December 2004), pp. 9-20, ISSN 0304-3835

Macek, C. (1984). East meets West to balance immunologic yin and yang. *Journal of American Medical Association*, Vol.251, No.4, (Januray 1984), pp. 433-439, ISSN 0098-7484

Mak, D.H., Chiu, P.Y., Poon, M.K., Ng, T.T., Chung, Y.K., Lam, B.Y., Du, Y., & Ko, K.M. (2004). A yang-promoting Chinese herbal suppository preparation enhances the antioxidant status of red cells in male human subjects. *Phytotherapy Research*, Vol.18, No.7, (July 2004), pp. 525-530, ISSN 0951-418X

Mann, D.L. (2001). Interleukin-6 and viral myocarditis: the Yin-Yang of cardiac innate immune responses. *Journal of Molecular and Cellular Cardiology*, Vol.33, No.9, (September 2001), pp. 1551-1553, ISSN 0022-2828

Mills, R. & Bhatt, D.L. (2004). The Yin and Yang of arterial inflammation. *Journal of American College of Cardiology*, Vol.44, No.1, (July 2004), pp. 50-52, ISSN 0735-1097

Min, X., Xiaohui, Z., Zhaixiang, D., & Ming, O. (1998). Effect of the Yang tonifying herbs on myocardial beta-adrenoceptors of hypothyroid rabbits. *Journal of Ethnopharmacology*, Vol.60, No.1, (February 1998), pp. 43-51, ISSN 0378-8741

Mizuno, T., Wang, G.Y., Zhang, J., Kawagishi, H., Nishitoba, T., & Li, J.X. (1995). Reishi, Ganoderma lucidum and Ganoderma tsugae - Bioactive Substances and Medicinal Effects. *Food Reviews International*, Vol.11, No.1, (November 2009), pp. 151-166, ISSN 8755-9129

Molassiotis, A., Potrata, B., & Cheng, K.K. (2009). A systematic review of the effectiveness of Chinese herbal medication in symptom management and improvement of quality of life in adult cancer patients. *Complementary Therapies Medicine*, Vol.17, No.2, (April 2009), pp. 92-120, ISSN 0965-2299

Ou, B., Huang, D., Hampsch-Woodill, M., & Flanagan, J.A. (2003). When east meets west: the relationship between yin-yang and antioxidation-oxidation. *The FASEB Journal*, Vol.17, No.2, (October 2002), pp. 127-129, ISSN 0892-6638

Palaszynski, K.M., Smith, D.L., Kamrava, S., Burgoyne, P.S., Arnold, A.P., & Voskuhl, R.R. (2005). A yin-yang effect between sex chromosome complement and sex hormones on the immune response. *Endocrinology*, Vol.146, No.8, (August 2005), pp. 3280-3285, ISSN 0013-7227

Paterson, R.R. (2008). Cordyceps: a traditional Chinese medicine and another fungal therapeutic biofactory? *Phytochemistry*, Vol.69, No.7, (May 2008), pp. 1469-1495, ISSN 0031-9422

Paton, J.F., Boscan, P., Pickering, A.E., & Nalivaiko, E. (2005). The yin and yang of cardiac autonomic control: vago-sympathetic interactions revisited.*Brain Research Reviews.*, Vol.49, No.3, (Novermber 2005), pp. 555-565, ISSN 0165-0173

Peng, X., Zhao, Y., Liang, X., Wu, L., Cui, S., Guo, A., & Wang, W. (2006). Assessing the quality of RCTs on the effect of beta-elemene, one ingredient of a Chinese herb, against malignant tumors. *Contemporary Clinical Trials*, Vol.27, No.1, (February 2006), pp. 70-82, ISSN 1551-7144

Pyo, S.H., Cho, J.S., Choi, H.J., & Han, B.H. (2007). Evaluation of paclitaxel rearrangement involving opening of the oxetane ring and migration of acetyl and benzoyl groups. *Journal of Pharmaceutical and Biomedical Analysis*, Vol.43, No.3, (February 2007), pp. 1141-1145, ISSN 0731-7085

Rabah, S. O. (2010). Acute taxol nephrotoxicity: Histological and ultrastructural studies of mice kidney parenchyma. *Saudi Journal of Biological Sciences*, *Vol.*17, No.2, (April 2010), pp. 105-114, ISSN 1319-562X

Robinson, M. M. & Zhang, X. 2011, *The World Medicine situation 2011: Traditional medicine: Global situation, issues and challenges*, WHO Press, Geneva, Retrieved from http://www.who.int/medicines/areas/policy/world_medicines_situation/WMS_ch18_wTraditionalMed.pdf

Samenuk, D., Link, M.S., Homoud, M.K., Contreras, R., Theoharides, T.C., Wang, P.J., & Estes, N.A., III (2002). Adverse cardiovascular events temporally associated with ma huang, an herbal source of ephedrine. *Mayo Clinic Proceedings*, Vol.77, No.1, (January 2002), pp. 12-16, ISSN 0025-6196

Schaneberg, B.T., Crockett, S., Bedir, E., & Khan, I.A. (2003). The role of chemical fingerprinting: application to Ephedra. *Phytochemistry*, Vol.62, No.6, (March 2003), pp. 911-918, ISSN 0031-9422

Shekelle, P.G., Hardy, M.L., Morton, S.C., Maglione, M., Mojica, W.A., Suttorp, M.J., Rhodes, S.L., Jungvig, L., & Gagne, J. (2003). Efficacy and safety of ephedra and ephedrine for weight loss and athletic performance: a meta-analysis. *Journal of American Medical Association*, Vol.289, No.12, (March 2003), pp. 1537-1545, ISSN 0098-7484

Shiang, E. & Li, F.P. (1971). The Yin-Yang (cold-hot) theory of disease. *Journal of American Medical Association*, Vol.217, No.8, (August 1971), pp. 1108, ISSN 0098-7484

Shouqin, Z., Junjie, Z., & Changzhen, W. (2004). Novel high pressure extraction technology. *International Journal of Pharmaceuticals*, Vol.278, No.2, (July 2004), pp. 471-474, ISSN 1811-7775

Siow, Y.L., Gong, Y., Au-Yeung, K.K., Woo, C.W., Choy, P.C., & O K (2005). Emerging issues in traditional Chinese medicine. *Canadian Journal of Physiology and Pharmacology*, Vol.83, No.4, (April 2005), pp. 321-334, ISSN 0008-4212

Siu, K.M., Mak, D.H., Chiu, P.Y., Poon, M.K., Du, Y., & Ko, K.M. (2004). Pharmacological basis of 'Yin-nourishing' and 'Yang-invigorating' actions of Cordyceps, a Chinese tonifying herb. *Life Science*, Vol.76, No.4, (December 2004), pp. 385-395, ISSN 1730-413X

Song, J., Yao, H., Li, Y., Li, X., Lin, Y., Liu, C., Han, J., Xie, C., & Chen, S. (2009). Authentication of the family Polygonaceae in Chinese pharmacopoeia by DNA barcoding technique. *Journal of Ethnopharmacology*, Vol.124, No.3, (July 2009), pp. 434-439, ISSN 0378-8741

World Health Organization Special Programme for Research and Training in Tropical Diseases (WHO-TDR). 2005. *Operational guidance: Information needed to support clinical trials of herbal products*, WHO Press, Geneva, Switcerland, Retrived from http://whqlibdoc.who.int/hq/2005/TDR_GEN_Guidance_05.1_eng.pdf

Szeto, Y.T. & Benzie, I.F. (2006). Is the yin-yang nature of Chinese herbal medicine equivalent to antioxidation-oxidation? *Journal of Ethnopharmacology*, Vol.108, No.3, (December 2006), pp. 361-366, ISSN 0378-8741

Taitano, K., Schnyer, R., Allen, J. J. B., Manber, R., & Hitt, S. K. (2003). The psychophysiology of yin and yang. *Journal of Herbal Pharmacotherapy*, Vol.3, pp. 63 ISSN 1552-8940

Tam, J.C., Lau, K.M., Liu, C.L., To, M.H., Kwok, H.F., Lai, K.K., Lau, C.P., Ko, C.H., Leung, P.C., Fung, K.P., & Lau, C.B. (2011). The in vivo and in vitro diabetic wound healing effects of a 2-herb formula and its mechanisms of action. *Journal of Ethnopharmacology*, Vol.134, No.3, (April 2011), pp. 831-838, ISSN 0378-8741

Tang, F., Zhang, Q.L., Nie, Z., Chen, B., & Yao, S.Z. (2009). Sample preparation for analyzing traditional Chinese medicines. *Trends in Analytical Chemistry*, Vol.28, No.11, (December 2009), pp. 1253-1262, ISSN 0165-9936

Tistaert, C., Dejaegher, B., & Vander, H.Y. (2011). Chromatographic separation techniques and data handling methods for herbal fingerprints: a review. *Analytica Chimica Acta*, Vol.690, No.2, (April 2011), pp. 148-161, ISSN 0003-2670

Tong, W. (2010). Challenge from the Philosophy of Scientific Practice and New Empiricism. *Systems Research and Behavioral Science*, Vol.27, No.2, (February 2010), pp. 190-199, ISSN1712-851X

Unschuld, P.U. (2003). *Huangdi nei jing su wen: Nature, kowledge, imagery in an ancient Chinese medical text* (1st edition), University of California Press, ISBN 0585468583, Berkeley

van Wijk, R., van der Greef, J., & van Wijk, E. (2010). Human ultraweak photon emission and the yin yang concept of Chinese medicine. *Journal of Acupuncture and Meridian Studies*, Vol.3, No.4, (December 2010), pp. 221-231, ISSN 2005-2901

Varbiro, G., Veres, B., Gallyas, F., Jr., & Sumegi, B. (2001). Direct effect of Taxol on free radical formation and mitochondrial permeability transition. *Free Radical Biology and Medicie*, Vol.31, No.4, (August 2001), pp. 548-558, ISSN 0891-5849

Vegiopoulos, A. & Herzig, S. (2007). Glucocorticoids, metabolism and metabolic diseases. *Molecular and Cellular Endocrinology*, Vol.275, No.1-2, (September 2007), pp. 43-61, ISSN 0303-7207

Wachtel-Galor, S., Yuen, J., Buswell, J. A., & Benzie, I. F. F. (2011). Ganoderma lucidum (Lingzhi or Reishi): A medicinal mushroom, In: *Herbal medicine - Biomolecular and clinical aspects*, (2nd edition), I.F.F. Benzie & S. Wachtel-Galor, (Eds.), pp. 175-198, CRC Press, ISBN 978143980132, Boca Raton, London, New York

Wang, B.J., Won, S.J., Yu, Z.R., & Su, C.L. (2005). Free radical scavenging and apoptotic effects of Cordyceps sinensis fractionated by supercritical carbon dioxide. *Food and Chemical Toxicology*, Vol.43, No.4, (April 2005), pp. 543-552, ISSN 0278-6915

Wang, G., Mao, B., Xiong, Z.Y., Fan, T., Chen, X.D., Wang, L., Liu, G.J., Liu, J., Guo, J., Chang, J., Wu, T.X., & Li, T.Q. (2007). The quality of reporting of randomized controlled trials of traditional Chinese medicine: a survey of 13 randomly selected journals from mainland China. *Clinical Therapeutics*, Vol.29, No.7, (July 2007), pp. 1456-1467, ISSN 0149-2918

Wang, L., Zhang, R.M., Liu, G.Y., Wei, B.L., Wang, Y., Cai, H.Y., Li, F.S., Xu, Y.L., Zheng, S.P., & Wang, G. (2010). Chinese herbs in treatment of influenza: a randomized, double-blind, placebo-controlled trial. *Respiratory Medicine*, Vol.104, No.9, (September 2010), pp. 1362-1369, ISSN 0954-6111

Wang, X.M., Yang, M., Guan, S.H., Liu, R.X., Xia, J.M., Bi, K.S., & Guo, D.A. (2006). Quantitative determination of six major triterpenoids in Ganoderma lucidum and related species by high performance liquid chromatography. *Journal of Pharmaceutical and Biomedical Analysis*, Vol.41, No.3, (June 2006), pp. 838-844, ISSN 0731-7085

Wilczynski, J.R. (2005). Th1/Th2 cytokines balance-yin and yang of reproductive immunology. *European Journal of Obstetrics and Gynecology and Reproductive Biology*, Vol.122, No.2, (Oct 2005), pp. 136-143, ISSN 0301-2115

Witz, I.P. (2008). Yin-yang activities and vicious cycles in the tumor microenvironment. *Cancer Research*, Vol.68, No.1, (January 2008), pp. 9-13, ISSN 0008-5472

Wolsko, P.M., Solondz, D.K., Phillips, R.S., Schachter, S.C., & Eisenberg, D.M. (2005). Lack of herbal supplement characterization in published randomized controlled trials. The *American Journal of Medicine*, Vol.118, No.10, (October 2005), pp. 1087-1093, ISSN 0002-9343

Wong, H. S., Leung, H. Y., & Ko, K. M. (2011). 'Yang-invigorating' chinese tonic herbs enhance mitochondrial ATP generation in H9c2 cardiomyocytes. *Chinese Medicine*, Vol.2, No.1, (March 2011), pp. 1-5, ISSN 2151-1918

Xie, P.S., Yan, Y.Z., Guo, B.L., Lam, C.W., Chui, S.H., & Yu, Q.X. (2010). Chemical pattern-aided classification to simplify the intricacy of morphological taxonomy of Epimedium species using chromatographic fingerprinting. *Journal of Pharmaceutical and Biomedical Analysis*, Vol.52, No.4, (August 2010), pp. 452-460, ISSN 0731-7085

Yang, M., Sun, J., Lu, Z., Chen, G., Guan, S., Liu, X., Jiang, B., Ye, M., & Guo, D.A. (2009). Phytochemical analysis of traditional Chinese medicine using liquid chromatography coupled with mass spectrometry. *Journal of Chromatography A*, Vol.1216, No.11, (March 2009), pp. 2045-2062, ISSN 0021-9673

Yang, Q., Wang, S., Xie, Y., Sun, J., & Wang, J. (2010). HPLC analysis of Ganoderma lucidum polysaccharides and its effect on antioxidant enzymes activity and Bax, Bcl-2 expression. *International Journal of Biological Macromolecules*, Vol.46, No.2, March 2010, pp. 167-172, ISSN 0141-8130

Yang, S.Z. (2005). *The divine famer's materia; medica: a translation of the shen nong ben cao jing* (1st edition)., Blue Poppy Press, ISBN 0585105464, Boulder, Colorado

Yap, K.Y.L., Chan, S.Y., & Lim, C.S. (2008). The reliability of traditional authentication - A case of ginseng misfit. *Food Chemistry*, Vol.107, No.1, (March 2008), pp. 570-575, ISSN 0308-8146

Yuen, J.W. & Gohel, M.D. (2005). Anticancer effects of Ganoderma lucidum: a review of scientific evidence. *Nutrition and Cancer: An International Journal*, Vol.53, No.1, (November 2005), pp. 11-17, ISSN 0163-5581

Yuen, J.W. & Gohel, M.D. (2008). The dual roles of Ganoderma antioxidants on urothelial cell DNA under carcinogenic attack. *Journal of Ethnopharmacology*, Vol.118, No.2, (July 2008), pp. 324-330 ISSN 0378-8741

Yuen, J.W., Gohel, M.D., & Au, D.W. (2008). Telomerase-associated apoptotic events by mushroom ganoderma lucidum on premalignant human urothelial cells. *Nutrition and Cancer: An International Journal*, Vol.60, No.1, (January 2008), pp. 109-119, ISSN 0163-5581

Yuen, J.W., Gohel, M.D., & Ng, C.F. (2011). The differential immunological activities of Ganoderma lucidum on human pre-cancerous uroepithelial cells. *Journal of Ethnopharmacology*, Vol.135, No.3, (June 2011), pp. 711-718, ISSN 0378-8741

Zhang, J. (2007). Yin and yang interplay of IFN-gamma in inflammation and autoimmune disease. *The Journal of Clinical Investigations*, Vol.117, No.4, (April 2007), pp. 871-873, ISSN 0021-9738

Zhang, Y. S. (2011). Mathematical reasoning of treatment principle based on "yin yang wu xing" theory in traditional Chinese medicine. *Chinese Medicine*, Vol.2, (March 2011), pp. 6-15, ISSN 2151-1918

Zhao, Y.Y., Zhang, Y., Lin, R.C., & Sun, W.J. (2009). An expeditious HPLC method to distinguish Aconitum kusnezoffii from related species. *Fitoterapia*, Vol.80, No.6, (September 2009), pp. 333-338, ISSN 0367-326X

Zhong, Y., Fu, J., Liu, X., Diao, X., Mao, B., Fan, T., Yang, H., Liu, G., & Zhang, W. (2010). The Reporting Quality, Scientific Rigor and Ethics of Randomized Placebo-Controlled Trials of traditional Chinese Medicine Compound Formulations and the Differences Between Chinese and Non-Chinese Trials. *Current Therapeutic Research*, Vol.71, No.1, (February 2010), pp. 30-49, ISSN 0011-393X

2

JIN Formula Inhibits Tumorigenesis Pathways in Human Lung Carcinoma Cells and Tumor Growth in Athymic Nude Mice

Yuhui Zhou et al.*
*Nanjing University of Chinese Medicine,
Tianjing Medical University General Hospital,
Hongkong Baptist University, Hongkong,
China*

1. Introduction

Lung cancer as the most common cancer in the world represents a major public health problem (1). Worldwide it has the highest rate of cancer mortality, exceeding the mortality rates of colorectal, breast and prostate cancers combined (2). Despite major advances in the treatment and management of lung cancer, most patients with lung cancer eventually die of this disease. Because conventional therapies have failed to make a major impact on survival, newer approaches are necessary in the battle against lung cancer. The poor lung cancer survival figures argue powerfully for new approaches to control this disease through chemoprevention, which has been defined as the use of agents that could reverse, suppress or completely halt tumor development. Developing novel mechanism-based chemopreventive approaches for lung cancer which humans can accept has become an important goal.

Many traditional Chinese medicine (TCM) formulas have been used in cancer therapy. JIN formula, an ancient herbal formula from classical book JIN KUI YAO LUE (Golden Chamber) for the treatment of lung cancer, which is composed of Ophiopogon japonicus 30g, Prepared Rhizoma Pinelliae15g, Ginseng radix 30g, Glycyrrhiza radix 12g, Peach Kernel 15g, Unprepared Coix lachryma jobi seed 30g, Chinese waxgourd seed 30g, and Phragmititis Caulis 30g. TCM theory regarded that lung cancer is related with both deficiency of Qi and Yin, or Qi insufficiency of the Spleen and Lung, as well as pathological changes of Qi stagnation, blood stasis, and accumulation of phlegm and toxin. Whereas, JIN formula could replenish both Qi and Yin, strengthen the Spleen and Lung, clear lung, resolve phlegm, activate blood circulation and remove stasis.

* Fei Xiong[1], Zhenzhou Huang[1], Luyu Zheng[1], Miao Jiang[1], Ming Jiang[3], Yuping Tang[1], Jian Ma[1],
Zhen Zhan[1], Jinao Duan[1] and Xu Zhang[*,1],
[1]*Nanjing University of Chinese Medicine, China*
[2]*Tianjing Medical University General Hospital, China*
[3]*Hongkong Baptist University, Hongkong, China*
**Corresponding Author

We extracted JIN formula with different solvents, hereafter referred to as JIN formula extracts (JFE). It is hypothesized that JFE may afford chemopreventive as well as chemotherapeutic effects against lung cancer. In the present study, we first demonstrated the antiproliferative effects of JFE (including E1 to E8) in A549 cells. This involves the tumorigenesis network of cells. Next, we determined the chemopreventive potential of JFE on regulation of PI3K/Akt, MAPK, NF-kB pathways in A549 and H157 human lung carcinoma cells. Based on the results of our in vitro data, we next carried out in vivo study in mice. We found that oral administration of a human acceptable dose of JIN formula (3%, wt/vol) to athymic nude mice implanted with A549 and H157 cells resulted in significant inhibition of tumor growth.

2. Materials and methods

2.1 Materials
Akt, JNK, and p38 antibodies were obtained from Cell Signaling Technology. The polyclonal antibodies NF-kB/p65, ERK1/2 were procured from Santa Cruz Biotechnology Inc. Anti-mouse and anti-rabbit secondary antibody horseradish peroxidase (HRP) conjugate was obtained from Amersham Life Science Inc.

2.2 Methods
2.2.1 Preparation of JFE
Fresh JIN formula was decocted in distilled water. As shown in Figure 1, different solvents were applied to acquire the following eight extracts: Water extraction concentrate (E1), Ethanol precipitation (E2), Precipitates in ethanol recovery (E3), Ethanol concentration (E4), Cyclohexane extract (E5), Ethyl acetate extract (E6), N-butanol extract (E7) and Water solution (E8). The extracts were condensed and freeze dried. The freeze-dried extracts were stored at 4°C to be used for various treatments.

2.2.2 Cell culture and treatment
The human lung carcinoma A549 and H157 cells were obtained from American Type Culture Collection and cultured in DMEM medium, supplemented with 10% fetal bovine serum, 1% penicillin/streptomycin (P-S) in a 5% CO_2 atmosphere at 37°C. The extracts were dissolved in dimethyl sulfoxide (DMSO) and were used for the treatment of cells. A total of 50-60% confluent cells were treated with the extracts (1–100 µg/ml) for 72 h in complete growth medium.

2.2.3 Cell viability (MTT assay)
The effect of JFE on the viability of cells was determined by 3-[4,5-dimethylthiazol-2-yl]-2,5-diphenyl tetrazoliumbromide assay. The cells were plated at 1×10^4 cells/well in 200 µl of complete culture medium containing 1–100 µg/ml concentrations of JFE in 96-well microtiter plates for 72 h. After incubation for specified times at 37°C in a humidified incubator, 3-[4,5-dimethylthiazol-2-yl]-2,5-diphenyl tetrazoliumbromide (5 mg/ml in PBS) was added to each well and incubated for 4 h, after which the plate was centrifuged at 1800g for 5 min at 4°C. The absorbance was recorded on a microplate reader at the wavelength of 540 nm. The effect of JFE on growth inhibition was assessed as percent cell viability where DMSO-treated cells were taken as 100% viable. DMSO at the concentrations used was without any effect on cell viability.

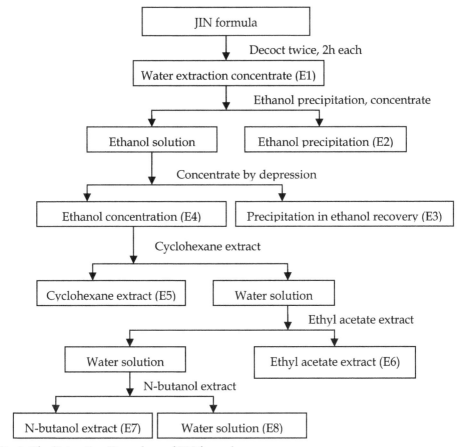

Fig. 1. The Extracting Procedure of JIN formula

2.2.4 Protein extraction and western blotting

Following the treatment of cells as described above, the media was aspirated, the cells were washed with cold PBS (pH 7.4), and ice-cold lysis buffer (50 mM Tris–HCl, 150 mM NaCl, 1 mM EGTA, 1 mM EDTA, 20 mM NaF, 100 mM Na_3VO_4, 0.5% NP-40, 1%Triton X-100, 1 mM PMSF (pH 7.4) with freshly added protease inhibitor cocktail (Protease Inhibitor Cocktail Set III; Calbiochem) over ice for 30 min. The cells were scraped and the lysate was collected in a microfuge tube and passed through needle to break up the cell aggregates. The lysate was cleared by centrifugation at 14 000g for 15 min at 4°C and the supernatant (whole cell lysate) was used or immediately stored at -80°C.

For western blotting, 30-50 mg protein was resolved over 8-12% polyacrylamide gels and transferred to a nitrocellulose membrane. The blot was blocked in blocking buffer (5% non-fat dry milk/1% Tween 20; in 20 mM TBS, pH 7.6) for 1 h at room temperature, incubated with appropriate monoclonal or polyclonal primary antibody in blocking buffer for 1.5 hours to overnight at 4°C, followed by incubation with anti-mouse or anti-rabbit secondary antibody HRP conjugate obtained from Amersham Life Science Inc. Densitometric measurements of the band detected by chemiluminescence in western blot analysis were performed using digitalized scientific software program Quantity One.

2.2.5 In vivo tumor xenograft model

Balb/c athymic (nude) mice (male, 6−8 weeks) weighing 21−25 g were purchased from Animal Center, Academy of Military Medical Sciences, (Beijing, China) and were housed under specific pathogen-free conditions according to the guidelines of Animal Care, Nanjing University of Chinese Medicine. The animal room was controlled for temperature (22 ±2°C), light (12 hour light/dark cycle) and humidity (50±10%). All laboratory feed pellets and bedding was autoclaved.

The tumor regression model in nude mice has been successfully applied to evaluate antitumor activity. This model was therefore used to evaluate suppression of solid tumor growth in JIN Formula (JIN). A total of 1×10^7 A549, H157 cells in 0.2 ml culture medium were injected subcutaneously into the flank of each mouse using a 26-gauge needle. After 7 days observation, an apparently solid tumor mass was excised from mice inoculated with lung cancer cells. When the tumor volume reached about 50 mm^3 in the nude mice, xenografted tumor model were randomly distributed into normal group, model group, Jin group, after sacrifice of animals with oral administration of JIN formula (3%, wt/vol) for 16 days, tumor inhibiting rate was recorded to show the effects of drugs on tumor growth.

Tumor inhibiting rate= (average of tumor weight in model group-average of tumor weight in JIN group) /average of tumor weight in model group ×100%.

2.3 Statistical analysis

Results were analyzed using a two-tailed Student's t-test to assess statistical significance and P-values<0.05 were considered significant.

3. Result

3.1 Inhibition of cell growth by JFE in A549 cells

This study was designed to show the chemopreventive/chemotherapeutic potential of JIN formula against lung cancer. Initially in our study, we investigated the antiproliferative effects of JFE treatment on human lung carcinoma A549 cells. Therefore, using A549 cells, we first evaluated the effect of JFE on the growth of these cells by MTT assay. We compared the antiproliferative effects of JFE (including E1 to E8) on A549 cells. As shown in Figure 2, treatment of JFE (1–100 μg/ml) for 72 h was found that E6 and E7 could decrease the viability of A549 cells.

3.2 Inhibition of tumorigenesis pathways by JFE in A549 and H157 cells

To explore the mechanism of antiproliferative effects of JIN formula against lung cancer, we investigated the involvement of Akt, ERK1/2, JNK1/2, p38 and NF-κB machinery during the inhibition of tumorigenesis by JFE in A549 and H157 cells.

Akt, also known as protein kinase B, which is a serine or threonine kinase, has been identified as an important component of tumorigenesis signaling pathway. The PI3K/Akt promotes cell survival by activating the NF-kB signaling pathway (3). Studies have shown that Akt plays an important role in carcinogenesis. We first investigated the effect of JFE on Akt protein expression in human lung carcinoma cells. In our study, we have demonstrated that the treatment of A549 and H157 cells with JFE (E1–E8) resulted in different degree inhibition of Akt pathways on tumor promotion processes as shown in Figure 3.

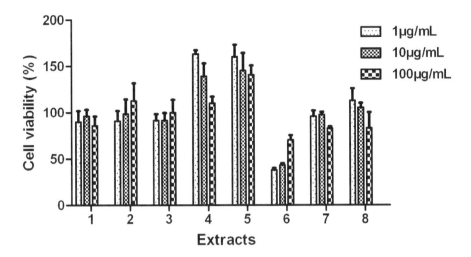

Fig. 2. The effects of JFE (including E1 to E8) on A549 cells growth

The MAP kinase superfamily (MAPKs) has been characterized into three groups which include extracellular signal-regulated kinase p44/42 (ERK), JNK/SAPK (c-jun N-terminal kinase/stress activated protein kinase) and p38 MAP kinase. MAPKs, a group of serine/threonine-specific, proline-directed protein kinases are known to modulate transcription factor activities. (4, 5). The involvement of the MAPK pathway in tumor proliferation is well documented. Transient activation of ERK is responsible for proliferation and differentiation and has also been shown to be involved in tumor promotion processes (3). Stimulation of JNK/SAPK and p38 can mediate differentiation, inflammatory responses and cell death (6). In the present study, we assessed the effect of JFE on MAPK pathway in A549 and H157 human lung carcinoma cells. The immunoblot analysis demonstrated that the treatment of cells with JFE inhibited ERK1/2, JNK1/2 and p38 proteins, and this inhibition of JNK1/2 and p38 in A549 cells was stronger than in H157 (Figure 3). Several studies have shown that JNK pathway plays a major role in cellular function, such as cell proliferation and transformation, whereas the ERK pathway suppresses apoptosis and enhances cell survival or tumorigenesis (4). ERK1/2 and p38 are also involved in the transcriptional activation of NF-kB (7, 8).

NF-kB is a sequence specific transcription factor that is known to be involved in the inflammatory and innate immune responses (9, 10). NF-kB is sequestered in the cytoplasm in an inactive form through interaction with IkB. Phosphorylation of IkB by IkB kinase (IKK) causes ubiquitination and degradation of IkB, thus releasing NF-kB which then translocates to the nucleus, where it binds to specific kB binding sites in the promoter regions of several genes (11). Studies have shown that NF-kB activation plays an important role in cell survival, by its ability to block or reduce apoptosis (12). In the present study, we further investigated the effect of JFE on the pattern of NF-kB activation and whether treatment with JFE inhibits nuclear translocation of NF-kB/p65 in A549 and H157 cells. As is evident from western blot analysis data and the relative density of bands, we found that JFE (E2, E3, E7) treatment of A549 cells resulted in inhibition of translocation of NF-kB/p65, meanwhile, we demonstrated that NF-kB is activated in H157 human lung carcinoma cells treated with JFE (E2, E3, E7) and is translocated to the nucleus when measured by western blot analysis (Figure 3).

(A)

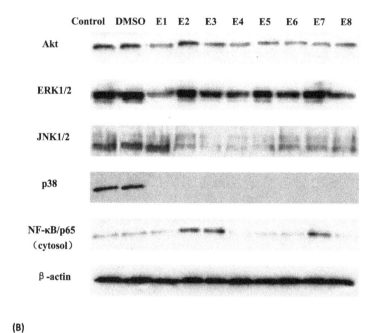

(B)

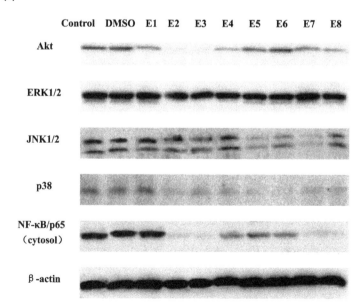

Fig. 3. (A) Inhibitory effects of JFE on tumorigenesis pathways in human lung carcinoma A549 cells (B) Inhibitory effects of JFE on tumorigenesis pathways in human lung carcinoma H157cells

The immunoblot analysis demonstrated that JFE (E1–E8) treatment could induce (i) inhibition of AKt, (ii) inhibition of ERK1/2 (p44 and p42), (iii) inhibition of JNK1/2 (p54 and p46), (iv) inhibition of p38 protein and (v) regulation of NF-kB.

3.3 Inhibition on the growth of human lung carcinoma A549 and H157 cells by JIN formula in nude mice

JFE inhibits the development of lung tumorigenesis by modulating and inhibiting PI3K/Akt, MAPK, and NF-kB signaling. To establish the relevance of these in vitro findings to in vivo situation, athymic nude mice were implanted with human lung carcinoma A549 and H157 cells. Compared with model group, Jin formula could significantly inhibit volume growth of A549 and H157 xenografted tumors. The inhibiting rate could reach to 28.5% and 25% in A549 and H157 tumor-bearing mice respectively (p < 0.05). We found that the oral administration of JIN formula significantly slowed the progression of A549 and H157 tumor growth in nude mice.

4. Discussion

Lung cancer as the most common cancer in the world represents a major public health problem. Worldwide it accounts for 1.18 million cancer-related deaths and is the most common cause of cancer death in both men and women (13). Lung carcinogenesis is a chronic and multistep process resulting in malignant lung tumors. This progression from normal to neoplastic pulmonary cells or tissues could be arrested or reversed through pharmacological treatments. These therapeutic interventions should reduce or avoid the clinical consequences of lung cancer by treating early neoplastic lesions before the development of clinically evident signs or symptoms of malignancy. Preclinical, clinical and epidemiological findings relating to different classes of candidate chemopreventive agents provide strong support for lung cancer prevention as a therapeutic strategy (14). Cancer chemoprevention is an attractive approach to reduce lung cancers by treating early steps in lung carcinogenesis. There is a convergence of basic scientific and clinical findings in lung cancer chemoprevention. Pharmacological interventions also can be used to reverse or arrest the progression of lung carcinogenesis. For this reason, additional clinical trials are needed that emphasize a mechanistic approach in which mechanisms identified in vitro can be validated in vivo.

This study was designed to show the chemopreventive/chemotherapeutic potential of JIN formula against lung cancer. we assessed the efficacy of the JIN formula, which is an ancient herbal formula from classical book JIN KUI YAO LUE (Golden Chamber) for the treatment of lung cancer and explored its probable molecular mechanisms. Initially, employing human lung carcinoma A549 cells, we compared the growth inhibitory effects of JIN formula extracts (JFE, including E1 to E8). The results showed that E6 and E7 could decrease the viability of A549 cells by the MTT assays. To explore the mechanism of antiproliferative effects of JIN formula against lung cancer, we investigated the involvement of Akt, ERK1/2, JNK1/2, p38 and NF-κB pathway during the inhibition of tumorigenesis by JFE in A549 and H157 cells. The immunoblot analysis demonstrated that JFE treatment could result in different degree inhibition of above signaling pathways on tumor promotion processes. Oral administration of JIN formula (3%, wt/vol) to athymic nude mice implanted with A549 and H157 cells resulted in a significant inhibition in tumor growth.

In conclusion, the present study demonstrates that human non small cell lung cancer A549 and H157 cells are highly sensitive to JIN formula both in vitro and in vivo experimental models. JIN formula inhibits the development of lung tumorigenesis by modulating the imbalance of proliferative and apoptotic signaling network. Based on the present study it is tempting to suggest that JIN formula and its effective extracts have strong potential for development as a chemopreventive and possibly as a chemotherapeutic agent against lung cancer.

5. Acknowledgements

This study was supported by National Science & Technology Pillar Program in the 11th Five year Plan of China (2006BAI11B08−01) and the Priority Academic Program Development (PAPD) of Jiangsu Higher Education Institutions.

6. References

[1] Parkin, D.M., Bray,F., Ferlay,J. and Pisani,P. (2001) Estimating the world lung cancer burden: Globocan 2000. Int. J. Cancer, 94, 153–156.

[2] Parkin, D.M., Bray,F., Ferlay,J. and Pisani,P. (2005) Global cancer statistics, 2002. CA Cancer J. Clin., 55, 74–108.

[3] Adhami, V.M., Siddiqui,I.A., Ahmad,N., Gupta,S. and Mukhtar,H. (2004) Oral consumption of green tea polyphenols inhibits insulin-like growth factor-I-induced signaling in an autochthonous mouse model of prostate cancer. Cancer Res., 64, 8715–8722.

[4] Afaq, F., Ahmad,N. and Mukhtar,H. (2003) Suppression of UVB-induced phosphorylation of mitogen-activated protein kinases and nuclear factor kappa B by green tea polyphenol in SKH-1 hairless mice. Oncogene, 22, 9254–9264.

[5] Katiyar, S.K., Afaq, F., Azizuddin, K. and Mukhtar, H. (2001) Inhibition of UVB-induced oxidative stress-mediated phosphorylation of mitogen-activated protein kinase signaling pathways in cultured human epidermal keratinocytes by green tea polyphenol (-) -epigallocatechin-3-gallate. Toxicol. Appl. Pharmacol., 176, 110–117.

[6] Cobb, M.H. and Goldsmith, E.J. (1995) How MAP kinases are regulated. J. Biol. Chem., 270, 14843–14846.

[7] Adderley, S.R. and Fitzgerald, D.J. (1999) Oxidative damage of cardiomyocytes is limited by extracellular regulated kinases 1/2-mediated induction of cyclooxygenase-2. J. Biol. Chem., 274, 5038–5046.

[8] Carter, A.B., Knudtson, K.L., Monick, M.M. and Hunninghake,G.W. (1999) The p38 mitogen-activated protein kinase is required for NF-kappaB- dependent gene expression: the role of TATA-binding protein (TBP). J. Biol. Chem., 274, 30858–30863.

[9] Baldwin, A.S. Jr. (1996) The NF-kappa B and I kappa B proteins: new discoveries and insights. Annu. Rev. Immunol., 14, 649–683.

[10] Maniatis, T. (1997) Catalysis by a multiprotein IkappaB kinase complex. Science, 278, 818–819.

[11] Gupta, S., Hastak, K., Afaq, F., Ahmad, N. and Mukhtar, H. (2004) Essential role of caspases in epigallocatechin-3-gallate-mediated inhibition of nuclear factor kappa B and induction of apoptosis. Oncogene, 23, 2507–2522.

[12] Kaufman, C.K. and Fuchs, E. (2000) It's got you covered. NF-kappaB in the epidermis. J. Cell Biol., 149, 999–1004.

[13] Peto, R., Darby, S., Deo, H., Silcocks, P., Whitley, E. and Doll, R. (2000) Smoking, smoking cessation and lung cancer in the UK since 1950: combination of national statistics with two case-control studies. Br. Med.J., 321, 323–329.

[14] Cohen, V. and Khuri, F.R. (2002) Chemoprevention of lung cancer: current status and future prospects. Cancer Metastasis Rev., 21, 349–362.

3

The Serotonergic System and Neuroplasticity are Implicated in the Effect of Phytochemicals on Mood and Cognitive Disorders

Ying Xu[1*], Chong Zhang[1*] and William O. Ogle[2]
[1]Department of Behavioral Medicine and Psychiatry, West Virginia University, WV,
[2]Crayton Pruitt Family Department of Biomedical Engineering and
Evelyn F. & William L. Mcknight Brain Institute, University of Florida, Gainesville, FL,
USA

1. Introduction

Studies has been established in the 1930s that any environmental changes, whether internal or external, that disturbs the maintenance of homeostasis can cause stress response, including psychological, neuronal, endocrine and immune system reactivity (B E Leonard, 2005). During chronic stress or long-term exposure to external stress, glucocorticosteroids induce the hyperactivity of the Hypothalamic-Pituitary-Adrenal (HPA) axis, which produces an increase in plasma glucocorticoid level that then impairs the negative feedback mechanism, causing psychological disorders (Croes, Merz, & Netter, 1993; Henry, 1992). In stress-induced emotional and cognitive disorders, such as depression, anxiety and learning and memory impairment, the serotonergic system mainly exerts its regulatory functions through different subtypes of receptors. Research over the past decades have found that serotonin receptors, such as $5-HT_{1A}$, $5-HT_{1B}$, $5-HT_{2A}$, $5-HT_{2C}$, $5-HT_4$, $5-HT_6$, and $5-HT_7$ subtypes, are closely related to depression and memory deficits. Moreover, clinical investigation suggests that some of the agonists or antagonists of the 5-HT receptor subtypes can be used for treatment of depression. However, the detailed roles of serotonin receptors in these disorders remain unclear.

Neuroplasticity has been described as the ability of the brain to reorganize itself and form new neuronal connections throughout life. Depression is associated with a neuronal loss in specific brain regions, which has been proven by functional brain imaging and other neurobiological techniques. The dendritic abnormalities seen in the hippocampus in animal models of depression and in patients with depression and Alzheimer's suggest changes in hippocampal circuitry are involved in disorders involving depression, anxiety and learning and memory impairment. The morphological and functional changes of neurons may be reversed after treatment with antidepressants, such as some natural compounds. In this review, a connection between neuroplasticity and the antidepressant-like effects of phytochemicals that are currently being studied is brought into attention. Some phytochemicals, such as curcumin, are found to reverse impaired hippocampal

---

* Equal contribution

neuroplasticity in chronically stressed rats by, for instance, increasing the dendritic length and the number of dendrites and axons. Compelling evidence now suggests a close relation between serotonin system and neuroplasticity in depression. For example, the reduced neuronal plasticity in chronically stressed rats is accompanied by down-regulation of 5-HT_{1A} receptor mRNA expression, which can be prevented by the administration of curcumin. Other intriguing findings suggest that 5-HT_7 receptor can even differentially regulate neuroplasticity in different brain regions after treatment with corticosterone and curcumin. With these findings, there has been a remarkable increase in interest regarding the use of phytochemicals in repairing the neuroplasticity related to central nervous system dysfunction.

Phytochemicals, particularly anti-oxidative natural compounds, are considered promising alternatives to conventional drugs, such as tricyclic antidepressants, monoamine oxidase inhibitors, serotonin reuptake inhibitors (SSRI), and norepinephrine and dopamine reuptake inhibitors. This is not only because they are extracted from fruits and vegetables and affect biological activities with high potency and low systemic toxicity, but also because they can bind to multiple targets. Studies in the early 90s had a general focus on long-term dietary supplementation. For example, foods supplemented with strawberry extracts and spinach had beneficial effects in retarding functional age-related mood and neurodegenerative diseases, due to their potent anti-oxidative properties. In the following years, phytochemicals have been isolated from the antioxidant-rich foods and their biological activities are gradually being elucidated. Typical phytochemicals that are being studied include curcumin, resveratrol, fisetin, and berberine.

This review summarizes the series of studies on the involvement of serotonin system and neuronal plasticity in treatment of mood and cognitive disorders using Chinese medicine.

2. The 5-HT system in mood and cognitive diseases

Serotonin (5-hydroxytryptamine, 5-HT) is an important neurotransmitter in the central nervous system (CNS). Through activation or inhibition of its receptor subtypes, studies have demonstrated that 5-HT has multiple physiological functions and dysregulation of serotonergic system can cause stress-related diseases such as Alzheimer's Diseases (AD), anxiety, depression and cognitive disorders (Goddard et al., 2010; Ramanathan & Glatt, 2009). The neurons of the raphe nuclei release the majority of 5-HT in the brain and project onto many other regions of the brain, exerting the regulatory function of 5-HT on physiology. 5-HT expression in developing raphe nuclei neurons and the preferential generation of the nerve fiber projecting terminals during the formation of neuronal synapses demonstrated that 5-HT affects not only morphology and neural activity of embryonic neurons, but also neurogenesis and neuroplasticity after neuronal maturation, including proliferation, translocation, differentiation and synapse formation (Veenstra-VanderWeele et al., 2000). 5-HT is also involved in the development of cerebral cortex in mammals; during the early stages of sensory cortex development, temporary serotonergic fiber projections were detected, indicating that 5-HT might be helpful in conjugation and integration of the developing cortex (Nayyar et al., 2009). Brain serotonin synthesis, packaging, transportation, targeting, release, reuptake and degradation all affect the concentration of 5-HT and its functions. Proteins and related genes that are involved in regulating these physiological functions include speed-limiting enzyme TPH-1 and TPH-2 (Illi et al., 2009), Vmat2 (Fukui et al., 2007; Zucker, Weizman, & Rehavi, 2005), serotonin transporter (SERT or 5-HTT),

The Serotonergic System and Neuroplasticity are Implicated in the Effect of Phytochemicals
on Mood and Cognitive Disorders

41

monoamine oxidase A (MAO-A) and 5-HT pre and post synaptic receptors (Paaver et al., 2007).

5-HT receptors are assigned to one of seven receptor families, 5-HT$_{1-7}$, comprising a total of fourteen structurally and pharmacologically distinct mammalian 5-HT receptor subtypes. With the exception of 5-HT$_3$ receptor, a ligand-gated ion channel, all receptors (5-HT$_{1A-E}$, 5-HT$_{2A-C}$, 5-HT$_4$, 5-HT$_5$, 5-HT$_6$, 5-HT$_7$) are G protein-coupled receptors (GPCR) that activate an intracellular second messenger cascade to produce an excitatory or inhibitory response. Activation of the specific G-protein can affect enzymes, such as adenylate cyclase, phospholipase A and C, mitogen-activated protein kinase, and cation channels, especially K$^+$ and Ca^{2+} (Kushwaha & Albert, 2005). Recent literature has shown, in intact brain, the unequivocal participation of 5-HT receptors in specific physiological responses, ranging from modulation of neuronal activity and transmitter release to behavioral change, especially in psychological disorders like depression, anxiety, obsessive-compulsive disorder, and panic disorder (Ayala, 2009). Among the receptor subtypes, 5-HT$_{1A}$, 5-HT$_{1B}$, 5-HT$_{2A}$, 5-HT$_{2C}$, 5-HT$_4$, 5-HT$_6$, 5-HT$_7$ are associated with chronic stress-induced neural diseases, inhibition of learning and memory, and cognitive disorders (King et al., 2008; Meneses, 2007; Pérez-García et al., 2006).

3. Role of neuroplasticity in mood and cognitive disabilities: Protective effects of herbal medicines

Neuroplasticity is referred to as the ability of the nervous system to respond and adapt to environmental challenges as a result of one's experiences. It encompasses a series of functional and structural adaptation mechanisms that may lead to neuronal remodeling, including adding, removing or changing the strength of connections between nerve cells and glial cells. Failure of such adaptations might enhance the susceptibility to environmental challenges and ultimately lead to psychopathology. The brain may become more vulnerable by losing the ability to maintain homeostasis. In the case of depression, it is now well accepted to be characterized by profound alterations in brain function and responsiveness, which might be closely linked with neuroplasticity and the ability to modulate a cascade of events from intracellular signaling mechanisms to gene expression.

3.1 Structure change in mood and cognitive disorders

Recent neuroimaging and post-mortem morphometric studies of several brain regions, including limbic and non-limbic circuits, in individuals with mood disorders have begun to demonstrate that depression is accompanied by morphological changes at both the macro-anatomical and histological levels (Miguel-hidalgo & Rajkowska, 2002). Some researchers applying the most sensitive structural neuroimaging techniques to the brains of patients with major depressive disorder (MDD) or bipolar disorder have shown that they are associated with an enlargement of the lateral ventricles, reduction in the volume of grey and white matter in the prefrontal cortex, shrinkage of the hippocampus and decreased volume of the amygdala. Due to the scant access to post-mortem studies on patients, whether treated or untreated, with mood disorders, information on possible morphological alterations of brain regions is limited. Instead, cytomorphological changes associated with mood disorders in animal models, such as the number of neurons, the size and shape of their cell bodies, as well as dendritic and axonal components, have been greatly studied.

Studies in rodents and nonhuman primates demonstrate that exposure to stress can cause alterations in cytomorphology of neurons. Layer II/III pyramidal neurons in the medial prefrontal cortex showed dendritic retraction and reduction in spine number after several weeks of glucocorticoid administration or restraint stress (S. C. Cook & Wellman, 2004). In the hippocampus, repeated stress is reported to cause atrophy of CA3 pyramidal neurons and dentate gyrus. This is supported by a decrease in the number and length of apical tree, but not base tree (R S Duman, 2002). Volume reduction and, more importantly, a shift from neuronal processes to glial processes to make up for the volume decrease have also been observed. Distinct from the CA3 hippocampal region, 24 hr after a single forced swim stress rather than a 3-week period, apical dendrites showed fewer branches in medial prefrontal cortex (mPFC) (Izquierdo, Wellman, & Holmes, 2006). Moreover, the hippocampus is one of the first brain regions to suffer damage from Alzheimer's disease. The comparison of multiple brain regions provides an even more convincing proof of the relationship between neuroplasticity and stress-induced mood disorders: while chronic stress induces significant regression of the apical dendrites in both hippocampus and prefrontal cortex (PFC), it enhances synaptic plasticity in amygdala (Pittenger & Ronald S Duman, 2008). The latter change could both result from and contribute to over-activation of neuronal circuits within amygdala that control fear, anxiety, and emotion. These findings in the animal models with regard to cytomorphological alterations are consistent with several structural imaging studies in human patients with major depression or anxiety.

In learning and memory, synaptic plasticity is even more thoroughly studied. The theory postulating that changes at synapses within the brain underlie learning and memory was formalized in the 1950s. Two crucial terms involved in this theory are long-term potentiation (LTP) and long-term depression (LTD) (Howland & Y. T. Wang, 2008). LTP is a long-lasting enhancement in signal transmission between two neurons that results from stimulating them synchronously. LTD, on the other hand, is an activity-dependent reduction in the efficacy of neuronal synapses lasting hours or longer and occurs in many areas of the CNS. Both of them describe the ability of chemical synapses to change their strength, which is considered one of the major cellular mechanisms that underlies learning and memory. Cytomorphology of individual neurons and macro-morphology of brain support the normal functioning of synaptic plasticity which plays a direct role in regulating cognitive functions. The underlying mechanisms of morphological alterations during the onset and treatment of mood and cognitive disorders have not yet been clearly understood. However, a few studies show that in patients with MDD and bipolar disorder, there are changes in synaptic proteins that might be associated with morphological changes in related brain regions (Jørgensen & Riederer, 1985). It has also been revealed that antidepressant treatment have a reversing effect on the intracellular signaling, transcription factors and target genes. Neurotophic factors (NTFs), particularly the neurotrophin family such as BDNF, are one of the activity-regulated gene expressions responsive to neuronal activity. It is possible that these treatments could oppose the adverse cellular effects, which may be regarded as a loss of neural plasticity, by blocking or reversing the atrophy of neurons and by increasing cell survival and function.

3.2 Herbal medicines able to restore neuroplasticity in some CNS malfunction

Antidepressant medications may act by correcting the dysfunction of neuronal adaptive responses, namely neuroplasticity. The most likely immediate cause of depressive

The Serotonergic System and Neuroplasticity are Implicated in the Effect of Phytochemicals on Mood and Cognitive Disorders

43

symptoms turns out to be changes in the synaptic availability of the monoamines such as noradrenaline (norepinephrine), serotonin and dopamine, or in the activity of their receptors. As a result, the best accepted pharmacological treatments for depression have been those that increase the availability of monoamines, particularly serotonin.These antidepressants also greatly correct dendritic abnormalities of patients with mood disorders. Dendrites and their spines undergo morphological changes after treatment with some antidepressants. For example, treatment with the selective serotonin reuptake inhibitors (SSRIs) produces a significant increase in dendritic spine density and total length of secondary dendrites in the CA1 region and dentate gyrus of the hippocampus (Norrholm & Ouimet, 2000).

Beyond the classical antidepressants, herbal medicines have been receiving mounting attention due to their ability to reverse or halt impaired neuroplasticity. A wide variety of herbal plants, including Panax ginseng, Zukomei-to (ZMT), Gongjin-dan (GJD), their extracts, compounds and so on have, to date, already presented beneficial results when tested against known pathological neuronal morphology in some mood and cognitive disorders.

Ginsenosides are extracts from Panax ginseng root that are widely used as a tonic medicine throughout the world and in the treatment of amnesia. In animal models, such as brain-damaged rats and aged rats, a significant improvement in learning and memory has been observed using ginseng powder, which contains the major ginseng saponins, ginsenoside Rb1 and Rg1 (Zhong et al., n d). Beyond all doubt, change of neuronal cells morphology underlies the above-mentioned beneficial effects of ginseng saponins. In the 1980s, Sugaya et al. was one of the earliest groups to show that ginseng saponins can improve neurite extension (A. Sugaya et al.,1988). In their study, rat cerebral cortex neurons were cultured. Cytochalasin-B induced disappearance of the growth cone and looping phenomenon were both blocked by administration of crude saponin extract. A proliferative effect of neurite extension, about 1.5 fold in ganglioside content, of cultured neurons was observed, indicating that ginsenosides can promote neurite extension and protect neurons against cytochalasin-B-induced cell lesion. However, this study did not clarify which component within the crude saponin extract of ginseng roots played the most significant role. Later studies screened out ginsenoside Rb1, Rb3, notoginsenosideR4 and Fa as the active compounds that caused the outgrowth and maturation of neurites and they could possibly recover the function of degenerated brains (Nishiyama, Cho, Kitagawa, & Saito, 1994; Tohda, N. Matsumoto, Zou, Meselhy, & Komatsu, 2002).

Zukomei-to (ZMT, or Xu Ming Tan in Chinese), composed of traditional Chinese and Japanese herbal drugs, has long been used in treating postapopletic sequelae, clinically indicating that it might reactivate neuronal function in degenerated neuronal circuits. Based on this speculation, the effects of ZMT on memory impairment and synaptic loss in an Alzheimer's mouse model were investigated (Tohda et al., 2003). In this study, synaptophysin, a vesicle protein located at the presynaptic membrane, was used as a marker for synaptic loss. Mice brain slices stained with anti-synaptophysin antibody showed that ZMT prevented synaptic loss induced by Aβ (25-35) in the CA1 region and dentate gyrus of the hippocampus and the parietal cortex. Neuron densities were also measured in CA1, CA3, and dentate gyrus of the hippocampus and the parietal cortex of mice brains treated with Aβ (25-35) only or both AMT and Aβ (25-35). However, no significant difference was observed, suggesting that synaptic reconstruction rather than neuronal death was involved here.

Gongjin-dan (GJD) is a multi-herbal formula containing different parts of up to six botanicals. It has been used clinically in Korea as an anti-fatigue and anti-aging agent for hundreds of years. GJD was proven to have beneficial effects not only on promoting neurite outgrowth but also on preventing neuronal cell death (Moon et al., 2009). GJD was used on PC12 cells and stressed mice models either as a mimetic or inducer of nerve growth factor (NGF), a small protein commonly reported to stimulate cholinergic neurons, improve memory loss, and increase long-term potentiation and learning tasks. PC12 cells exhibited extended neurite outgrowth after treatment with GJD, although not as obvious as after treatment with NGF. Moreover, NGF level in the cell culture media was elevated. The effect of GJD on survival of neurons was examined by immunostaining microtubule-associated protein-2 (MAP-2), which is a key player in neurogenesis. In the hippocampus of immobilization stressed rats, neuronal cell death was greatly triggered, and GJD was able to decrease this neuronal loss. Since NGF is also required for the survival of the neurons, it is highly possible that GJD exert its neuroprotective function, both in neuroplasticity and neuronal cell survival, by activating the secretion of NGF or simply acting as a mimetic of NGF.

Herbal medicines that have similar effects on the shape and structure of the CNS are not limited to the above-mentioned examples. In later sections of this chapter, more natural compounds, such as curcumin, resveratrol and others, will be discussed with respect to their tonic effects on CNS and operating mechanisms, especially when the 5-HT system is involved. Most of them appear to prevent morphological alterations induced by stress insults. Even though individual studies might have slightly different outcomes due to different cell types or animal models, herbal medicine generally proves to be a promising in treating CNS-related disorders.

4. The antioxidative effects of neuroprotective natural compounds

4.1 Oxidative stress and the 5-HT system

Oxidative stress is a result of a build-up of reactive oxygen species (ROS) due to reduced ability of a biological system to detoxify the reactive intermediates or to repair the resulting damage. ROS are a group of chemically-reactive molecules containing oxygen. They are generated by enzymatic and non-enzymatic reactions in the mitochondria and cytoplasm. In humans, oxidative stress is involved in many diseases including those in the CNS. Oxygen radicals initiate neurotoxicity such as build up of Abeta, leading to neurodegenerations. For example, neurodegenerative diseases, such as Alzheimer's disease (AD), Parkinson's disease (PD), and stroke, are commonly accompanied by oxidative stress markers. Environmental stress can lead the body into pathological conditions, in which ROS levels can increase dramatically, activating enzymes including proteases, phospholipases, and nucleases that result in significant damage to cell morphology. As a result, there is increasing attention to develop nutritional therapies to combat these age-related oxidative processes. Mounting focus has been placed on compounds extracted from botanicals in vegetables, fruits, grains, roots, flowers and so on. Polyphenolics, like resveratrol from grape and red wine and curcumin from turmeric, are becoming recognized for their antioxidative effects against neurodegenerative diseases, possibly by restoring the neuronal cell morphology, as mentioned earlier in this chapter.

The 5-HT system is involved with the oxidative process in several aspects. First, the process interferes with 5-HT system's precursor tryptophan. ROS and reactive nitrogen species (RNS), excluding NO, oxygen and superoxide anion, rapidly react with many tryptophan

The Serotonergic System and Neuroplasticity are Implicated in the Effect of Phytochemicals
on Mood and Cognitive Disorders

45

derivatives, thus gradually eliminating the important neurotransmitter serotonin (Peyrot & Ducrocq, 2008). Second, serotonin and oxidative stress have a counterbalance effect in synthesizing NO. NO, as an endothelium-derived relaxing factor, is synthesized by the endothelial isoform of nitric oxide synthase (eNOS). This process involves pertussis-toxin-sensitive G protein that responses to serotonin and can be inhibited by oxidative stress (Michel & Vanhoutte, 2010). Third, 5-HT receptor subtypes interact with components of the oxidative process. For example, NADPH oxidase is necessary for the activation of 5-HT_2 receptors (MacFarlane et al., 2011). NADPH oxidase is recognized for its dual-edge roles in health and disease. Altered NADPH oxidase function has been linked to neurological disorders such as AD, as it is present in Abeta-induced ROS production (Lambeth, 2007). Superoxide produced by NADPH oxidase may interact with NO to form the toxic peroxynitrite, which is normally associated with neuronal death (Brown, 2007). All in all, oxidative stressors impair neuronal plasticity while concurrently altering neurotransmission, contributing to CNS diseases.

4.2 Natural compounds as antioxidants

Plant-derived supplements for improving mental health are gradually gaining popularity because they are natural and thus considered to be safer and produce fewer side effects than chemically synthesized antioxidants. One of the most commonly studied type is the polyphenols, which have a wide array of phenol ring structures, as one of the first antioxidative natural compounds to catch attention. They are divided into different groups according to the number of phenol rings and the chemical groups attached to them, among which flavonoids are the largest and most well-known group. The capacity of flavonoids to act as an antioxidant, i.e. scavenging free radicals, depends on their molecular structure. In general, polyphenols are rapidly converted to their glucuronide derivatives upon ingestion and transported to the circulatory system, where they can cross the blood brain barrier.

4.2.1 Resveratrol

Dietary supplement of polyphenols extracted from grape skin and seeds had been reported to ameliorate oxidative damage in synaptic membrane of brain cells (G. Y. Sun et al., 1999). Later on, trans-resveratrol was found to be the most effective extract from grape skin and seed, as well as a variety of other plants such as peanuts and berries, that produces beneficial health effects. To assess its role as an antioxidant, resveratrol was compared with the classical antioxidative vitamins C and E in a 1977 study (Chanvitayapongs et al., 1997). In this study, oxidative stress was induced by addition of $Fe2+$ and t-butyl hydroperoxide to the cultured PC12 cell medium. Even though the combination of the three antioxidants exhibited the greatest effect, when used alone, resveratrol is more effective than vitamins C and E combined.

Several studies have demonstrated the ability of resveratrol to protect neurons against Abeta-induced oxidative toxicity in vitro. In a rat model of sporadic AD induced by intracerebroventricular streptozotocin, in which both oxidative stress and cognitive impairment were present, trans-resveratrol significantly prevented the cognitive deficits (Sharma & Gupta, 2002). Red wine, with a high content of resveratrol, was also reported to markedly attenuate AD-type deterioration of spatial memory function and Abeta neuropathology (Jun Wang et al., 2006). The mechanism by which resveratrol fights against Abeta-induced oxidative stress mainly lies in its ability to inhibit not only the secretion of

Abeta, but also formation and extension of Abeta fibrils and to destabilize the fibrilized Abeta (Marambaud et al., 2005; Ono et al., 2006).

The antidepressant-like activity of resveratrol, which involves the inhibition of monoamine oxidase (MAO) isoform activity, also attributes to its potent antioxidative effects (Ying Xu et al., 2010). MAOs are mitochondrial-bound isoenzymes that catalyze the oxidative deamination of dietary amines and monoamine neurotransmitters, such as 5-HT, noradrenaline, dopamine and other trace amines. In a PCPA-induced serotonin-depleted mice model, treatment with resveratrol significantly improved the performance of mice in forced swimming and tail suspension tests. In the meantime, serotonin levels were dramatically increased, accompanied by inhibition of MAO-B activity. The involvement of 5-HT system in neuroprotective effects of resveratrol was also confirmed by an electrophysiological study (Lee et al., 2011). It was reported that resveratrol is able to mediate current flow in the cell by regulating $5-HT_3$ receptor activity, possibly through interactions with the N-terminal domain of the receptor.

There are different modes of administration of resveratrol, such as i.p. injection or supplemention with grape powder formulation. Studies to examine bioavailability indicate that resveratrol is rapidly conjugated to its glucuronide derivative and can be transported to the circulatory system. Once in the circulatory system, it can pass through the blood brain barrier. This renders a possibility that resveratrol can be developed into drugs for use in clinical trials.

4.2.2 Curcumin

The learning and memory deficits associated with chronic stress may be alleviated by novel therapeutic strategies involving dietary and medicinal phyto-antioxidants. One such nutraceutical is turmeric, which has been used throughout Asia as a food additive and a traditional herbal medicine. The active substance in turmeric is curcumin, the yellow pigment extracted from the rhizoma of Curcuma longa (Ying Xu et al., 2009). In this study, the effects of curcumin on restraint stress-induced spatial learning and memory dysfunction in a water maze task were investigated, and related neuroendocrine and plasticity changes were measured. The results showed that memory deficits were reversed with curcumin in a dose-dependent manner, as were stress-induced increases in serum corticosterone levels. These effects were similar to those seen with positive antidepressant imipramine. Additionally, curcumin prevented adverse changes in the dendritic morphology of CA3 pyramidal neurons in the hippocampus, as assessed by the changes in branch points and dendritic length. Moreover, curcumin protected primary hippocampal neurons against corticosterone-induced toxicity.

Curcumin supplementation has also been recently considered as an alternative approach to reduce oxidative damage associated with AD (Wu et al., 2006). High-fat diet has been shown to induce oxidative stress as an intrinsic component that can exacerbate the damage caused by traumatic brain injury (TBI). The group of rats feeding on curcumin supplemented high-fat diet performed better in the cognition tests than the group of rats feeding on high-fat diet only, when both groups were subjected to a mild fluid percussion injury. Synaptic plasticity also changed in accordance with the cognition results. Brain-derived neurotrophic factor (BDNF) was shown involved in this neuroprotective effect of curcumin. Detailed mechanisms by which curcumin regulate the expression of BDNF will be discussed in a later section of this chapter. Moreover, curcumin, but not ibuprofen, a conventional non-steroidal

The Serotonergic System and Neuroplasticity are Implicated in the Effect of Phytochemicals
on Mood and Cognitive Disorders

47

anti-inflammatory drug, was also able to prevent the synaptic loss related to Abeta-induced oxidative damage (Frautschy et al., 2001).

The impact of curcumin on the 5-HT system has been extensively studied. One study showed that curcumin protected against arsenic-induced neurobehavioral toxicity by modulating oxidative stress and dopaminergic functions in rats; the serotonin level was restored to normal if the rats were treated with both curcumin and arsenic, compared with the group of rats treated with arsenic only (Yadav et al., 2010). A similar phenomenon was found in a stressed mice model (Ying Xu et al., 2005): neurochemical assays showed that curcumin produced a marked increase in serotonin levels at 10 mg/kg in both the frontal cortex and hippocampus.

Alterations in 5-HT transmission are associated with changes in adult cell proliferation, since 5-HT depletion results in significant decreases in the number of newborn cells in the hippocampus. In order to further clarify the mechanism by which curcumin interacts with the 5-HT system and affects neuronal cells morphology, different 5-HT receptor subtypes were studied. A study aimed to investigate the effects of curcumin on hippocampal neurogenesis in chronically stressed rats used an unpredictable chronic stress paradigm (Ying Xu et al., 2007). It found that 5, 10 and 20 mg/kg, p.o. chromic treatment for 20 days could alleviate or reverse the effects of stress on adult hippocampal neurogenesis, denoted by BrdU labeling. This result was similar to 10 mg/kg, i.p. classic antidepressant imipramine treatment. In addition, curcumin significantly prevented the stress-induced decrease in 5-HT$_{1A}$ mRNA and BDNF protein levels in the hippocampal subfields. These results suggest that curcumin treatment overcomes the stress-induced behavioral abnormalities and hippocampal neuronal damage by increasing cell proliferation and neuronal populations.

Moving on to neuroplasticity, the 5-HT system also plays a significant role in the neuroprotective effects of curcumin. In a 2011 study, exposure of cortical neurons to corticosterone resulted in decreased mRNA levels for the 5-HT receptor subtypes 5-HT$_{1A}$, 5-HT$_{2A}$ and 5-HT$_{4}$, but no change for the 5-HT$_{1B}$, 5-HT$_{2B}$, 5-HT$_{2C}$, 5-HT$_{6}$ and 5-HT$_{7}$. Pretreatment with curcumin reversed this decreased mRNA level for the 5-HT$_{1A}$ and 5-HT$_{4}$ receptors, but not the 5-HT$_{2A}$ receptor. Moreover, curcumin exerted a neuroprotective effect against corticosterone-induced neuronal death. This observed effect was partially blocked with the separate application of 5-HT$_{1A}$ receptor antagonist p-MPPI and 5-HT$_{4}$ receptor antagonist RS 39604, and completely blocked with the simultaneous application of the two antagonists. Curcumin was also found to regulate corticosterone-induced morphological changes, such as increases in soma size, dendritic branching and dendritic spine density, as well as elevate synaptophysin expression in cortical neurons. Again, p-MPPI and RS 39604 reversed these effects of curcumin to prevent the morphological changes of neurons (Ying Xu et al., 2011).

4.2.3 EGCG

Green tea polyphenols (GTPs) are the most active antioxidative constituents in green tea. Among the 5 isoforms of GTPs, EGCG has the greatest potential beneficial effects in the CNS. In male Wistar rats undergoing restraint stress for 3 weeks, EGCG-treated groups performed better in the open field test and step-through test than the stress group. Similar results were observed in the crude GTP-treated group. Moreover, plasma levels of serotonin in both EGCG- and GTP- treated groups were elevated closer to the normal groups, compared to the stress group (Chen et al., 2010). This supports the involvement of the 5-HT system in the mechanism of the antioxidative effects of many neuroprotective herbals.

4.2.4 Other herbal supplements

Ginkgo biloba, also known as the maiden tree, contains compounds with antioxidant properties that protect neuron membranes, regulate neurotransmitters and retard cell degeneration. Standardized Ginkgo biloba extract EGb 761 was shown to improve neurogenesis and cognitive function in both young and old transgenic mice model TgAPP/PS1 with AD (Tchantchou et al., 2007). Later studies however suggested that Ginkgo biloba aids cognition only when subjects have AD rather than preventing AD. The neuroprotective effects of EGb 761 pertaining to the serotonin system and depression were also examined (P. Rojas et al., 2011). Not surprisingly, EGb 761 exerted its antidepressant property, as assessed by the forced swimming test, via its antioxidative effects. Moreover, serotonin level in the midbrain was increased in the EGb 761-treated group of mice, compared to the stress group. This indicates that ginkgo biloba can modulate serotonergic neurotransmission. A recent study suggests that ginkgo biloba is able to block the 5-HT3 receptor channel, further attesting to its function on the serotonin system (Thompson et al., 2011).

Huperzine A (HupA) is an alkaloid compound extracted from the Chinese moss Huperzia serrata. Besides its role as a natural acetylcholinesterase inhibitor in treating AD, HupA also has potent antioxidative effects. It has been found to protect against Abeta-induced cell lesion and abnormal morphology in the primary cultured rat cortical neurons (Xiao et al., 2002) HupA treatment reduced ROS formation and caspase 3 (a protein regulating cell apoptosis) activity in a dose-dependent manner in cortical neurons. In PC12 cells, cell death triggered by oxygen-glucose deprivation (OGD) was alleviated by HupA treatment as well (Zhou et al., 2001). Moreover, it prevented the change in cell morphology caused by OGD. After 30 min OGD exposure, PC12 cells developed a mild cell body swelling and neurites retraction or even complete loss. Cells pre-treated with HupA, however, maintained their morphology almost at the same level as normal control. Regarding cognitive behavior, HupA also exhibited beneficial effects. For instance, daily administration of HupA produced significant reversals of the Abeta-induced deficit in learning and memory tasks (R. Wang et al., 2001).

There are other natural antioxidants outside of the above-mentioned ones that are being used to treat or prevent some CNS diseases, such as withania somnifera from a small evergreen shrub; apocynin from Picrorhiza kurroa, a creeping plant native to the mountains of India, Nepal, Tibet and Pakistan; and Coenzyme Q, enriched in a number of diets, all of which have neuroprotective effects via oxidative stress reduction in mammalian brains. Natural antioxidants are advantageous for use, because they can cross the blood brain barrier, have low toxicity to the overall health being, and can be easily administered. Many antioxidant studies have indicated their interactions with the 5-HT system, including serotonin and the 5-HT receptor subtypes. More attention to these interactions may bring promise to the development of drugs treating depression and neurodegenerative diseases caused by oxidative stress.

5. Beyond the antioxidants

Even though the biological actions of most neuroprotective natural compounds have been attributed to their antioxidant properties, namely their abilities to scavenge free radicals or

The Serotonergic System and Neuroplasticity are Implicated in the Effect of Phytochemicals
on Mood and Cognitive Disorders

49

through their impact on the intracellular redox status, studies have also argued that at least some of these compounds' bioactivity in vivo is not due to their classical H-donating antioxidant property. This is mainly because of their relatively low level in the brain. Instead, the neuroprotective actions might be exerted through the modulation of the expression of genes that control neuronal survival, death and differentiation; interactions with mitochondria; structural similarities to other hormones in the body and so on.

5.1 Natural compounds used as estrogen replacement

Natural estrogen, also known as the female sex hormone, is a group of compounds belonging to the steroid hormones that exist in humans and other animals. The actions of estrogen are mediated by the estrogen receptors (ER). One of the key functions of estrogen in women is the maintenance of mental health. Withdrawal and fluctuating or low levels of estrogen correlate with significant mood lowering. For example, animal behavioral studies have shown that ovariectomy may lead to the development of cognitive dysfunction, accompanied by changes in neuronal architecture. And estrogen replacement can prevent these changes (Birge, 1996). As a result, there has been increasing interest in the cognitive preserving effects of soybean isoflavones, mainly in post-menopausal women, due to their structural similarity to estrogen and ability to mimic the actions of estrogen in the brain (Henderson, 2006; Kritz-Silverstein et al., 2003). Resveratrol, like soy products and other polyphenols, has free hydroxyl groups and phenolic ring structures that are important for estrogen receptor binding. Indeed, resveratrol can ameliorate neuronal damage induced by acute and chronic stress in different neuronal cell types by interacting directly with both estrogen receptors alpha and beta, though stronger with ER-beta (Robb & Stuart, 2010). Ginsenoside Rb1 also proved to have comparable effects with estrogen on improving behavioral performance in ovariectomized mice (K. Hao et al., 2011). After treatment with ginsenoside Rb1, there were increased TPH (an enzyme in the synthesis of 5-HT) level, decreased MAO activities, and finally elevated 5-HT levels in the mice brains, all to a similar extent observed using estrogen treatment. Additionally, estrogen receptor clomiphene blocked the effects of both ginsenoside Rb1 and estrogen, confirming that ginsenoside Rb1 shares similar pathways with estrogen.

5.2 Increase in the expression of growth factors

Neurotrophic factors are a family of proteins responsible for the growth and survival of developing neurons, thus maintaining the normal function and integral plasticity of the brain. There are three families involved: neurotrophins, glial cell-line derived neurotrophic factor family ligands (GFLs), and neuropoietic cytokines, among which neurotrophins is the most commonly studied. In this family, nerve growth factor (NGF), brain-derived neurotrophic factor (BDNF), neurotrophin-3 (NT-3), and neurotrophin-4/5 (NT 4/5) are basic components. Regulated by the transcriptional factor CREB, BDNF plays a central role in brain development and plasticity by opposing neuronal damage and promoting neurogenesis and cell survival. Similar to classical antidepressant imipramine, chronic curcumin treatment prevented stress-induced decreases in BDNF levels and neurogenesis across all hippocampal subfields (Y. Xu et al., 2007). Malonylginsenoside Rb1 (GRb1-m) extracted from dried root of Panax ginseng C.A. Meyer and ginsenoside Rb1 had a synergizing effect on NGF (Nishiyama et al., 1994). They potentiated the effect of NGF on promoting the neurite outgrowth, eliminating the glial cells when they are co-cultured with neurons, and prolonging the duration of neuronal survival.

Vascular endothelial growth factor (VEGF) is an important signaling molecule that induces proliferation and migration and reduces apoptosis of endothelial cells. It has also gained attention for its beneficial effect on the physiological function of the brain, such as increasing angiogenesis in the ischemic area and enhancing neurogenesis in the hippocampus, which leads to improved cognitive performances (Q. Zhao et al., 2010). Kangen-karyu, a traditional Chinese medicine prescription consisting of six different herbs, upregulates not only BDNF, but also VEGF levels in SAMP8 mice brains. As a result, anxiety-like behaviors as observed in the elevated plus-maze test and impairment in learning and memory as measured in the object recognition/location tests were reduced.

5.3 Increase in blood flow

Learning and memory have long been connected with neurogenesis, i.e. new neuronal growth, increases in the spine density and morphology, especially in the hippocampal area. New hippocampal cells are not only observed to be stimulated by neurotrophic factors, but also cluster near blood vessels, where they proliferate in response to vascular growth factors (Palmer et al., 2000). A brain imaging study showed that cocoa flavanol are able to enhance the cortical blood flow, indicating its potential ability to increase angiogenesis and neurogenesis (Dinges, 2006). Indeed, though flavanol (-)epicatechin did not increase the number of new born cells in the dentate gyrus of the hippocampus in this case, it was reported to increase angiogenesis and neural spine density (H. van Praag et al., 2007). In this study, behavioral tests were also conducted to confirm the effects of neurogenesis. Retention of spatial memory in the water maze test increased in both sedentary and wheel-running performance. Cognition, too, was enhanced, though to a greater extent in the wheel-running group.

6. The signaling pathways

Synaptic plasticity is often involved in stress-induced brain injury, neuroinflammation, and neurocognitive performances. There are several signaling pathways linked with the neuroprotective effects of natural compounds that preserve normal synaptic plasticity. It is likely that the neuroprotection process is carried through selective activation or inhibition of different components, as well as change of gene expression, within a number of protein kinase and lipid kinase signaling pathways, including the mitogen-activated protein kinase (MAPK), protein kinae A (PKA), phosphatidylinositol-3 kinase (PI3K), protein kinase C (PKC) and CaMK pathways. The activation of these pathways commonly result in the activation of the cAMP response element-binding protein (CREB) and a variety of downstream responses, including neurotrophin expression, dendritic spine remodeling and synaptic plasticity such as LTP. Moreover, most flavonoids can bind to the ATP-binding sites of a large number of proteins (Conseil et al., 1998), such as mitochondrial ATPase and Ca2+ plasma membrane ATPase. This binding leads to a three-dimensional structural change, followed by series of kinase inactivation, thus preventing the formation of pro-apoptotic proteins in the neurons.

6.1 Mitogen-activated protein kinase (MAPK) signaling cascade

MAPK is mainly responsible for transducing various extracellular stimuli into intracellular responses. There are three levels of regulation: a MAP kinase kinase kinase (MAPKKK), a

The Serotonergic System and Neuroplasticity are Implicated in the Effect of Phytochemicals
on Mood and Cognitive Disorders

51

MAP kinase kinase (MAPKK) and a MAPK, each regulating the following element. Each MAPKK can be activated by more than one MAPKKK, thus increasing the complexity and diversity of MAPK signaling. The three best characterized pathways involved in the neuroprotective effects of most natural compounds are: the mitogenic extracellular signal-regulated protein kinase (ERK) pathway, the stress activated, c-Jun N-terminal kinase (JNK) pathway, and the p38 pathway (Schroeter et al., 2002). The activation of these MAP kinases phosphorylates their downstream proteins and transcription factors, leading to change in gene expression, as well as neuronal activities.

6.1.1 ERK1/2

ERK1/2 are usually associated with pro-survival signaling such as upregulation of the anti-apoptotic protein Bcl-2. ERK1/2 are activated by upstream MAPKKs, such as MEK1/2, and MAPKKKs, such as c-Raf. Phosphorylation of ERK usually occurs at 2 sites, threonin 202 and tyrosin 204, within the tripeptide motif TEY, and activates a series of transcription factors that regulate neuronal cell differentiation, survival and plasticity. Flavonoids have not only been reported to modulate the phosphorylation state of ERK1/2, but also to have an effect on upstream kinases and membrane receptors. This might be due to their structural homology to specific inhibitors of the ERK signaling. For example, PD 098059 is a flavone that has the ability to bind to the inactive MEK, preventing its activation by upstream MAPKKK and thus inhibiting the pro-survival process (Alessi et al., 1995). Compared to the neurotoxic properties of flavones through the ERK1/2 pathway, the neuroprotective effects are even more intriguing. Curcumin, mentioned multiple times previously, also has an influence on the ERK1/2 pathway. Adminstration of curcumin alleviated corticosterone-induced cytotoxicity in PC12 cells, with an increase in the ERK1/2 phosphorylation (H. Zhou et al., 2009). Moreover, elevation of phosphorylated ERK1/2 was only visible at a certain time period, 15-90 min in this case, indicating that other mechanisms are also involved in the ERK-regulated cell morphology. There is also evidence of the involvement of 5-HT system in this pathway: serotonin was able to increase ERK1/2 phosphorylation, possibly involving 5-HT1A, 5-HT2B and 5-HT2C receptors (Debata et al., 2010; B. Li et al., 2010).

6.1.2 JNK

JNK is considered to oppose the effects of ERK, in that they generally promote neuronal apoptosis rather than neuronal survival. JNK cascade is strongly activated by stress signals such as oxidative stress, inflammatory cytokines and UV radiation. Regulated by GTPases such as Rac1, MAPKKKs such as MEKK1/4 and ASK1 activate MAPKKs, such as MKK4/7, which go on to regulate the JNK1/2/3. Activated JNK then enters the nucleus and activates or inhibit a series of downstream gene expression, including c-jun and AP-1 proteins that transduce the apoptotic signaling. Similar to ERK, JNK is dually phosphorylated at threonin138 and tyrosine185 within the motif pTPpY. Since changes in the cellular redox status may result in the activation of JNK, and oxidative stress can more or less be alleviated by many antioxidative plant extracts, massive studies are investigating whether JNK pathway is involved in the neuroprotective process of these plant extracts. Oxidized low-density lipoprotein (oxLDL) can be used to induce oxidative stress in cultured striatal neurons (H Schroeter et al., 2001). The neurotoxicity was characterized by the activation of JNK, which phosporylates c-jun, as measured by western blots. Flavonoid epicatechin strongly inhibited this activation. JNK is also necessary for the serotonin-induced cell proliferation, for this was blocked with exposure to a specific JNK inhibitor. Furthermore, 10min of serotonin addition maximally activated of JNK. Blockade of 5-HT1B and 2A receptors abolished the stimulatory effect of serotonin in JNK (Wei et al., 2010).

6.1.3 P38
p38 shares some of the upstream MAPKKKs with the JNK, i.e. MEK1/4 and ASK1, which regulates MKK3/4/6 (MAPKKs). Downstream transcription factors include ATF-2, Max and MEF2. p38 MAP kinase is activated by cellular stresses, including osmotic shock, inflammatory cytokines, UV radiation and growth factors. An isoflavonoid from soybean, genistein, was found to induce the activation of p38, followed by downregulation of Cdc25C, thus preventing the dividing MCF-10F, a nonmalignant human mammary epithelia cell line, from entering mitosis. In other words, genistein can inhibit cell proliferation by activating p38, indicating that it may be able to induce neural effects via this pathway (Frey & Singletary, 2003). However, the precise sites of action within the p38 pathway and the specific elements involved in regulating stress-induced neuronal death remain unknown.

6.2 PKA pathway
PKA is a family of enzymes that have several functions in the cell by phosphorylating other proteins and altering their function. It is also known as cAMP-dependent protein kinase, because its activity is only dependent on the level of cyclic AMP (cAMP). In the activation process, activated alpha subunit of G-protein binds to the enzyme adenylyl cyclase (AC), which catalyzes the conversion of ATP into cAMP, which further leads to the activation of PKA. Once PKA is activated, a series of proteins gets phosphorylated, including the transcription factor CREB. Since PKA exists in different types of cell, where they exert different biological functions, it is plausible that the same compound may have different regulatory effects on the activity of PKA. Curcumin was reported to inhibit the growth of several tumor cell types, in which hyperactivated PKA might play an important role in unlimited cell division, prompting a study on the mechanism by which curcumin may inhibit different types of phosphatases (Reddy & Aggarwal, 1994). Indeed, curcumin was able to inhibit the activity of PKA in tumor cells, even though not to a very high extent. However, in neurons, curcumin activated the PKA pathway rather than inhibited it,and this effect involved the 5-HT system (Y Xu et al., 2011). Treatment of the primary cortical cultured neurons with curcumin significantly increased the cAMP level, PKA activity and pCREB level, compared with the corticosterone-treated only group. Cell morphology parameters, including the soma size, total number of branching points, dendritic length and spine density, were also positively regulated by curcumin compare with the corticosterone-treated group. Addition of 5-HT4 receptor antagonist, RS 39604, blocked the elevation of cAMP level, while 5-HT1A antagonist, p-MPPI, inhibited the increase in PKA activity and pCREB. These findings suggest that the neuroprotection and modulation of neuroplasticity exhibited by curcumin might be mediated, at least in part, via the 5-HT receptor-cAMP-PKA-CREB signal pathway.

6.3 PI3K/Akt signaling cascade (PKB pathway)
PI3Ks are a family of enzymes involved in cellular functions, such as cell survival, growth, proliferation, differentiation and motility. Activation of PI3K by extracellular signals

The Serotonergic System and Neuroplasticity are Implicated in the Effect of Phytochemicals
on Mood and Cognitive Disorders

53

catalyzes the production of phosphatidylinositol-3,4,5-triphosphate (PIP3), phosphatidylinositol-4-phosphate (PIP) and phosphatidylinositol-4,5-bisphosphate (PIP2). PIP3 then activates phosphoinositide-dependent protein (PDK1/2), which plays a role in many signal transduction pathways by activating Akt (also known as protein kinase B, or PKB). Akt can promote cell survival mainly by inhibiting some important apoptosis-inducing proteins such as Bad (Cardone et al., 1998; Zha et al., 1996). Querctin has been reported to dose dependently regulate neuronal cell fate. At lower doses, quercetin may activate the MAPK pathway and exert its protective mechanism. However, high concentrations of quercetin inhibit the PI3K pathway and thus stimulate the pro-apoptotic pathway (Kong et al., 2000). The relationship between serotonin and PI3K/Akt signaling has also been studied. 5-HT-induced phosphorylation of Akt in different cell types was blocked either by PI3K inhibitors or 5-HT$_{1A}$ antagonist, indicating the necessary presence of both elements in the proliferation and migration activities of cells (Dizeyi et al., 2011).

6.4 PKC pathway

PKC is a family of enzymes responsible for phosphorylating other proteins at the hydroxyl groups of serine and threonin residues, and plays an important role in several signal transduction cascades that regulate growth, differentiation and tumorigenesis. Signals such as an increase in the diacylglycerol or Ca^{2+} levels can initiate this signal cascade. The PKC pathway shares some components with the PI3K/Akt pathway, such as the intracellular signaling molecules PI3K and PDK1. Flavonoids have been reported only to have an inhibitory effect on the PKC activity, rather than activation or a dual effect. TPA is a potent tumor promoter often employed to activate PKC, and consequently PKC is considered as a cellular receptor for TPA. In a brain-purified mixture of PKC isoenzymes, flavonols, in particular fisetin, quercetin and myricetin, and flavones, in particular luteolin, were found to be the most potent inhibitors for PKC. They also inhibited PI3K activity (Agullo et al., 1997; Ferriola et al., 1989). Since PKC is expressed in different cell types, the same compound may have varying extent of inhibitory effects on its activity (Y. T. Huang et al., 1996).

6.5 CaMK pathway

Ca^{2+}/calmodulin-dependent protein kinases II or CaM kinases II are serine/threonine-specific protein kinases that are regulated by the Ca^{2+}/calmodulin complex. CaMKII is intricately involved in memory formation and synaptic plasticity in the hippocampus. The phosphorylation of CaMKII at Thr286 switches the kinase into an active biochemical state required for synaptic plasticity and learning, including spatial learning. However, CaMKII over phosphorylation may produce some degree of neurotoxicity to the cells and alter some biochemical pathways involved in memory processing. It should be noted that mice that expressed a constitutively active CaMKII lacked low frequency LTP and were not able to form stable place cells within the hippocampus (Ying Xu et al., 2009). In hippocampal neurons, pCaMKII levels were significantly increased in response to corticosterone exposure, though no changes were found in total CaMKII levels. These results are similar to the changes elicited by the immobilization stress, which was previously reported (Suenaga et al., 2004). This elevation of pCaMKII was reversed by curcumin administration at different dose ranges from 0.62 to 2.5 mM (Ying Xu et al., 2009).

6.6 Other cascades

Signaling cascades involved in the neuroprotection effect of natural compounds may not be limited to the above-mentioned pathways. Besides the common transcription factor CREB of these pathways, there is FoxO1, an important target for insulin and growth factor signaling in the regulation of metabolism and cell proliferation. FoxO1 can mediate an autofeedback loop regulating SIRT1 expression (Xiong et al., 2011), a protein previously discussed to be regulated by resveratrol as well. A lot of the flavonoids also modulate the functions of the mitochondria by binding to the ATP-binding sites (Conseil et al., 1998). More or less, these pathways involve the 5-HT system, as well as its different receptor subtypes, and together they regulate gene expressions that are responsible for neuronal cell survival or inhibition of abnormal cell proliferation under stress insults. Other than behavioral tests, the most effective way to observe their function is to assess the cell morphology. Indeed, most neuroprotective natural compounds are able to morphologically restore the neurons close to normal conditions.

7. References

Acker, S. A. van, Berg, D. J. van den, Tromp, M. N., Griffioen, D. H., Bennekom, W. P. van, Vijgh, W. J. van der, et al. (1996). Structural aspects of antioxidant activity of flavonoids. *Free radical biology & medicine*, 20(3), 331-42.

Agullo, G., Gamet-Payrastre, L., Manenti, S., Viala, C., Rémésy, C., Chap, H., et al. (1997). Relationship between flavonoid structure and inhibition of phosphatidylinositol 3-kinase: a comparison with tyrosine kinase and protein kinase C inhibition. *Biochemical pharmacology*, 53(11), 1649-57.

Alessi, D. R., Cuenda, A., Cohen, P., Dudley, D. T., & Saltiel, A. R. (1995). PD 098059 is a specific inhibitor of the activation of mitogen-activated protein kinase kinase in vitro and in vivo. *The Journal of biological chemistry*, 270(46), 27489-94.

Ayala, M. E. (2009). Brain serotonin, psychoactive drugs, and effects on reproduction. *Central nervous system agents in medicinal chemistry*, 9(4), 258-76.

Birge, S. J. (1996). Is there a role for estrogen replacement therapy in the prevention and treatment of dementia? *Journal of the American Geriatrics Society*, 44(7), 865-70.

Brown, G. C. (2007). Mechanisms of inflammatory neurodegeneration: iNOS and NADPH oxidase. *Biochemical Society transactions*, 35(Pt 5), 1119-21.

Cardone, M. H., Roy, N., Stennicke, H. R., Salvesen, G. S., Franke, T. F., Stanbridge, E., et al. (1998). Regulation of cell death protease caspase-9 by phosphorylation. *Science (New York, N.Y.)*, 282(5392), 1318-21.

Chanvitayapongs, S., Draczynska-Lusiak, B., & Sun, A. Y. (1997). Amelioration of oxidative stress by antioxidants and resveratrol in PC12 cells. *Neuroreport*, 8(6), 1499-502.

Chen, W.-Q., Zhao, X.-L., Wang, D.-L., Li, S.-T., Hou, Y., Hong, Y., et al. (2010). Effects of epigallocatechin-3-gallate on behavioral impairments induced by psychological stress in rats. *Experimental biology and medicine (Maywood, N.J.)*, 235(5), 577-83.

Conseil, G., Baubichon-Cortay, H., Dayan, G., Jault, J. M., Barron, D., & Di Pietro, A. (1998). Flavonoids: a class of modulators with bifunctional interactions at vicinal ATP- and steroid-binding sites on mouse P-glycoprotein. *Proceedings of the National Academy of Sciences of the United States of America*, 95(17), 9831-6.

Cook, S. C., & Wellman, C. L. (2004). Chronic stress alters dendritic morphology in rat medial prefrontal cortex. *Journal of neurobiology*, 60(2), 236-48.

The Serotonergic System and Neuroplasticity are Implicated in the Effect of Phytochemicals
on Mood and Cognitive Disorders

55

Croes, S., Merz, P., & Netter, P. (1993). Cortisol reaction in success and failure condition in endogenous depressed patients and controls. *Psychoneuroendocrinology, 18*(1), 23-35.

Debata, P. R., Ranasinghe, B., Berliner, A., Curcio, G. M., Tantry, S. J., Ponimaskin, E., et al. (2010). Erk1/2-dependent phosphorylation of PKCalpha at threonine 638 in hippocampal 5-HT(1A) receptor-mediated signaling. *Biochemical and biophysical research communications, 397*(3), 401-6.

Dinges, D. F. (2006). Cocoa flavanols, cerebral blood flow, cognition, and health: going forward. *Journal of cardiovascular pharmacology, 47 Suppl 2*, S221-3.

Dizeyi, N., Hedlund, P., Bjartell, A., Tinzl, M., Austild-Taskén, K., & Abrahamsson, P.-A. (n.d.). Serotonin activates MAP kinase and PI3K/Akt signaling pathways in prostate cancer cell lines. *Urologic oncology, 29*(4), 436-45.

Dröge, W., & Schipper, H. M. (2007). Oxidative stress and aberrant signaling in aging and cognitive decline. *Aging cell, 6*(3), 361-70.

Duman, R S. (2002). Pathophysiology of depression: the concept of synaptic plasticity. *European psychiatry : the journal of the Association of European Psychiatrists, 17 Suppl 3*(October), 306-10.

Ferriola, P. C., Cody, V., & Middleton, E. (1989). Protein kinase C inhibition by plant flavonoids. Kinetic mechanisms and structure-activity relationships. *Biochemical pharmacology, 38*(10), 1617-24.

Frautschy, S. A., Hu, W., Kim, P., Miller, S. A., Chu, T., Harris-White, M. E., et al. (n.d.). Phenolic anti-inflammatory antioxidant reversal of Abeta-induced cognitive deficits and neuropathology. *Neurobiology of aging, 22*(6), 993-1005.

Frey, R. S., & Singletary, K. W. (2003). Genistein activates p38 mitogen-activated protein kinase, inactivates ERK1/ERK2 and decreases Cdc25C expression in immortalized human mammary epithelial cells. *The Journal of nutrition, 133*(1), 226-31.

Fukui, M., Rodriguiz, R. M., Zhou, Jiechun, Jiang, S. X., Phillips, L. E., Caron, M. G., et al. (2007). Vmat2 heterozygous mutant mice display a depressive-like phenotype. *The Journal of neuroscience : the official journal of the Society for Neuroscience, 27*(39), 10520-9.

Goddard, A. W., Ball, S. G., Martinez, J., Robinson, M. J., Yang, C. R., Russell, J. M., et al. (2010). Current perspectives of the roles of the central norepinephrine system in anxiety and depression. *Depression and anxiety, 27*(4), 339-50.

Hao, K., Gong, P., Sun, S.-Q., Hao, H.-P., Wang, G.-J., Dai, Y., et al. (2011). Beneficial estrogen-like effects of ginsenoside Rb1, an active component of Panax ginseng, on neural 5-HT disposition and behavioral tasks in ovariectomized mice. *European journal of pharmacology.* [Epub ahead of print]

Henderson, V. W. (2006). Estrogen-containing hormone therapy and Alzheimer's disease risk: understanding discrepant inferences from observational and experimental research. *Neuroscience, 138*(3), 1031-9.

Henry, J. P. (n.d.). Biological basis of the stress response. *Integrative physiological and behavioral science : the official journal of the Pavlovian Society, 27*(1), 66-83.

Howland, J. G., & Wang, Y. T. (2008). *Synaptic plasticity in learning and memory : stress effects in the hippocampus. Progress in Brain Research* (Vol. 169, pp. 145-158). Elsevier.

Inhibitions of protein kinase C and proto-oncogene expressions in NIH 3T3 cells by apigenin. *European journal of cancer (Oxford, England : 1990), 32A*(1), 146-51.

Izquierdo, A., Wellman, C. L., & Holmes, A. (2006). Brief uncontrollable stress causes dendritic retraction in infralimbic cortex and resistance to fear extinction in mice. *The Journal of neuroscience : the official journal of the Society for Neuroscience, 26*(21), 5733-8.

Jørgensen, O. S., & Riederer, P. (1985). Increased synaptic markers in hippocampus of depressed patients. *Journal of neural transmission, 64*(1), 55-66.

Kaneda, Y. (2009). Verbal working memory and functional outcome in patients with unipolar major depressive disorder. *The world journal of biological psychiatry : the official journal of the World Federation of Societies of Biological Psychiatry, 10*(4 Pt 2), 591-4.

King, M. V., Marsden, C. A., & Fone, K. C. F. (2008). A role for the 5-HT(1A), 5-HT4 and 5-HT6 receptors in learning and memory. Trends in pharmacological sciences, 29(9), 482-92.

Kong, A. N., Yu, R., Chen, C., Mandlekar, S., & Primiano, T. (2000). Signal transduction events elicited by natural products: role of MAPK and caspase pathways in homeostatic response and induction of apoptosis. *Archives of pharmacal research, 23*(1), 1-16.

Kritz-Silverstein, D., Von Mühlen, D., Barrett-Connor, E., & Bressel, M. A. B. (n.d.). Isoflavones and cognitive function in older women: the SOy and Postmenopausal Health In Aging (SOPHIA) Study. *Menopause (New York, N.Y.), 10*(3), 196-202.

Kushwaha, N., & Albert, P. R. (2005). Coupling of 5-HT1A autoreceptors to inhibition of mitogen-activated protein kinase activation via G beta gamma subunit signaling. *The European journal of neuroscience, 21*(3), 721-32.

Lambeth, J. D. (2007). Nox enzymes, ROS, and chronic disease: an example of antagonistic pleiotropy. *Free radical biology & medicine, 43*(3), 332-47.

Le Poul, E., Laaris, N., Hamon, M., & Lanfumey, L. (1997). Fluoxetine-induced desensitization of somatodendritic 5-HT1A autoreceptors is independent of glucocorticoid(s). *Synapse (New York, N.Y.), 27*(4), 303-12.

Lee, B.-H., Hwang, S.-H., Choi, S.-H., Shin, T.-J., Kang, J., Lee, S.-M., et al. (2011). Resveratrol enhances 5-hydroxytryptamine type 3A receptor-mediated ion currents: the role of arginine 222 residue in pre-transmembrane domain I. *Biological & pharmaceutical bulletin, 34*(4), 523-7.

Lee, B.-H., Lee, Jun-Ho, Yoon, I.-S., Lee, Joon-Hee, Choi, S.-H., Shin, T.-J., et al. (2007). Mutations of arginine 222 in pre-transmembrane domain I of mouse 5-HT(3A) receptor abolish 20(R)- but not 20(S)-ginsenoside Rg(3) inhibition of 5-HT-mediated ion currents. *Biological & pharmaceutical bulletin, 30*(9), 1721-6.

Leonard, B E. (2005). The HPA and immune axes in stress: the involvement of the serotonergic system. *European psychiatry : the journal of the Association of European Psychiatrists, 20 Suppl 3*, S302-6.

Li, B., Zhang, S., Li, M., Hertz, L., & Peng, L. (2010). Serotonin increases ERK1/2 phosphorylation in astrocytes by stimulation of 5-HT2B and 5-HT2C receptors. *Neurochemistry international, 57*(4), 432-9.

MacFarlane, P. M., Vinit, S., & Mitchell, G. S. (2011). Serotonin 2A and 2B receptor-induced phrenic motor facilitation: differential requirement for spinal NADPH oxidase activity. *Neuroscience, 178*, 45-55.

Marambaud, P., Zhao, Haitian, & Davies, P. (2005). Resveratrol promotes clearance of Alzheimer's disease amyloid-beta peptides. *The Journal of biological chemistry, 280*(45), 37377-82.

Meneses, A. (2007). Stimulation of 5-HT1A, 5-HT1B, 5-HT2A/2C, 5-HT3 and 5-HT4 receptors or 5-HT uptake inhibition: short- and long-term memory. *Behavioural brain research, 184*(1), 81-90.

Michel, T., & Vanhoutte, P. M. (2010). Cellular signaling and NO production. *Pflügers Archiv : European journal of physiology, 459*(6), 807-16.

Miguel-hidalgo, J. J., & Rajkowska, G. (2002). Morphological Brain Changes in Depression Can Antidepressants Reverse Them ? *CNS Drugs, 16*(6), 361-372.

Moon, E., Her, Y., Lee, J. B., Park, J.-H., Lee, E. H., Kim, S.-H., et al. (2009). The multi-herbal medicine Gongjin-dan enhances memory and learning tasks via NGF regulation. *Neuroscience letters, 466*(3), 114-9.

Morikawa, H., Manzoni, O. J., Crabbe, J. C., & Williams, J. T. (2000). Regulation of central synaptic transmission by 5-HT(1B) auto- and heteroreceptors. *Molecular pharmacology, 58*(6), 1271-8.

Nayyar, T., Bubser, M., Ferguson, M. C., Neely, M. D., Shawn Goodwin, J., Montine, T. J., et al. (2009). Cortical serotonin and norepinephrine denervation in parkinsonism: preferential loss of the beaded serotonin innervation. *The European journal of neuroscience, 30*(2), 207-16.

Nishiyama, N., Cho, S. I., Kitagawa, I., & Saito, H. (1994). Malonylginsenoside Rb1 potentiates nerve growth factor (NGF)-induced neurite outgrowth of cultured chick embryonic dorsal root ganglia. *Biological & pharmaceutical bulletin, 17*(4), 509-13.

Norrholm, S. D., & Ouimet, C. C. (2000). Chronic fluoxetine administration to juvenile rats prevents age-associated dendritic spine proliferation in hippocampus. *Brain research, 883*(2), 205-15.

Ono, K., Naiki, H., & Yamada, M. (2006). The development of preventives and therapeutics for Alzheimer's disease that inhibit the formation of beta-amyloid fibrils (fAbeta), as well as destabilize preformed fAbeta. Current pharmaceutical design, 12(33), 4357-75.

Paaver, M., Nordquist, N., Parik, J., Harro, M., Oreland, L., & Harro, J. (2007). Platelet MAO activity and the 5-HTT gene promoter polymorphism are associated with impulsivity and cognitive style in visual information processing. *Psychopharmacology, 194*(4), 545-54.

Palmer, T. D., Willhoite, A. R., & Gage, F H. (2000). Vascular niche for adult hippocampal neurogenesis. *The Journal of comparative neurology, 425*(4), 479-94.

Peyrot, F., & Ducrocq, C. (2008). Potential role of tryptophan derivatives in stress responses characterized by the generation of reactive oxygen and nitrogen species. *Journal of pineal research, 45*(3), 235-46.

Pittenger, C., & Duman, Ronald S. (2008). Stress, depression, and neuroplasticity: a convergence of mechanisms. *Neuropsychopharmacology : official publication of the American College of Neuropsychopharmacology, 33*(1), 88-109.

Praag, H. van, Lucero, M. J., Yeo, G. W., Stecker, K., Heivand, N., Zhao, C., et al. (2007). Plant-derived flavanol (-)epicatechin enhances angiogenesis and retention of spatial memory in mice. *The Journal of neuroscience : the official journal of the Society for Neuroscience, 27*(22), 5869-78.

Pérez-García, G., Gonzalez-Espinosa, C., & Meneses, A. (2006). An mRNA expression analysis of stimulation and blockade of 5-HT7 receptors during memory consolidation. *Behavioural brain research, 169*(1), 83-92.

Ramanathan, S., & Glatt, S. J. (2009). Serotonergic system genes in psychosis of Alzheimer dementia: meta-analysis. *The American journal of geriatric psychiatry : official journal of the American Association for Geriatric Psychiatry, 17*(10), 839-46.

Reddy, S., & Aggarwal, B. B. (1994). Curcumin is a non-competitive and selective inhibitor of phosphorylase kinase. *FEBS letters, 341*(1), 19-22.

Ribes, D., Colomina, M. T., Vicens, P., & Domingo, J. L. (2010). Impaired spatial learning and unaltered neurogenesis in a transgenic model of Alzheimer's disease after oral aluminum exposure. *Current Alzheimer research, 7*(5), 401-8.

Robb, E. L., & Stuart, J. A. (2010). trans-Resveratrol as a neuroprotectant. *Molecules (Basel, Switzerland), 15*(3), 1196-212.

Rojas, P., Serrano-García, N., Medina-Campos, O. N., Pedraza-Chaverri, J., Ogren, Sven O, & Rojas, C. (2011). Antidepressant-like effect of a Ginkgo biloba extract (EGb761) in the mouse forced swimming test: Role of oxidative stress. *Neurochemistry international.*

Schroeter, H, Spencer, J. P., Rice-Evans, C, & Williams, R J. (2001). Flavonoids protect neurons from oxidized low-density-lipoprotein-induced apoptosis involving c-Jun N-terminal kinase (JNK), c-Jun and caspase-3. The Biochemical journal, 358(Pt 3), 547-57.

Schroeter, Hagen, Boyd, C., Spencer, J. P. E., Williams, Robert J, Cadenas, E., & Rice-Evans, Catherine. (n.d.). MAPK signaling in neurodegeneration: influences of flavonoids and of nitric oxide. *Neurobiology of aging, 23*(5), 861-80.

Sharma, M., & Gupta, Y. K. (2002). Chronic treatment with trans resveratrol prevents intracerebroventricular streptozotocin induced cognitive impairment and oxidative stress in rats. *Life sciences, 71*(21), 2489-98.

Suenaga, T., Morinobu, S., Kawano, K.-I., Sawada, T., & Yamawaki, S. (2004). Influence of immobilization stress on the levels of CaMKII and phospho-CaMKII in the rat hippocampus. *The international journal of neuropsychopharmacology / official scientific journal of the Collegium Internationale Neuropsychopharmacologicum (CINP), 7*(3), 299-309.

Sugaya, A., Yuzurihara, M., Tsuda, T., Yasuda, K., Kajiwara, K., & Sugaya, E. (n.d.). Proliferative effect of ginseng saponin on neurite extension of primary cultured neurons of the rat cerebral cortex. *Journal of ethnopharmacology, 22*(2), 173-81.

Sun, G. Y., Xia, J., Xu, J., Allenbrand, B., Simonyi, A., Rudeen, P. K., et al. (1999). Dietary supplementation of grape polyphenols to rats ameliorates chronic ethanol-induced changes in hepatic morphology without altering changes in hepatic lipids. *The Journal of nutrition, 129*(10), 1814-9.

Tchantchou, F., Xu, Yanan, Wu, Y., Christen, Y., & Luo, Y. (2007). EGb 761 enhances adult hippocampal neurogenesis and phosphorylation of CREB in transgenic mouse model of Alzheimer's disease. *The FASEB journal : official publication of the Federation of American Societies for Experimental Biology, 21*(10), 2400-8.

Thompson, A. J., Jarvis, G. E., Duke, R. K., Johnston, G. A. R., & Lummis, S. C. R. (n.d.). Ginkgolide B and bilobalide block the pore of the 5-HT(3) receptor at a location that overlaps the picrotoxin binding site. *Neuropharmacology, 60*(2-3), 488-95.

Tohda, C., Matsumoto, N., Zou, K., Meselhy, M. R., & Komatsu, K. (2002). Axonal and dendritic extension by protopanaxadiol-type saponins from ginseng drugs in SK-N-SH cells. *Japanese journal of pharmacology, 90*(3), 254-62.

Tohda, C., Tamura, T., & Komatsu, K. (2003). Repair of amyloid beta(25-35)-induced memory impairment and synaptic loss by a Kampo formula, Zokumei-to. *Brain research, 990*(1-2), 141-7.

Uc, E. Y., McDermott, M. P., Marder, K. S., Anderson, S. W., Litvan, I., Como, P. G., et al. (2009). Incidence of and risk factors for cognitive impairment in an early Parkinson disease clinical trial cohort. *Neurology, 73*(18), 1469-77.

The Serotonergic System and Neuroplasticity are Implicated in the Effect of Phytochemicals
on Mood and Cognitive Disorders

59

Veenstra-VanderWeele, J., Anderson, G. M., & Cook, E. H. (2000). Pharmacogenetics and the serotonin system: initial studies and future directions. *European journal of pharmacology, 410*(2-3), 165-181.

Wang, Jun, Ho, L., Zhao, Z., Seror, I., Humala, N., Dickstein, D. L., et al. (2006). Moderate consumption of Cabernet Sauvignon attenuates Abeta neuropathology in a mouse model of Alzheimer's disease. *The FASEB journal : official publication of the Federation of American Societies for Experimental Biology, 20*(13), 2313-20.

Wang, R., Zhang, H Y, & Tang, X C. (2001). Huperzine A attenuates cognitive dysfunction and neuronal degeneration caused by beta-amyloid protein-(1-40) in rat. *European journal of pharmacology, 421*(3), 149-56.

Wei, L., Liu, Y., Kaneto, H., & Fanburg, B. L. (2010). JNK regulates serotonin-mediated proliferation and migration of pulmonary artery smooth muscle cells. *American journal of physiology. Lung cellular and molecular physiology, 298*(6), L863-9.

Wu, A., Ying, Z., & Gomez-Pinilla, F. (2006). Dietary curcumin counteracts the outcome of traumatic brain injury on oxidative stress, synaptic plasticity, and cognition. *Experimental neurology, 197*(2), 309-17.

Xiao, X. Q., Zhang, Hai Yan, & Tang, Xi Can. (2002). Huperzine A attenuates amyloid beta-peptide fragment 25-35-induced apoptosis in rat cortical neurons via inhibiting reactive oxygen species formation and caspase-3 activation. *Journal of neuroscience research, 67*(1), 30-6.

Xiong, S., Salazar, G., Patrushev, N., & Alexander, R. W. (2011). FoxO1 mediates an autofeedback loop regulating SIRT1 expression. *The Journal of biological chemistry, 286*(7), 5289-99.

Xu, Y, Zhang, C., Wang, R., Govindarajan, S S, Barish, P A, Vernon, M M, et al. (2011). Corticosterone induced morphological changes of hippocampal and amygdaloid cell lines are dependent on 5-HT7 receptor related signal pathway. *Neuroscience, 182*, 71-81.

Xu, Ying, Ku, B.-S., Yao, H.-Y., Lin, Y.-H., Ma, X., Zhang, Y.-H., et al. (2005). The effects of curcumin on depressive-like behaviors in mice. *European journal of pharmacology, 518*(1), 40-6.

Xu, Ying, Ku, B., Cui, L., Li, Xuejun, Barish, P. a, Foster, T. C., et al. (2007). Curcumin reverses impaired hippocampal neurogenesis and increases serotonin receptor 1A mRNA and brain-derived neurotrophic factor expression in chronically stressed rats. *Brain research, 1162*, 9-18.

Xu, Ying, Li, S., Vernon, Matthew M, Pan, Jianchun, Chen, Ling, Barish, Philip A, et al. (2011). Curcumin prevents corticosterone-induced neurotoxicity and abnormalities of neuroplasticity via 5-HT receptor pathway. *Journal of neurochemistry*

Xu, Ying, Lin, Dan, Li, S., Li, G., Shyamala, S. G., Barish, P. a, et al. (2009). Curcumin reverses impaired cognition and neuronal plasticity induced by chronic stress. *Neuropharmacology, 57*(4), 463-71.

Xu, Ying, Wang, Z., You, W., Zhang, X., Li, S., Barish, P. a, et al. (2010). Antidepressant-like effect of trans-resveratrol: Involvement of serotonin and noradrenaline system. *European neuropsychopharmacology : the journal of the European College of Neuropsychopharmacology, 20*(6), 405-13.

Yadav, R. S., Shukla, R. K., Sankhwar, M. L., Patel, D. K., Ansari, R. W., Pant, A. B., et al. (2010). Neuroprotective effect of curcumin in arsenic-induced neurotoxicity in rats. *Neurotoxicology, 31*(5), 533-9.

Yamada, N., Araki, H., & Yoshimura, H. (2011). Identification of antidepressant-like ingredients in ginseng root (Panax ginseng C.A. Meyer) using a menopausal depressive-like state in female mice: participation of 5-HT(2A) receptors. *Psychopharmacology*, , 216(4): 589-99.

Zha, J., Harada, H., Yang, E., Jockel, J., & Korsmeyer, S. J. (1996). Serine phosphorylation of death agonist BAD in response to survival factor results in binding to 14-3-3 not BCL-X(L). *Cell*, *87*(4), 619-28.

Zhao, Haifeng, Li, Q., Zhang, Z., Pei, X., Wang, Junbo, & Li, Y. (2009). Long-term ginsenoside consumption prevents memory loss in aged SAMP8 mice by decreasing oxidative stress and up-regulating the plasticity-related proteins in hippocampus. *Brain research*, *1256*, 111-22.

Zhao, Q., Yokozawa, T., Yamabe, N., Tsuneyama, K., Li, Xiaohan, & Matsumoto, K. (2010). Kangen-karyu improves memory deficit caused by aging through normalization of neuro-plasticity-related signaling system and VEGF system in the brain. *Journal of ethnopharmacology*, *131*(2), 377-85.

Zhong, Y. M., Nishijo, H., Uwano, T., Tamura, R., Kawanishi, K., & Ono, T. (n.d.). Red ginseng ameliorated place navigation deficits in young rats with hippocampal lesions and aged rats. *Physiology & behavior*, *69*(4-5), 511-25.

Zhou, H., Li, Xuejun, & Gao, M. (2009). Curcumin protects PC12 cells from corticosterone-induced cytotoxicity: possible involvement of the ERK1/2 pathway. *Basic & clinical pharmacology & toxicology*, *104*(3), 236-40.

Zhou, J, Fu, Y., & Tang, X C. (2001). Huperzine A and donepezil protect rat pheochromocytoma cells against oxygen-glucose deprivation. *Neuroscience letters*, *306*(1-2), 53-6.

Zucker, M., Weizman, A., & Rehavi, M. (2005). Repeated swim stress leads to down-regulation of vesicular monoamine transporter 2 in rat brain nucleus accumbens and striatum. *European neuropsychopharmacology : the journal of the European College of Neuropsychopharmacology*, *15*(2), 199-201.

4

Effects of Vasoactive Chinese Herbs on the Endothelial NO System

Huige Li

Department of Pharmacology, University Medical Center,
Johannes Gutenberg University, Mainz,
Germany

1. Introduction

In the vasculature, nitric oxide (NO) is produced from the endothelium mainly by endothelial NO synthase (eNOS), which is activated by agonists such as bradykinin and acetylcholine or by shear stress produced by the flowing blood. NO is a potent vasodilator and protects blood vessels from thrombosis by inhibiting platelet aggregation and adhesion. In addition, endothelial NO possesses multiple anti-atherosclerotic properties, which include (i) prevention of leukocyte adhesion to the vascular endothelium and leukocyte migration into the vascular wall; (ii) decreased endothelial permeability, reduced influx of lipoproteins into the vascular wall and inhibition of low density lipoprotein (LDL) oxidation; and (iii) inhibition of DNA synthesis, mitogenesis, and proliferation of vascular smooth muscle cells [1, 2]. Recent studies suggest that eNOS is also involved in mitochondrial biogenesis, anti-aging effects and extension of lifespan in mammals [3, 4].

Based on the abovementioned protective effects of eNOS-derived NO, a pharmacological enhancement of NO production is of therapeutic interest. Indeed, numerous Chinese medicinal plants, herbal preparations, or isolated compounds thereof have been shown to stimulate endothelial NO production, which is likely to be a contributing mechanism for their therapeutic effects.

2. Regulation of endothelial NO production

Endothelial NO production is regulated at different levels, including

- Regulation of eNOS expression: expression of the eNOS enzyme is regulated at both the transcriptional and post-transcriptional levels. Estrogens, for example, increase eNOS expression by stimulating eNOS promoter activity. TNFα, on the other hand, reduces eNOS expression by destabilizing eNOS mRNA [5, 6]. Several Chinese herbal products have been shown to enhance eNOS expression (Table 1).
- Regulation of eNOS activity by post-translational modifications: the enzymatic activity of eNOS is regulated by different cellular events such as increased intracellular Ca^{2+}, interactions with substrates, co-factors, adaptors and regulatory proteins, and through shuttling between distinct subcellular domains [7]. In addition, eNOS activity is also regulated by post-translational modification of the eNOS protein. For example, phosphorylation of serine 1177 enhances eNOS activity, whereas phosphorylation of

threonine 495 decreases eNOS activity [7]. Recent studies indicate that eNOS activity can be also enhanced by SIRT1-mediated deacetylation of lysine residues in the calmodulin-binding domain [8].

- Regulation of eNOS activity by changing the intracellular concentration of asymmetric dimethylarginine (ADMA): elevated plasma levels of ADMA have been shown to be associated with cardiovascular events and mortality. ADMA is believed to be an endogenous eNOS inhibitor, although NO-independent effects of ADMA have also been reported [9]. ADMA is formed during proteolysis and is degraded by the intracellular enzyme dimethylarginine dimethylaminohydrolase (DDAH). Decreased DDAH expression/activity is evident in disease states associated with endothelial dysfunction [10].

- Regulation of eNOS functionality: under a number of pathological conditions, the enzymatic reduction of molecular oxygen by eNOS is no longer coupled to L-arginine oxidation, resulting in production of superoxide rather than NO. This phenomenon is referred to as "eNOS uncoupling" [1, 5]. A number of potential mechanisms have been reported to contribute to eNOS uncoupling. Among all of these mechanisms, a deficiency of the NOS cofactor tetrahydrobiopterin (BH_4) seems to be the primary cause for eNOS uncoupling in pathophysiology. In BH_4 deficiency, the reduction of molecular oxygen still occurs at the heme site of eNOS, but oxidation of the guanidine nitrogen of L-arginine is prevented, so that the reduced oxygen comes off the enzyme as superoxide [11, 12]. eNOS-mediated superoxide production has been observed in animal models of atherosclerosis, hypertension, diabetes mellitus and nitroglycerin tolerance, and also in patients with endothelial dysfunction resulting from hypercholesterolemia, diabetes mellitus, or essential hypertension, in chronic smokers, and in nitroglycerin-treated patients [11, 12]. Thus, eNOS uncoupling turns eNOS from a NO-producing protective enzyme into a superoxide-generating deleterious molecule. It is therefore of therapeutic interest to reverse eNOS uncoupling and restore eNOS functionality. An elevation of endothelial BH_4 levels (by enhancing BH_4 biosynthesis and/or by preventing oxidative stress-mediated BH_4 oxidation) may reverse eNOS uncoupling [13]. Chinese herbs containing large amounts of polyphenolic compounds with antioxidant properties may have the potential to prevent BH_4 oxidation and eNOS uncoupling.

- Regulation of NO bioactivity by reducing the levels of reactive oxygen species (ROS): NO can be rapidly inactivated by superoxide. A reduction of oxidative stress (by downregulating ROS-producing enzymes, upregulating antioxidant enzymes, or by ROS scavenging activities) may enhance NO bioactivity by two means: prevention of eNOS uncoupling and reduction of superoxide-mediated NO inactivation [1].

3. Searching for eNOS-enhancing Chinese herbs

Numerous Chinese herbs have been shown to enhance endothelial NO production. These reports are summarized in Table 1. This chapter focuses on our own findings.

EA.hy 926 cells are an immortalized endothelial cell line derived from human umbilical vein endothelial cells (HUVEC). This cell line has been generated by fusing HUVEC with the permanent human alveolar epithelial cell line A549 [14]. We cloned the 5'-flanking region (3.5 kb in length) of the human eNOS gene into pGL3-neo, which contains a promoterless luciferase reporter gene and a neomycin resistance gene [15]. Stable transfection of EA.hy 926 cells with this construct (selection using G418) resulted in an immortalized human endothelial cell line (termed "stable EA.hy cells" for simplicity) that expresses the luciferase gene driven by the human eNOS promoter. Luciferase activity in cell homogenates, which can be easily measured in a luminometer or on a chemiluminescence plate reader, is used as a determinant of promoter activity of the human eNOS gene.

To search for eNOS-regulating Chinese herbs, we generated aqueous extracts of 17 herbs possessing "circulation-improving" effects according to traditional Chinese medicine (TCM) [16]. These were:

- Angelicae sinensis radix
- Astragali radix
- Carthami flos
- Celosiae semen
- Chrysanthemi indici flos
- Eucommiae cortex
- Ligustici radix
- Metaphyreum roseum
- Moutan radicis cortex
- Paeoniae rubrae radix
- Panacis notoginseng radix
- Persicae semen
- Prunella vulgaris L.
- Puerariae radix
- Salviae miltiorrhizae radix
- Uncariae ramulus et unci
- Zizyphi spinosae semen

Human EA.hy 926 endothelial cells stably transfected with a 3.5 kb fragment of the human eNOS promoter (stable EA.hy cells) were treated with each extract (corresponding to 5 g of raw plant extract per ml) at dilutions of 1:100000 to 1:300 for 18 hours to study their effects on eNOS promoter activity. Ten herbal extracts increased eNOS promoter activity in a concentration-dependent manner with a maximal effect over 150%: *Carthami flos, Chrysanthemi indici flos, Eucommiae cortex, Ligustici radix, Paeoniae rubrae radix, Prunella vulgaris L., Puerariae radix, Uncariae ramulus et unci, Salviae miltiorrhizae radix* and *Zizyphi spinosae semen.*

These ten herbal extracts were further analyzed in a second screening (RNase protection assay) for their effect on eNOS mRNA levels in normal EA.hy 926 cells. In this experiment, only *Prunella vulgaris L., Salviae miltiorrhizae radix* and *Zizyphi spinosae semen* significantly increased eNOS mRNA expression [16].

Our screening procedure using stable EA.hy cells has some limitations: (i) it is based on eNOS promoter activity and the positive results must be verified by additional methods for analyses of mRNA expression to exclude false positive hits. (ii) Herbs/compounds that regulate NO production via mechanisms other than modulating eNOS expression will provide false negative results. For example, *Astragali radix* had no effect on eNOS expression and was negative in our screening. However, *Astragali radix* can stimulate NO production from eNOS by enhancing eNOS enzymatic activity [17]. Despite of its limitations, this screening procedure has the advantages of being a low-cost method of relatively high efficiency which is easy to perform. Because of these strengths, it has also been used by pharmaceutical companies in the screening for eNOS enhancers [18]. Based on this screening, we have identified *Prunella vulgaris L.*, *Salviae miltiorrhizae radix* and *Zizyphi spinosae semen* as eNOS-regulating Chinese herbs.

Plant	Compounds / extracts	Cells / models	Effects on eNOS	Additional effects	References
Astragali radix	extract	HUVEC	eNOS activity↑	VEGF↑, PI3K-Akt↑, angiogenesis↑	[17]
Epimedii herba	icariin	coronary artery isolated from canine	eNOS activity↑	vasodilation	[74]
Ginseng	ginsenosides	I/R in Langendorff hearts; HAEC	eNOS-P↑	cardiac function↑, coronary perfusion flow↑, prostacyclin↑, PI3K-Akt↑	[75]
Ginseng (Korean red ginseng)	saponin fraction	Hypertensive rats	eNOS activity↑	blood pressure↓	[76]
Magnolia officinalis	honokiol	oxLDL-treated HUVEC	eNOS protein expression↑	adhesion molecules↓, EC-monocyte interaction↓, LDL-oxidation↓, ROS↓	[77]
Panax notoginseng	saponin extract	HUVEC / zebrafish	eNOS-P↑	angiogenesis↑, VEGF↑, PI3K-Akt↑	[78]
Polygonum multiflorum	TSG	aorta isolated from fat-fed rats	eNOS expression↑	endothelial function↑, intimal remodeling↓, iNOS↓	[79]
Pueraria lobata	puerarin	fat-fed rats	eNOS expression↑	cholesterol↓	[80]
Prunella vulgaris	extract	EA.hy / HUVEC	eNOS expression↑	NO↑	[16]
Salvia miltiorrhiza (Danshen)	crypto-tanshinone	HUVEC	eNOS expression↑	ET-1↓, NF-κB↓	[81]
	magnesium lithospermate B	HUVEC (hyperglycemia) / OLETF rats	eNOS-P↑	Endothelial function↑ Akt↑, Nrf-2↑, HO-1↑	[82]
	tanshinone IIA	angiotensin II-treated rat cardiac fibroblasts	eNOS-P↑	ET-1↓, ROS↓, fibroblast proliferation ↓	[83]
	tanshinone IIA	renovascular hypertension model in hamsters	eNOS expression↑ eNOS -P↑	Vasodilation, blood pressure↓	[84]
	extract / ursolic acid	EA.hy 926 / HUVEC	eNOS expression↑	NADPH oxidase↓	[24]
	extract	rat hypoxic pulmonary hypertension	eNOS expression↑	media thickening↓, iNOS↓	[85]
Seabuckthorn	flavonoids	EA.hy 926	eNOS expression↑	LOX-1↓, cell death↓	[86]

Plant	Compounds / extracts	Cells / models	Effects on eNOS	Additional effects	References
Sophora flavescens roots	matrine	RIMEC	eNOS expression↑	IL-6, IL-8 & sICAM-1↓	[87]
Szechwan lovage rhizome	TMP	Cerebral vasospasm in rabbit	eNOS expression↑	cerebral vasospasm↓	[88]
Xanthoceras sorbifolia	ethanol extract	Rat aorta	eNOS activity↑	vasodilation	[89]
Zizyphi Spinosi semen	betulinic acid	EA.hy / HUVEC	eNOS expression↑	ROS↓	[62]
Combinations & compounds					
A&A	decoction	obstructed rat kidney	eNOS activity↑	renal fibrosis↓, ROS↓	[90]
ELCAS	extract	H_2O_2-treated ECV304	eNOS expression↑	SOD↑, CAT↑, GPx↑	[91]
Qing Huo Yi Hao	TMP	glucose-treated bEnd.3	eNOS-P↑	ROS↓, Akt↑, UCP2↑	[92]
Refined Qing Kai Ling	injection	MCAO in rats	eNOS expression↑	infarct size↓	[93]
Shen-fu	injection	myocardial I/R in diabetic rats	eNOS-P↑	infarct size↓, Akt↑	[94]
Tongxinluo	compound	HUVEC / aortic rings from rats on a methionine-rich diet	eNOS expression↑	Endothelial function↑, PI3K- Akt↑	[95]
		myocardial no-reflow and I/R in minipigs	eNOS-P↑	PKA↑, infarct size↓	[96]

A&A, a combination of roots Astragalus membranaceus var. mongholicus and Angelica sinensis; bEnd.3, mouse brain microvascular cells; CAT, catalase; EA.hy 926, an immortalized human endothelial cell line derived from HUVEC; ECV 304, a misidentified (as endothelial cells) human bladder cell line of epithelial origin; ELCAS, an extract of Ligusticum chuanxiong and Angelica sinensis; eNOS-P, eNOS phosphorylation at serine 1177; GPx, glutathione peroxidase; HAEC, human aortic endothelial cells; HO-1, heme oxygenase-1; H/R, hypoxia/reoxygenation; HUVEC, human umbilical vein endothelial cells; I/R, ischemia-reperfusion injury; MCAO, middle cerebral artery occlusion; Nrf-2, nuclear factor erythroid 2-related factor-2; OLETF, Otsuka Long-Evans Tokushima Fatty rats; RIMEC, rat intestinal microvascular endothelial cells; ROS, reactive oxygen species; SOD, superoxide dismutase; TMP, tetramethylpyrazine; TSG, 2,3,4',5-tetrahydroxystilbene 2-O-beta-D-glucoside; UCP2, uncoupling protein 2.

Table 1. Effects of Chinese herbs on endothelial NO production.

3.1 *Prunella vulgaris L.* (PVL)

PVL is used in TCM as well as in Western herbal medicine. In the West, the plant has been used primarily as a remedy to alleviate pains in the throat, to treat fevers and to accelerate wound healing. Modern pharmacological studies have revealed a wide array of biological effects and numerous therapeutic possibilities for the herb, including anti-viral and anti-bacterial effects, immunomodulatory, anti-allergy and anti-cancer potential, as well as antioxidant activity [16].

In TCM, PVL (fruiting spikes) is used as an anti-microbial, anti-inflammatory and anti-tumor drug [19], but it is also commonly used as a component in combination therapy for hypertension. PVL extracts relax isolated epinephrine-precontracted rabbit aorta [20]. Intravenous injection of PVL saponins results in a reduction of both systolic and diastolic blood pressures in anesthetized rats [21]. A PVL-containing Chinese herb combination (consisting of *Crataegus pinnatifida Bge, Uncariae ramulus et uncis, Alisma orientalis radix* and PVL at 1:1:1:1, w/w) reduces blood pressure and lowers cholesterol and triglyceride in hypertensive and hypercholesterolemic patients [22].

Our study demonstrated that PVL is an effective eNOS-upregulating herb; it significantly increases eNOS promoter activity, eNOS mRNA and protein expression and NO production in human endothelial cells [16].

PVL extracts contain a variety of chemical constituents, including triterpenoids (such as ursolic acid, betulinic acid, oleanolic acid, vulgarsaponins), steroids (such as β-sitosterol, stigmasterol, α-spinasterol), flavonoids (such as rosmarinic acid, luteolin, cynaroside, homoorientin, quercetin), coumarins (such as umbelliferone, scopoletin, esculetin), organic acids (such as caffeic acid, palmitic acid, stearic acid, oleic acid, arachidic acid, lauric acid, myristic acid), sugars, as well as essential oils [23].

Importantly, our studies have demonstrated that ursolic acid (also present in *Salviae miltiorrhizae radix*) [24], betulinic acid (also a constituent of *Zizyphi spinosae semen*) [24], luteolin and cynaroside (also constituents of artichoke, *Cynara scolymus L.*) [25] are eNOS-upregulating compounds. Ursolic acid and betulinic acid are two of the main PVL triterpenoids; luteolin and cynaroside are two of the main PVL flavonoids [23]. Therefore, these four compounds, possibly in combination with other yet unidentified compounds, may be responsible for the observed eNOS-upregulating effect of PVL.

Our recent experience indicates that the effects of PVL on eNOS may vary significantly from batch to batch. With the last two batches of PVL products we bought recently, we could not find any eNOS-enhancing activities. This might be due to concentration variation of the active constituents in the PVL plant.

3.2 *Salviae miltiorrhizae radix* (Danshen)

Danshen, the dried root of *Salvia miltiorrhiza* Bunge (Lamiaceae), is one of the most commonly used TCM remedies. A Danshen-containing preparation was the first TCM product approved for phase II and III clinical trials by the Food and Drug Administration (FDA) [26]. Ancient TCM books describe Danshen as a drug "improving circulation" and "removing blood stasis". Today, Danshen is available in China, Japan, the United States, and also in many European countries and is used for the treatment of angina pectoris, hyperlipidemia, and acute ischemic stroke [26]. Clinical trials have indicated that Danshen preparations are superior to nitroglycerin or isosorbide dinitrate for the treatment of stable angina pectoris, with respect to efficacy and side effects [27, 28].

Various *in vitro* and *in vivo* studies have demonstrated that several constituents of Danshen can improve microcirculation, dilate coronary arteries, increase blood flow, and prevent myocardial ischemia. Aqueous Danshen extracts and purified active principles of Danshen (tanshinones) have been shown to cause vasodilation of coronary, renal, femoral, and mesenteric arteries, and suppress systemic blood pressure in rats and rabbits [29, 30]. In a rat acute myocardial infarction model, Danshen extracts increased the survival rate and reduced the infarct size to an extent comparable with that of the angiotensin converting enzyme inhibitor ramipril [31]. Tanshinone IIA, a pharmacologically active component isolated from Danshen, reduced myocardial infarct size by about 50% in a rabbit ischemia-reperfusion model [32].

Interestingly, the cardiovascular protective effects of Danshen resemble the action profile of endothelium-derived NO. Danshen extracts and constituents inhibit platelet aggregation [33] and attenuate neutrophil-endothelial adhesion [34]. Danshen also lowers plasma cholesterol levels, enhances smooth muscle apoptosis and attenuates neointimal hyperplasia in the balloon-injured abdominal aorta of hypercholesterolemic rabbits [35]. Danshen has also been shown to reduce lipid peroxidation, inhibit LDL oxidation, and reduce atherosclerosis in cholesterol-fed rabbits [36].

In stable EA.hy cells we have identified Danshen as an eNOS-enhancer. Danshen extracts increase eNOS promoter activity, eNOS mRNA and protein expression, as well as endothelial NO production [24]. Danshen extracts contain large amounts of polyphenolic compounds with antioxidant properties [26, 37]. This may prevent BH_4 oxidation and eNOS uncoupling.

So far, more than 100 compounds have been isolated and identified from Danshen. Most of the lipophilic compounds are diterpene chinone compounds of the tanshinone type, including tanshinone I, IIA, and IIB, cryptotanshinone, dihydrotanshinone, and other related compounds [26, 37]. Hydrophilic constituents include polyphenolic acids (such as various salvianolic acids) and related compounds (such as danshensu, i.e. salvianic acid A, protocatechuic aldehyde, and protocatechuic acid); but also rosmarinic acid and isoferulic acid. Baicalin and ursolic acid have been isolated from alcohol extracts of Danshen [26].

In EA.hy 926 cells, an aqueous extract of Danshen and a methanol extract of the plant increase eNOS promoter activity, eNOS mRNA and protein expression. On the contrary, a dichloromethane extract does not change eNOS gene expression [24]. Thus, hydrophilic and alcohol-soluble, but not lipophilic constituents of Danshen seem to be responsible for its eNOS-upregulating effect. Accordingly, the commercially available lipophilic compounds (tanshinone I, tanshinone IIA, cryptotanshinone and dihydrotanshinone) of Danshen have no effect on eNOS expression in EA.hy 926 cells [24]. We have also tested several commercially available hydrophilic compounds, including protocatechuic acid, protocatechuic aldehyde, rosmarinic acid, isoferulic acid, salvianic acid A, and salvianolic acid B. They show no significant effects on eNOS expression [24]. Therefore, the hydrophilic compounds that are responsible for the eNOS-upregulating effect of Danshen still remain to be identified. Among the alcohol-soluble compounds, we have found that ursolic acid, but not baicalin, significantly enhances eNOS mRNA and protein expression [24] Therefore, ursolic acid is likely to represent one of the compounds responsible for enhanced eNOS expression in response to Danshen.

3.3 Ursolic acid

Ursolic acid is a secondary plant metabolite not only found in Danshen [38], but also widespread in some other plants including apple pomace, rosemary leaves, and sage leaves (*Salvia officinalis*) [39]. This pentacyclic triterpenoid has emerged as a multifunctional compound with diverse pharmacological properties, including anticancer, antioxidant, anti-inflammatory, anti-HIV, antimicrobial, and hepatoprotective activities. Currently, ursolic acid is in human clinical trials for treating cancer and skin wrinkles [40, 41]. In addition, ursolic acid possesses anti-obestic and anti-diabetic effects. It prevents abdominal adiposity

[42, 43], improves pancreatic beta-cell function [44], ameliorates glucose intolerance [45], inhibits hepatic glucose production in diabetic mice [46], and inhibits diabetic nephropathy [47, 48].

Also in the cardiovascular system, ursolic acid shows therapeutic effects. In rat models of hypertension, ursolic acid prevents the development of severe hypertension which may be attributed to a potent diuretic/saluretic activity and a negative chronotropic effect. In addition, ursolic acid shows antihyperlipidemic (reduction of LDL and triglycerides), antioxidant (upregulation of glutathione peroxidase, GPx, and superoxide dismutase, SOD), and hypoglycemic effects [49].

The reported effects of ursolic acid on atherogenesis are controversial. TNFα-induced E-selectin expression is shown to be suppressed by ursolic acid via the inhibition of NF-κB [50]. In the rat carotid artery injury model, ursolic acid has been demonstrated to inhibit neointima formation [51]. In contrast, a recent study has shown that oral treatment of apolipoprotein E-knockout mice with ursolic acid for 24 weeks accelerates atherosclerotic plaque formation in a dose-dependent manner [52]. In the latter study, ursolic acid inhibited endothelial proliferation and induced endothelial cell death. Ursolic acid caused DNA damage, followed by the activation of a p53-, BAK-, and caspase-dependent cell-death pathway [52]. Further studies are needed to clarify this controversy.

We have provided the first evidence that ursolic acid enhances eNOS mRNA and protein expression in human endothelial cells [24]. This leads to increased NO production and improved endothelial cell function. In a recent study by Lee et al., treatment of human coronary artery endothelial cells with ursolic acid increased tube formation, endothelial cell migration capacities and the expression of allograft inflammatory factor-1 (AIF-1, a mediator of vasculogenesis) through an NO-related mechanism [53]. In a mouse hind limb ischemia model, ursolic acid enhanced eNOS and AIF-1 expression, and increased collateral blood flow and capillary density through the induction of neovascularization [53].

In addition to this stimulatory effect on gene expression observed at concentrations of 1-10 μM, ursolic acid at higher concentrations also stimulated eNOS activity. In organ chamber experiments with isolated rat aorta, ursolic acid (and a methanolic extract of *Lepechinia caulescens*) induced an endothelium-dependent, NO-mediated vasodilation (EC$_{50}$ for ursolic acid 44 μM) [54].

Ursolic acid also possesses anti-oxidative effects. It has been shown to reduce endothelial superoxide production by suppressing the expression of NOX4 [24], which is the predominant NADPH oxidase isoform in endothelial cells [55]. In addition, ursolic acid also enhances ROS inactivation by upregulating the expression/activity of antioxidant enzymes, e.g., GPx and SOD [49]. Thus, ursolic acid may also have the potential to prevent BH$_4$ oxidation and eNOS uncoupling.

3.4 *Zizyphi spinosae semen* (ZSS)

ZSS is a sedative and hypnotic drug with additional effects on the cardiovascular system [19]. ZSS protects cardiomyocytes from ischemic injury, and oxygen and glucose deprivation-induced damage of cultured neonatal rat myocardial cells can be markedly reduced by ZSS total saponins [56]. Anoxia/reoxygenation of cultured neonatal rat myocardial cells results in increased intracellular malondialdehyde and lipid peroxides, increased intercellular calcium concentration and decreased SOD activity. All of these parameters can be reversed by ZSS total saponins [56, 57].

ZSS has also antihypertensive effects. Intravenous injection of an aqueous solution of ZSS extract markedly decreases blood pressure in anesthetized rats, dogs, and cats without any significant effect on coronary blood flow, heart rate, or myocardial contractility [58]. Oral treatment of spontaneously hypertensive rats with ZSS jujubosides resultes in a reduction in blood pressure [59]. Blood pressure reduction can be observed as early as 30 min and lasted for at least 3.5 h; the effect declined after 7.5 h [59]. Moreover, treatment of hypercholesterolemic rabbits with ZSS for three months leads to a reduction in total cholesterol, LDL cholesterol and triglycerides, an increase in HDL and a decrease in atherosclerotic lesions [60].

The molecular mechanisms underlying these cardiovascular effects are poorly understood. Interestingly, treatment of rats with ZSS resulted in increased plasma levels of NO through unknown mechanisms [61]. We have found that ZSS increases eNOS promoter activity, eNOS mRNA and protein expression, as well as NO production in human endothelial cells [62].

The active constituents of ZSS include saponins, triterpenoids, flavonoids, alkaloids, and fatty acids [19, 63, 64]. The most important ZSS saponins are triterpenoid oligoglycosides, such as jujubosides A and B. Triterpenoids found in ZSS include betulin and betulinic acid [63, 65].

Jujuboside A, B and betulin show no effect on eNOS promoter activity or eNOS mRNA expression. Interestingly, treatment of human endothelial cells with betulinic acid results in a significant up-regulation of eNOS mRNA and protein expression [62]. The content of betulinic acid in ZSS is approximately 7 mg/kg [63]. When cells are treated with this ZSS extract (concentration of 5 g/ml) at a 1:100 dilution, the estimated final concentration of betulinic acid is in the low micromolar range. In our study, betulinic acid increases eNOS mRNA expression even at 1 μM. Thus, betulinic acid is likely to be one of the compounds responsible for the eNOS up-regulation induced by ZSS [62].

3.5 Betulinic acid

The pentacyclic triterpenoid betulinic acid is not only found in ZSS, but is also widespread in fruit peel, leaves and stem bark of several species of plants, including white birch bark (*Betula pubescens*), plane bark (*Plantanus acerifolia*), rosemary leaves (*Rosmarinus officinalis*), Ber tree (*Ziziphus mauritiana*) and selfheal (*Prunella vulgaris*) [39, 66]. The compound is mainly known for its anti-tumor, anti-viral and anti-inflammatory activities [66, 67]. Our study has identified betulinic acid as an eNOS-stimulating compound [62].

Interestingly, accumulating data in the recent years support a protective effect of betulinic acid in the cardiovascular system. In a rat renal ischemia/reperfusion (I/R) injury model, betulinic acid attenuates I/R-induced oxidant responses, inhibits microscopic damage, and improves renal function by regulating the apoptotic function of leukocytes and inhibiting neutrophil infiltration [68]. Recently, betulinic acid and ursolic acid have been identified as selective agonists of the G protein-coupled receptor TGR5, which plays an important role in the control of energy metabolism. This suggests the therapeutic potential of betulinic acid and ursolic acid for metabolic diseases [69].

In HUVEC, betulinic acid has been shown to inhibit TNFα-induced ROS production and NF-κB activation. The resulting inhibition of endothelial activation and leukocyte adhesion points to a protective role of the compound against vascular inflammation [70].

We have found that betulinic acid upregulates eNOS expression in endothelial cells [62]. As mentioned above, upregulation of eNOS does not necessarily result in an increase in bioactive NO. Under pathological conditions of oxidative stress, eNOS is often uncoupled and dysfunctional. The primary cause of eNOS uncoupling is a deficiency of its cofactor BH_4 due to oxidative stress-mediated oxidation (e.g. by peroxynitrite) [1, 12]. Importantly, betulinic acid also reduces the expression of NADPH oxidases (NOX4 and p22phox) [62], a major source of ROS in the vasculature [71]. We have demonstrated that betulic acid reduces the levels of peroxynitrite in the mouse *in vivo* [72]. These results suggest the potential of betulinic acid to reverse eNOS uncoupling. In a mouse stroke model, betulinic acid upregulates eNOS and downregulated NADPH oxidases, events which are associated with a reduction in infarct size [72].

Our recent results indicate that betulinic acid not only enhances eNOS expression but also enhances eNOS enzymatic activity. Treatment of human endothelial cells with betulinic acid leads to phosphorylation of eNOS at serine 1177 and dephosphorylation of eNOS at threonine 495, and an increase in NO production [Hohmann N, Xia N, Forstermann U and Li H, unpublished data]. This is consistent with a recent report demonstrating that betulinic acid induces an endothelium-dependent, NO-mediated relaxation of isolated rat aorta [73].

4. Conclusion

Numerous vasoactive Chinese herbs possess stimulating effects on endothelial NO production, e.g. by enhancing eNOS expression and/or by modulating eNOS phosphorylation status. Such molecular events are likely to be contributing mechanisms for the therapeutic effects of these herbs described in traditional Chinese medicine.

5. References

[1] Li H, Forstermann U. Prevention of atherosclerosis by interference with the vascular nitric oxide system. *Curr Pharm Des*. 2009; 15: 3133-3145.

[2] Li H, Forstermann U. Nitric oxide in the pathogenesis of vascular disease. *J Pathol*. 2000; 190: 244-254.

[3] Csiszar A, Labinskyy N, Pinto JT, Ballabh P, Zhang H, Losonczy G, Pearson K, de Cabo R, Pacher P, Zhang C, Ungvari Z. Resveratrol induces mitochondrial biogenesis in endothelial cells. *Am J Physiol Heart Circ Physiol*. 2009; 297: H13-20.

[4] Nisoli E, Tonello C, Cardile A, Cozzi V, Bracale R, Tedesco L, Falcone S, Valerio A, Cantoni O, Clementi E, Moncada S, Carruba MO. Calorie restriction promotes mitochondrial biogenesis by inducing the expression of eNOS. *Science*. 2005; 310: 314-317.

[5] Li H, Wallerath T, Munzel T, Forstermann U. Regulation of endothelial-type NO synthase expression in pathophysiology and in response to drugs. *Nitric Oxide*. 2002; 7: 149-164.

[6] Li H, Wallerath T, Forstermann U. Physiological mechanisms regulating the expression of endothelial-type NO synthase. *Nitric Oxide*. 2002; 7: 132-147.

[7] Fleming I. Molecular mechanisms underlying the activation of eNOS. *Pflugers Arch*. 2010; 459: 793-806.

[8] Mattagajasingh I, Kim CS, Naqvi A, Yamamori T, Hoffman TA, Jung SB, DeRicco J, Kasuno K, Irani K. SIRT1 promotes endothelium-dependent vascular relaxation by

activating endothelial nitric oxide synthase. *Proc Natl Acad Sci USA.* 2007; 104: 14855-14860.

[9] Maas R, Boger R, Luneburg N. ADMA and the role of the genes: lessons from genetically modified animals and human gene polymorphisms. *Pharmacol Res.* 2009; 60: 475-480.

[10] Pope AJ, Karuppiah K, Cardounel AJ. Role of the PRMT-DDAH-ADMA axis in the regulation of endothelial nitric oxide production. *Pharmacol Res.* 2009; 60: 461-465.

[11] Forstermann U, Li H. Therapeutic effect of enhancing endothelial nitric oxide synthase (eNOS) expression and preventing eNOS uncoupling. *Br J Pharmacol.* 2010: DOI: 10.1111/j.1476-5381.2010.01196.x.

[12] Forstermann U, Munzel T. Endothelial nitric oxide synthase in vascular disease: from marvel to menace. *Circulation.* 2006; 113: 1708-1714.

[13] Xia N, Daiber A, Habermeier A, Closs EI, Thum T, Spanier G, Lu Q, Oelze M, Torzewski M, Lackner KJ, Münzel T, Förstermann U, Li H. Resveratrol reverses endothelial nitric-oxide synthase uncoupling in apolipoprotein E knockout mice. *J Pharmacol Exp Ther.* 2010; 335: 149-154.

[14] Edgell CJ, McDonald CC, Graham JB. Permanent cell line expressing human factor VIII-related antigen established by hybridization. *Proc Natl Acad Sci USA.* 1983; 80: 3734-3737.

[15] Li H, Oehrlein SA, Wallerath T, Ihrig-Biedert I, Wohlfart P, Ulshofer T, Jessen T, Herget T, Forstermann U, Kleinert H. Activation of protein kinase C alpha and/or epsilon enhances transcription of the human endothelial nitric oxide synthase gene. *Mol Pharmacol.* 1998; 53: 630-637.

[16] Xia N, Bollinger L, Steinkamp-Fenske K, Forstermann U, Li H. Prunella vulgaris L. Upregulates eNOS expression in human endothelial cells. *Am J Chin Med.* 2010; 38: 599-611.

[17] Zhang Y, Hu G, Lin HC, Hong SJ, Deng YH, Tang JY, Seto SW, Kwan YW, Waye MM, Wang YT, Lee SM. Radix Astragali extract promotes angiogenesis involving vascular endothelial growth factor receptor-related phosphatidylinositol 3-kinase/Akt-dependent pathway in human endothelial cells. *Phytother Res.* 2009; 23: 1205-1213.

[18] Wohlfart P, Xu H, Endlich A, Habermeier A, Closs EI, Hubschle T, Mang C, Strobel H, Suzuki T, Kleinert H, Forstermann U, Ruetten H, Li H. Antiatherosclerotic effects of small-molecular-weight compounds enhancing endothelial nitric-oxide synthase (eNOS) expression and preventing eNOS uncoupling. *J Pharmacol Exp Ther.* 2008; 325: 370-379.

[19] Huang KC. *The pharmacology of Chinese herbs.* Second edition ed. Boca Raton: CRC Press; 1999.

[20] Sun H, Yuan B, Liu B, Zhang C. The effect of Prunella vulgaris L. extracts on isolated rabbit artery. *Xi'an Jiao Tong Da Xue Xue Bao.* 2005; 26: 19-21.

[21] Wang HB, Zhang ZY, Su ZW, Li CG. [The effect of total saponins from common selfheal (Prunella vulgaris) on experimental myocardial infarction and hypertension of anesthetized rats]. *Zhong Cao Yao.* 1994; 25: 264-266.

[22] Heart-Disease-Group. [Clinical observation with Jiangya-Jiangzhi-chongji]. *Zhonghua Xin Xue Guan Bing Za Zhi.* 1976; 16: 54-56.

[23] Liu Y, Song S-J, Xu S-X. [Advances in the study on the chemical constituents and biological activities of Prunella vulgaris L.]. *Journal of Shenyang Pharmaceutical University.* 2003; 20: 55-59.

[24] Steinkamp-Fenske K, Bollinger L, Voller N, Xu H, Yao Y, Bauer R, Forstermann U, Li H. Ursolic acid from the Chinese herb danshen (Salvia miltiorrhiza L.) upregulates eNOS and downregulates Nox4 expression in human endothelial cells. *Atherosclerosis.* 2007; 195: e104-111.

[25] Li H, Xia N, Brausch I, Yao Y, Forstermann U. Flavonoids from artichoke (Cynara scolymus L.) up-regulate endothelial-type nitric-oxide synthase gene expression in human endothelial cells. *J Pharmacol Exp Ther.* 2004; 310: 926-932.

[26] Zhou L, Zuo Z, Chow MS. Danshen: an overview of its chemistry, pharmacology, pharmacokinetics, and clinical use. *J Clin Pharmacol.* 2005; 45: 1345-1359.

[27] Wang G, Wang L, Xiong ZY, Mao B, Li TQ. Compound salvia pellet, a traditional Chinese medicine, for the treatment of chronic stable angina pectoris compared with nitrates: a meta-analysis. *Med Sci Monit.* 2006; 12: SR1-7.

[28] Zhang JH, Shang HC, Gao XM, Zhang BL, Xiang YZ, Cao HB, Ren M, Wang H. Compound Salvia droplet pill, a traditional Chinese medicine, for the treatment of unstable angina pectoris: a systematic review. *Med Sci Monit.* 2008; 14: RA1-7.

[29] Lam FF, Yeung JH, Cheung JH. Mechanisms of the dilator action of Danshen (Salvia miltiorrhiza) on rat isolated femoral artery. *J Cardiovasc Pharmacol.* 2005; 46: 361-368.

[30] Lei XL, Chiou GC. Studies on cardiovascular actions of Salvia miltiorrhiza. *Am J Chin Med.* 1986; 14: 26-32.

[31] Ji X, Tan BK, Zhu YC, Linz W, Zhu YZ. Comparison of cardioprotective effects using ramipril and DanShen for the treatment of acute myocardial infarction in rats. *Life Sci.* 2003; 73: 1413-1426.

[32] Wu TW, Zeng LH, Fung KP, Wu J, Pang H, Grey AA, Weisel RD, Wang JY. Effect of sodium tanshinone IIA sulfonate in the rabbit myocardium and on human cardiomyocytes and vascular endothelial cells. *Biochem Pharmacol.* 1993; 46: 2327-2332.

[33] Wang Z, Roberts JM, Grant PG, Colman RW, Schreiber AD. The effect of a medicinal Chinese herb on platelet function. *Thromb Haemost.* 1982; 48: 301-306.

[34] Chen YH, Lin SJ, Ku HH, Shiao MS, Lin FY, Chen JW, Chen YL. Salvianolic acid B attenuates VCAM-1 and ICAM-1 expression in TNF-alpha-treated human aortic endothelial cells. *J Cell Biochem.* 2001; 82: 512-521.

[35] Chen YL, Yang SP, Shiao MS, Chen JW, Lin SJ. Salvia miltiorrhiza inhibits intimal hyperplasia and monocyte chemotactic protein-1 expression after balloon injury in cholesterol-fed rabbits. *J Cell Biochem.* 2001; 83: 484-493.

[36] Wu YJ, Hong CY, Lin SJ, Wu P, Shiao MS. Increase of vitamin E content in LDL and reduction of atherosclerosis in cholesterol-fed rabbits by a water-soluble antioxidant-rich fraction of Salvia miltiorrhiza. *Arterioscler Thromb Vasc Biol.* 1998; 18: 481-486.

[37] Wang X, Morris-Natschke SL, Lee KH. New developments in the chemistry and biology of the bioactive constituents of Tanshen. *Med Res Rev.* 2007; 27: 133-148.

[38] Kong DY. Chemical constituents of Salvia miltiorrhiza. *Zhongguo Yiyao Gongye Zazhi.* 1989; 20: 279-285.

[39] Jager S, Trojan H, Kopp T, Laszczyk MN, Scheffler A. Pentacyclic triterpene distribution in various plants - rich sources for a new group of multi-potent plant extracts. *Molecules.* 2009; 14: 2016-2031.

[40] Sultana N. Clinically useful anticancer, antitumor, and antiwrinkle agent, ursolic acid and related derivatives as medicinally important natural product. *J Enzyme Inhib Med Chem.* 2011.

[41] Shao JW, Dai YC, Xue JP, Wang JC, Lin FP, Guo YH. In vitro and in vivo anticancer activity evaluation of ursolic acid derivatives. *Eur J Med Chem.* 2011; 46: 2652-2661.

[42] Kim J, Jang DS, Kim H, Kim JS. Anti-lipase and lipolytic activities of ursolic acid isolated from the roots of Actinidia arguta. *Arch Pharm Res.* 2009; 32: 983-987.

[43] Rao VS, Melo CL, Queiroz MG, Lemos TL, Menezes DB, Melo TS, Santos FA. Ursolic acid, a pentacyclic triterpene from Sambucus australis, prevents abdominal adiposity in mice fed a high-fat diet. *J Med Food.* 2011; in press. doi:10.1089/jmf.2010.0267.

[44] Jang SM, Yee ST, Choi J, Choi MS, Do GM, Jeon SM, Yeo J, Kim MJ, Seo KI, Lee MK. Ursolic acid enhances the cellular immune system and pancreatic beta-cell function in streptozotocin-induced diabetic mice fed a high-fat diet. *Int Immunopharmacol.* 2009; 9: 113-119.

[45] Jayaprakasam B, Olson LK, Schutzki RE, Tai MH, Nair MG. Amelioration of obesity and glucose intolerance in high-fat-fed C57BL/6 mice by anthocyanins and ursolic acid in Cornelian cherry (Cornus mas). *J Agric Food Chem.* 2006; 54: 243-248.

[46] Jang SM, Kim MJ, Choi MS, Kwon EY, Lee MK. Inhibitory effects of ursolic acid on hepatic polyol pathway and glucose production in streptozotocin-induced diabetic mice. *Metabolism.* 2010; 59: 512-519.

[47] Zhou Y, Li JS, Zhang X, Wu YJ, Huang K, Zheng L. Ursolic acid inhibits early lesions of diabetic nephropathy. *Int J Mol Med.* 2010; 26: 565-570.

[48] Wang ZH, Hsu CC, Huang CN, Yin MC. Anti-glycative effects of oleanolic acid and ursolic acid in kidney of diabetic mice. *Eur J Pharmacol.* 2010; 628: 255-260.

[49] Somova LO, Nadar A, Rammanan P, Shode FO. Cardiovascular, antihyperlipidemic and antioxidant effects of oleanolic and ursolic acids in experimental hypertension. *Phytomedicine.* 2003; 10: 115-121.

[50] Takada K, Nakane T, Masuda K, Ishii H. Ursolic acid and oleanolic acid, members of pentacyclic triterpenoid acids, suppress TNF-alpha-induced E-selectin expression by cultured umbilical vein endothelial cells. *Phytomedicine.* 2010; 17: 1114-1119.

[51] Pozo M, Castilla V, Gutierrez C, de Nicolas R, Egido J, Gonzalez-Cabrero J. Ursolic acid inhibits neointima formation in the rat carotid artery injury model. *Atherosclerosis.* 2006; 184: 53-62.

[52] Messner B, Zeller I, Ploner C, Frotschnig S, Ringer T, Steinacher-Nigisch A, Ritsch A, Laufer G, Huck C, Bernhard D. Ursolic acid causes DNA-damage, p53-mediated, mitochondria- and caspase-dependent human endothelial cell apoptosis, and accelerates atherosclerotic plaque formation in vivo. *Atherosclerosis.* 2011: doi:10.1016/j.atherosclerosis.2011.1005.1025.

[53] Lee AW, Chen TL, Shih CM, Huang CY, Tsao NW, Chang NC, Chen YH, Fong TH, Lin FY. Ursolic acid induces allograft inflammatory factor-1 expression via a nitric oxide-related mechanism and increases neovascularization. *J Agric Food Chem.* 2010; 58: 12941-12949.

[54] Aguirre-Crespo F, Vergara-Galicia J, Villalobos-Molina R, Javier Lopez-Guerrero J, Navarrete-Vazquez G, Estrada-Soto S. Ursolic acid mediates the vasorelaxant activity of Lepechinia caulescens via NO release in isolated rat thoracic aorta. *Life Sci*. 2006; 79: 1062-1068.

[55] Xu H, Goettsch C, Xia N, Horke S, Morawietz H, Forstermann U, Li H. Differential roles of PKCalpha and PKCepsilon in controlling the gene expression of Nox4 in human endothelial cells. *Free Radic Biol Med*. 2008; 44: 1656-1667.

[56] Chen XJ, Yu CL, Liu JF. [Protective effects of total saponins of semen Ziziphi spinosae on cultured rat myocardial cells]. *Zhongguo Yao Li Xue Bao*. 1990; 11: 153-155.

[57] Wan HY, Ding L, Kong XP, Liu SJ, Chen XJ. [Effect of total saponins of semen Ziziphi spinosae on hypoxia-reoxygenation injury in myocardial cells]. *Zhongguo Bingli Shengli Za Zhi*. 1997; 13: 522-526.

[58] Gu WX, Liu JF, Zhang JX, Liu XM, Liu JS, Chen YR. [Blood pressure-lowering effect and mechanism of total saponins from Ziziphus Mill seeds]. *Di Yi Jun Yi Da Xue Xue Bao*. 1987; 7: 8-10.

[59] Zhang D, Yuang BX, Sun H. [The effect of jujuboside on rats with spontaneous hypertension]. *Xi'an Jiao Tong Da Xue Xue Bao*. 2003; 24: 59-60.

[60] Wu SX, Lang XC, Jia BY, Zhao SX, Li MX, Lan MY. [Effects of Ziziphus spinosa Hu on serum lipoprotein and experimental atherosclerosis]. *Zhongguo Zhong Yao Za Zhi*. 1989; 14: 434-451, 448.

[61] Wang X, Xie M. [Effects of suanzaoren decoction on serum NO and the Level of cytokines in rats]. *Beijing Zhong Yi Yao Da Xue Xue Bao*. 2004; 11: 16-18.

[62] Steinkamp-Fenske K, Bollinger L, Xu H, Yao Y, Horke S, Forstermann U, Li H. Reciprocal regulation of endothelial nitric-oxide synthase and NADPH oxidase by betulinic acid in human endothelial cells. *J Pharmacol Exp Ther*. 2007; 322: 836-842.

[63] Li L-M, Liao X, Peng S-L, Ding L-S. Chemical constituents from the seeds of Ziziphus jujuba var. spinosa (Bunge) Hu. *Journal of Integrative Plant Biology*. 2005; 47: 494-498.

[64] Zhao J, Li SP, Yang FQ, Li P, Wang YT. Simultaneous determination of saponins and fatty acids in Ziziphus jujuba (Suanzaoren) by high performance liquid chromatography-evaporative light scattering detection and pressurized liquid extraction. *J Chromatogr A*. 2006; 1108: 188-194.

[65] Zhang M, Zhang Y, Xie J. Simultaneous determination of jujuboside A, B and betulinic acid in semen Ziziphi spinosae by high performance liquid chromatography-evaporative light scattering detection. *J Pharm Biomed Anal*. 2008; 48: 1467-1470.

[66] Mullauer FB, Kessler JH, Medema JP. Betulinic acid, a natural compound with potent anticancer effects. *Anticancer Drugs*. 2010; 21: 215-227.

[67] Fulda S. Betulinic acid: a natural product with anticancer activity. *Mol Nutr Food Res*. 2009; 53: 140-146.

[68] Eksioglu-Demiralp E, Kardas ER, Ozgul S, Yagci T, Bilgin H, Sehirli O, Ercan F, Sener G. Betulinic acid protects against ischemia/reperfusion-induced renal damage and inhibits leukocyte apoptosis. *Phytother Res*. 2010; 24: 325-332.

[69] Genet C, Strehle A, Schmidt C, Boudjelal G, Lobstein A, Schoonjans K, Souchet M, Auwerx J, Saladin R, Wagner A. Structure-activity relationship study of betulinic acid, a novel and selective TGR5 agonist, and its synthetic derivatives: potential impact in diabetes. *J Med Chem*. 2010; 53: 178-190.

[70] Yoon JJ, Lee YJ, Kim JS, Kang DG, Lee HS. Protective role of betulinic acid on TNF-alpha-induced cell adhesion molecules in vascular endothelial cells. *Biochem Biophys Res Commun.* 2010; 391: 96-101.

[71] Forstermann U. Oxidative stress in vascular disease: causes, defense mechanisms and potential therapies. *Nat Clin Pract Cardiovasc Med.* 2008; 5: 338-349.

[72] Lu Q, Xia N, Xu H, Guo L, Wenzel P, Daiber A, Munzel T, Forstermann U, Li H. Betulinic acid protects against cerebral ischemia-reperfusion injury in mice by reducing oxidative and nitrosative stress. *Nitric Oxide.* 2011; 24: 132-138.

[73] Fu JY, Xia ML, Lu JF, Liu Q, Cai X, Yang J, Wang HP, Xia Q. [Betulinic acid ameliorates impairment of endothelium-dependent relaxation induced by oxidative stress in rat aorta]. *Zhejiang Da Xue Xue Bao Yi Xue Ban.* 2010; 39: 523-529.

[74] Xu HB, Huang ZQ. Vasorelaxant effects of icariin on isolated canine coronary artery. *J Cardiovasc Pharmacol.* 2007; 49: 207-213.

[75] Yi XQ, Li T, Wang JR, Wong VK, Luo P, Wong IY, Jiang ZH, Liu L, Zhou H. Total ginsenosides increase coronary perfusion flow in isolated rat hearts through activation of PI3K/Akt-eNOS signaling. *Phytomedicine.* 2010; 17: 1006-1015.

[76] Jeon BH, Kim CS, Kim HS, Park JB, Nam KY, Chang SJ. Effect of Korean red ginseng on blood pressure and nitric oxide production. *Acta Pharmacol Sin.* 2000; 21: 1095-1100.

[77] Ou HC, Chou FP, Lin TM, Yang CH, Sheu WH. Protective effects of honokiol against oxidized LDL-induced cytotoxicity and adhesion molecule expression in endothelial cells. *Chem Biol Interact.* 2006; 161: 1-13.

[78] Hong SJ, Wan JB, Zhang Y, Hu G, Lin HC, Seto SW, Kwan YW, Lin ZX, Wang YT, Lee SM. Angiogenic effect of saponin extract from Panax notoginseng on HUVECs in vitro and zebrafish in vivo. *Phytother Res.* 2009; 23: 677-686.

[79] Zhang W, Xu XL, Wang YQ, Wang CH, Zhu WZ. Effects of 2,3,4',5-tetrahydroxystilbene 2-O-beta-D-glucoside on vascular endothelial dysfunction in atherogenic-diet rats. *Planta Med.* 2009; 75: 1209-1214.

[80] Yan LP, Chan SW, Chan AS, Chen SL, Ma XJ, Xu HX. Puerarin decreases serum total cholesterol and enhances thoracic aorta endothelial nitric oxide synthase expression in diet-induced hypercholesterolemic rats. *Life Sci.* 2006; 79: 324-330.

[81] Zhou Z, Wang SQ, Liu Y, Miao AD. Cryptotanshinone inhibits endothelin-1 expression and stimulates nitric oxide production in human vascular endothelial cells. *Biochim Biophys Acta.* 2006; 1760: 1-9.

[82] Kim SH, Choi M, Lee Y, Kim YO, Ahn DS, Kim YH, Kang ES, Lee EJ, Jung M, Cho JW, Williams DR, Lee HC. Natural therapeutic magnesium lithospermate B potently protects the endothelium from hyperglycaemia-induced dysfunction. *Cardiovasc Res.* 2010; 87: 713-722.

[83] Chan P, Liu JC, Lin LJ, Chen PY, Cheng TH, Lin JG, Hong HJ. Tanshinone IIA inhibits angiotensin II-induced cell proliferation in rat cardiac fibroblasts. *Am J Chin Med.* 2011; 39: 381-394.

[84] Kim DD, Sanchez FA, Duran RG, Kanetaka T, Duran WN. Endothelial nitric oxide synthase is a molecular vascular target for the Chinese herb Danshen in hypertension. *Am J Physiol Heart Circ Physiol.* 2007; 292: H2131-H2137.

[85] Chen Y, Ruan Y, Li L, Chu Y, Xu X, Wang Q, Zhou X. Effects of Salvia miltiorrhiza extracts on rat hypoxic pulmonary hypertension, heme oxygenase-1 and nitric oxide synthase. *Chin Med J (Engl).* 2003; 116: 757-760.

[86] Bao M, Lou Y. Flavonoids from seabuckthorn protect endothelial cells (EA.hy926) from oxidized low-density lipoprotein induced injuries via regulation of LOX-1 and eNOS expression. *J Cardiovasc Pharmacol*. 2006; 48: 834-841.

[87] Suo Z, Liu Y, Ferreri M, Zhang T, Liu Z, Mu X, Han B. Impact of matrine on inflammation related factors in rat intestinal microvascular endothelial cells. *J Ethnopharmacol*. 2009; 125: 404-409.

[88] Shao Z, Li J, Zhao Z, Gao C, Sun Z, Liu X. Effects of tetramethylpyrazine on nitric oxide/cGMP signaling after cerebral vasospasm in rabbits. *Brain Res*. 2010; 1361: 67-75.

[89] Jin SN, Wen JF, Kim HY, Kang DG, Lee HS, Cho KW. Vascular relaxation by ethanol extract of Xanthoceras sorbifolia via Akt- and SOCE-eNOS-cGMP pathways. *J Ethnopharmacol*. 2010; 132: 240-245.

[90] Meng L, Qu L, Tang J, Cai SQ, Wang H, Li X. A combination of Chinese herbs, Astragalus membranaceus var. mongholicus and Angelica sinensis, enhanced nitric oxide production in obstructed rat kidney. *Vascul Pharmacol*. 2007; 47: 174-183.

[91] Hou YZ, Zhao GR, Yang J, Yuan YJ, Zhu GG, Hiltunen R. Protective effect of Ligusticum chuanxiong and Angelica sinensis on endothelial cell damage induced by hydrogen peroxide. *Life Sci*. 2004; 75: 1775-1786.

[92] Kang Y, Hu M, Zhu Y, Gao X, Wang MW. Antioxidative effect of the herbal remedy Qin Huo Yi Hao and its active component tetramethylpyrazine on high glucose-treated endothelial cells. *Life Sci*. 2009; 84: 428-436.

[93] Hua Q, Zhu X, Li P, Tang H, Cai D, Xu Y, Jia X, Chen J, Shen Y. Refined Qing Kai Ling, traditional Chinese medicinal preparation, reduces ischemic stroke-induced infarct size and neurological deficits and increases expression of endothelial nitric oxide synthase. *Biol Pharm Bull*. 2008; 31: 633-637.

[94] Wu Y, Xia ZY, Meng QT, Zhu J, Lei S, Xu J, Dou J. Shen-Fu injection preconditioning inhibits myocardial ischemia-reperfusion injury in diabetic rats: activation of eNOS via the PI3K/Akt pathway. *J Biomed Biotechnol*. 2011; 2011: 384627.

[95] Liang JQ, Wu K, Jia ZH, Liu C, Ding J, Huang SN, Yin PP, Wu XC, Wei C, Wu YL, Wang HY. Chinese medicine Tongxinluo modulates vascular endothelial function by inducing eNOS expression via the PI-3K/Akt/HIF-dependent signaling pathway. *J Ethnopharmacol*. 2011; 133: 517-523.

[96] Li XD, Yang YJ, Geng YJ, Jin C, Hu FH, Zhao JL, Zhang HT, Cheng YT, Qian HY, Wang LL, Zhang BJ, Wu YL. Tongxinluo reduces myocardial no-reflow and ischemia-reperfusion injury by stimulating the phosphorylation of eNOS via the PKA pathway. *Am J Physiol Heart Circ Physiol*. 2010; 299: H1255-1261.

5

Targeting Effect of Traditional Chinese Medicine

Rui-Zhi Zhao

Second Affiliated Clinical College, Guangzhou University of Chinese Medicine,
Nei Huan XiLu, Guangzhou Daxue Cheng, Guangzhou,
China

1. Introduction

Most drugs have a widespread distribution in vivo, and effects beyond the disease site need to be avoided. As to herbs, it contains many components with different structure and varied effects, how to achieve the desired effect at the required site is a great challange. In ancient China, people usually get this goal by co-administration of other drugs, and in thousands of years, the experience was summarized as meridian guide theory. Since meridian guide theory is based on meridian distribution and compatibility, therefore, we should give a brief review about meridian, meridian distribution, and meridian guide drug.

In ancient China, diseases were treated by many methods, such as acupuncture, stone needle, drug, medicated bath, application, fumigate, and surgery. Concept of meridian was raised with acupuncture. In <Huangdi's Internal Classics>, the first monograph of China published at about 200 BC, diseases were divided according to their meridian, "meridian belongs to entrails inside and artus outside". There are 12 meridians, named as lung meridian, large intestine meridian, pericardium meridian, San Jiao meridian, heart meridian, small intestine meridian, spleen meridian, stomach meridian, liver meridian, gallbladder meridian, kidney meridian and urinary bladder meridian. Name of meridian is based on the main entrails the disease correlate and the route it will pass. And in <Huangdi's Internal Classics>, there are descriptions about the position, shape and weight of liver, heart, spleen, lung, kidney, intestine, stomach, gallbladder and urinary bladder, which are similar to that of modern anatomy. However, in ancient times, the anatomy was rough, and some version is different from modern views. For example, kidney is the main organ in kidney meridian, the function of "kidney" in traditional Chinese medicine includes kidney and genitical gland located near kidney. At that time, disease diagnosis and treatment especially in acupuncture was based on their meridian, such as taiyang diseases, yangming diseases, etc.

In Han dynasty, the famous physician Zhang Zhong-Jing described a method of diagnose - analyse and differentiate febrile diseases in accordance with the theory of six pairs of channels in his book < Treatise on Febrile Diseases> (Fu, 1990). Thereafter, drug use was summarized according to syndrome- differentiation of the six meridians. For example, nutgrass galingale rhizome is used to treat liver diseases, therefore, its meridian belongs to liver; fritillariae tuber is used to treat lung diseases such as cough, asthma, therefore, its meridian belongs to Lung; borneol is used to treat heart diseases, its meridian distribution is heart, etc. Some drugs have a wide use, its meridian distribution may be two or three entrails. For example, bupleuriradix is used to treat diseases of liver, Sanjiao, arcula cordis, and it belonges to these three meridians. And this is the basis for the formation of meridian distribution theory. In Tang and Song dynasty, there were some descriptions about drug orient and site-direct effect in books <Shi Liao Ben Cao>, <Supplement to the Herbal>, <Amplification on Canon of Materia Medica> and <Su Shen Liang Fang>. Thereafter, in Jin and Yuan dynasty, the famous physician Zhang Jie-Gu summarized these results and combined with his own experiment, raised the concept of meridian distribution. In his book <Zhen Zhu Lang>, and <Yi Xue Qi Yuan>, he summarized the experience of drug use according to meridian channels, such as "drug used to remove fire in ZANG FU-organ", "Meridian Guide drug of channels", and described meridian distribution as an important item of drug property. He thought that drug effect is related to its channal, and when used properly, the effect would be great. For example, Coptis chinensis, schtellaria, paeoniae radix, anemarrhenae, caulis hocquartiae, phellodendricortex, and gypsum all had the effect of purging pathogenic fire, however, Coptis chinensis is mainly used to purge the sthenic heart-fire, scutellaria is mainly used to purte the White, paeoniaeradix is mainly used to purge the sthenic liver-fire, caulis hocquartiae is used to rush down the fire in small intestine, phellodendricortex is mainly used to purge the fire in bladder. His disciple, famous physician Li Dong-Yuan and Wang Hao-Gu inherited his theory and developed it. In the book <Yong Yao Fa Xiang> of Li Dong-Yuan and <Materia Medica of Decoction> of Wang Hao-Gu, meridian distribution theory was used and improved. In <Materia Medica of Decoction>, there were 242 different kinds of drugs, among them, 80 were described as drugs with meridian distribution. In this book, drugs with meridian distribution were summarized in a table, named as "Guide profiles of various meridians". Due to its effectiveness in choosing drugs to formulate prescription, as it appeared, it was accepted by many physicians and more and more experience about drug meridian distribution was summarized. Then, in Ming dynasty, two famous physicians Liu Wen-Tai and Jia Ru-Li described meridian distribution as an indispensable content of drug property in their book <Ben Cao Pin Hui Jing Yao> and <Yao Pin Hua Yi> respectively. Li Shi-Zhen, a famous physician and pharmacist in Ming dynasty, inherited and developed the theory of meridian distribution of Zhang Jie-Gu in his world-famous book <Compendium of Materia Medica>, and indicated that "Chinese lovage is TaiYang meridian drug", "gypsum is cold Yangming meridian drug" etc. The meridian distribution of herbs was introduced when discussing drug property, such as "ephedra herb is the herb for lung meridian specially, when treating lung diseases, it is usually used." "frenugreek, herbs of right kidney, when kidney-YANG is deficient, it is used when cold-QI incubate in body and could not return to Yuan", "gastrodiarhizome is Qifen herbs belonging to liver meridian, in <Huangdi's Internal Classics>, it was indicated that all kinds of dazzling belongs to liver meridian, therefore, gastrodiarhizome could treat dizzy." Afterwards, meridian distribution was extensively described in books <Ben Cao Jing Shu> of Liao Xi-Yong, <Lei Gong Pao Zhi Yao Xing Jie> and <Ben Cao Tu Jie> by Li Zhong-Zi, , and more and more people accepted meridian distribution theory.

Meridian guide theory is the combination of meridian distribution and compatibility. It is first proposed in Qin and Han dynasty, and was developed in Tang and Song dynasty, formed at Jin and Yuan dynasty, completed in Ming and Qing dynasty. At 200 BC, in the first herb book <Shennong's herbal>, there was description that "Jun Gui is the message of other drugs". In Wei and Jin dynasty, famous physician Tao Hong-Jing described in his book <Ming Yi Bie Lu> that "cinnamomicortex guides other drugs". In Bei Song dynasty, Kou Zong-Shuang described in his book <Amplification on Canon of Materia Medica> that "Zhang Zhong-Jing used *Alismae rhizoma* in "Ba Wei Wan", just used it to guide cinnamomicortex and aconite root into kidney meridian, and no other means". In Jin and Yuan dynasty, Zhang Jie-Gu raised the concept of meridian guide drug. In his book <Zhen Zhu Lang>, he called drugs which could enforce other drugs effect at the meridian of its own as meridian guide drug, and listed meridian guide drug for twelve meridians. His disciple Li Dong-Yuan developed this idea and the theory. And then, in the book <Compendium of Materia Medica>, Li Shi-Zhen summarized the work of previous physicians, combined his and his father's experience in treating diseases, and revised the meridian guide drug of twelve channels. Also in this book, it is said that "ramuluscinnamomi guides other drugs to arm", "achyranthisradix guides other drugs to the lower part of the body" etc. Afterwards, many physicians exercised this method for diseases treatment, and got good results.

The twelve meridian guide drugs are: platycodonradix, angelica root, cimicifugae for lung meridian, gypsum and angelica root for large intestine meridian, cortex moutan and bupleuriradix for pericardium meridian, forsythia suspensa and bupleuriradix for San Jiao meridian, coptis chinensis, asariradix and borneol for heart meridian, Chinese lovage and phellodendri for small intestine meridian, atractylodes and cimicifugae for spleen meridian, angelica root, gypsum and pueraria for stomach meridian, vinger-baked bupleuriradix, evodiaefructus, and green tangerine peel for liver meridian, green tangerine peel and bupleuriradix for bladder meridian, cassia and anemarrhenae for kidney meridian, and incised notopterygium rhizome for urinary bladder meridian. There are some crossovers in meridian guide drug among different channels, for example, bupleuriradix and cimicifugae are meridian guide drugs for four channels, angelica root is the meridian guide drug for three channels. Besides twelve meridian guide drugs, there are some drugs for site targeting, such as chuanxiong for headache; ramulus cinnamomi and mulberry twig for Brachialgia; achyranthisradix for melosalgia; notopterygiirhizoma for cervical part disease etc. Many physicians practised meridian guide method in treating diseases and had a good effect, and they recorded their thoughts in their books. You Zai-Jing, a famous physician, said in his book <Yi Xue Du Shu Ji> that "soldiers could not reach enemies' place if there is not a guide, and drugs could not reach the disease site if there is not a meridian guide drug". Another physician in Qing dynasty, Shen Shi-Pao said that " meridian guide drug could induce other drugs to the disease site, and a great effect could be achieved with less drug used". Many famous prescriptions contained meridian guide drug, such as bupleuriradix in "Xiao Chai Hu Tang", gypsum in "Bai Hu Tang", kudzuvine root in "Ge Gen Qin Lian Tang", platycodiradix in "Sen Ling Bai Zhu San", and evodiaefructus in "Zuo Jin Wan", achyranthisradix in "San Miao San" and "Hu Qian Wan". Even in modern times, many famous physicians indicated that using meridian guide drug is an effective way for drug targeting (R.Z. Zhao et al, 2005).

Nowdays, more and more drugs are found to have side effects, and these effects affected clinical results especially for cancer treatment, about 30% patients give up treatment due to serious side effects of anticancer drugs. Many technologies are used to increase the therapeutic effect and reduce the side effect. However, site-directed pharmaco-delivery is a desirable but elusive goal. Although there are great achievements in target delivery, the clinical results were beyond people's expectation due to the difference between animals and human beings. The concept of meridian guide drug is similar to that of target delivery system, may be a new way for targeting delivery. Therefore, some studies had been carried out to demonstrate the meridian guide theory by experiment.

2. Modern study of meridian guide drug

At present, two methods are usually used to study meridian guide theory. One is pharmacokinetics method. This method demonstrated the effect of meridian guide drug by comparing drug distribution before and after co-administration with meridian guide drugs. This method is based on the hypothesis that drug effect is dependent on its concentration. The second method is pharmacological method. Meridian guide effect was investigated by comparing the target site effect between drug and their co-administration with meridian guide drugs. This method is based on the clinical definition of meridian guide drug. Vinegar-baked bupleuriradix, meridian guide drug of liver, platycodiradix, meridian guide drug of lung, borneol, meridian guide of heart meridian, and achyranthisradix, meridian guide drug of legs have been studied.

2.1 Study of liver meridian guide drug: vinegar-baked bupleuriradix

Bupleuriradix, is the dry radix of *Bupleurum Chinense DC*, and *B. Scozoneri folium wide*. It tastes acrid, and belongs to liver, cholecyst, Sanjiao and pericardium meridian. It is usually used in the treatment of influenza, fever, malaria, hepatitis, jaundice, nephritis, dizziness, bitter taste in the mouth, lung disease, cancer, and menstrual disorders in China, Japan, and other Asia. Pharmacological study showed that it had the effect of anti-inflammatory (S.M.Chen et al, 2008), antiviral activities (Chiang, 2003), antioxidant and hepatoprotective effect (B.J. Wang et al, 2004) etc. It is the meridian guide drug of liver, pericardium, gall bladder and Sanjiao meridian. In traditional Chinese medicine theory, it is regarded that drugs with sour taste enters liver first, and when baked with vinegar, it is the liver meridian guide only. It is described in the book <Ben Cao Zheng Yi> that "...besides, there is stagnation in collaterals and subcollaterals of liver, add few of bupleuriradix, the effect is quick".

Li Xiao-Dong and Nie Sa et al studied the effect of vinegar on pharmacological and chemical of bupleuriradix. The results showed that both pharmacological effect and components in the drug changed a little bit due to the vinegar-baked procedure (X.D. Li, 2000; S.Nie et al; 2008). It was demonstrated that vinegar-baked bupleuriradix had a much stronger effect on acesodyne and bile secretion than that of the bupleuriradix (J.Wu, 2008; S.Q Nie et al; 2002). Therefore, vinegar-baked bupleuriradix was extensively used in the liver diseases treatment medicines (Kou et al, 2006), such as DA Chai Hu Tang, Xiao Yao San, Xiao Chai Hu Tang etc. The study method was pharmacokinetics based.

2.1.1 Vinegar-baked bupleuriradix affected drug distribution

Four components were chosen in studying the liver targeting effect of vinegar-baked bupleuriradix, these are resveratrol (R.Z. Zhao et al., 2009), rhein (R.Z. Zhao et al., 2010), oxymatrine (unpublished data), and gentiopicroside (unpublished data). Their structure belongs to chrysophenine glycoside, anthraquinone, alkaloid and iridoid glycode respectively. In these studies, except resveratrol, animals were divided into two large groups according to dose of the components, and in each large group, animals were divided into four groups based on the dose of vinegar-baked bupleuriradix. For resveastrol, there was only one large group, and subgroup was similar to that of the other studies.

The detail of the experiment is listed in Table 1. For oral administration, components were suspended in solutions containing 1% sodium carboxymethylcellulose or in vinegar-baked bupleuriradix solutions containing 1% sodium carboxymethylcellulose. At predetermined time points, six animals were taken out from each group and blood was collected via heart puncture. Tissues of interest (heart, liver, spleen, lung, and kidney) were collected immediately after cervical dislocation and were blotted dry with tissue paper. Plasma and tissue samples were frozen at -80°C until analysis.

Component	Animal	Detection method	Detected components	subgroups	Drug dose (mg/kg)	Dose of vinegar-baked bupleuriradix (mg/kg)
resveratrol	mice	HPLC	resveratrol	4	200	300, 600,1200
rhein	rats	HPLC	Rhein and conjugated rhein	8	80, 40	300, 600, 1200
oxymatrine	mice	HPLC-MS	Oxymatrine and matrine	8	80, 10	400, 800, 1200
gentiopicroside	mice	HPLC-MS	gentiopicroside	8	100, 50	400, 800,1200

Table 1. Experiment design of liver targeting effect of vinegar-baked bupleuriradix

In all the studied animal groups, vinegar-baked bupleuriradix showed liver targeting effects for all the components with different degree. This effect is dependent on the dose of vinegar-baked bupleuriradix, components and its structure. Table 2 listed the most effective group within the study.

Vinegar- baked bupleuriradix enhanced other drugs liver distribution by three ways. First, it increased the Cmax of other drugs in liver, this indicated that vinegar-baked bupleuriradix enhanced liver uptake of other drug. This effect is component structure related. Among these four components, rhein is the most sensitive drug to the effect of vinegar-baked bupleuriradix, the maximal increased Cmax ratio in liver was 565%; second sensitive component is oxymatrine, the maximal increased Cmax ratio in liver was 89%, the third is gentiopicroside, the maximal increased Cmax ratio was 21%; and resveratrol is the least sensitive to the effect of vinegar baked bupleuriradix, its Cmax had marginal change. AUC is a parameter determined by Cmax and elimination rate. When using AUC as the evaluation criteria, rhein is still the most sensitive component to the effect of vinegar-baked bupleuriradix, second is oxymatrine. However the third is resveratrol, the increased AUC in liver was 79%, and gentiopicroside was the most insensitive component to the effect of vinegar-baked bupleuriradix. It should be indicated that although vinegar-baked bupleuriradix had marginal effect on the uptake of resveratrol, it decreased the elimination rate of resveratrol in liver significantly, also induced an increase in AUC.

Second, vinegar-baked bupleuriradix decreased AUC and Cmax of these components in other tissues. Rhein is the most sensitive components to the effect of vinegar-baked bupleuriradix. Low dose of vinegar-baked bupleuriradix decreased the distribution of rhein in other tissues except liver, and the decreased AUC ratio was 82%, 57%, 30%, 25% and 15% for spleen, heart, blood, lung and kidney respectively. The second sensitive component was resveratrol, high dose of vinegar-baked bupleuriradix decreased the distribution of resveratrol in kidney, spleen, heart and lung significantly, the decreased AUC ratio was 30%, 30%, 32% and 30% respectively. The third sensitive component was oxymatrine, medium dose of vinegar-baked bupleuriradix decreased the distribution of oxymatrine in blood, spleen, heart, and lung, the decreased AUC ratio was 33%, 27%, 17% and 19%, the least sensitive components was gentiopicroside, medium dose of vinegar-baked bupleuriradix only decreased the AUC of gentiopicroside in blood and lung, the decreased ratio was 17% and 18% respectively.

Drugs	AUC Changed extent in liver	Cmax Changed extent in liver	AUC Changed extent in other tissues	Cmax Changed extent in other tissues	Drug distribution original
resveratrol	79%	No significance	-44% in lung, 58% in heart, and 42% in kidney	-46% in kidney, -23% in lung, and -16% in heart	Kidney> liver> lung> blood> heart> spleen
rhein	264%	226%	-72%, -57%, -30%, -25%, -15% in spleen, heart, blood, lung and kidney respectively	- 31% in heart, and -65% in spleen	Kidney> lung> blood> liver> spleen> heart
Conjugated rhein	21%	No significance	-53%, -48%, -43%, -39% and -30% in lung, heart, spleen, kidney, and blood respectively	-36% in heart, and -23% in kidney	Spleen> lung> kidney> heart > liver≈blood
oxymatrine	152%	89%	-33%, -17%, -27%, -19% in blood, heart, spleen and lung respectively	56% in kidney, -36% in lung, -15% in blood	Blood> lung> spleen> kidney> liver≈ blood
matrine	32%	20%	-73%,-37%, -35%, -16% in lung, blood, heart, and kidney respectively	-63%,-46%,-41%, 35%,-28% in heart, kidney, blood, spleen, and lung respectively	Blood> liver> kidney> spleen≈ heart≈ lung
Gentio-picroside	No significance	20%	-39%, -27%, -27%, -18% in kidney, heart, spleen, lung respectively	-35% ,-36% -15% in heart, spleen and kidney respectively	Kidney> blood> liver> lung> heart> spleen

Table 2. The results of vinegar-baked bupleuriradix on the AUC, Cmax of other components, listed results were the most effective groups when using relative targeting ratio as evaluation index.

Third, vinegar-baked bupleuriradix decreased the elimination rate of all these four components in liver, but increased their elimination rate in other tissues. This may be another reason for AUC increase in liver and AUC decrease in other tissues.

The liver targeting effect of vinegar-baked bupleuriradix also depended on drug and vinegar-baked bupleuriradix dose. For resveratrol and gentiopicroside, medium dose of vinegar-baked bupleuriradix had the strongest effect. For rhein, in high rhein dose group, low dose of vinegar-baked bupleuriradix had the strongest effect, but in low rhein dose group, high dose of vinegar-baked bupleuriradix had the strongest effect. For oxymatrine, in high oxymatrine dose group, high and medium dose of vinegar-baked bupleuriradix had the strongest effect. For gentiopicroside, rhein and oxymatrine, all components were sensitive to the effect of vinegar-baked bupleuriradix at their high dose than that at low dose.

In the study of rhein and oxymatrine, effects of vinegar-baked bupleuriradix on the distribution of their metabolites were also studied. Interestingly, similar phenomenon was observed when the index is conjugated rhein and matrine. Vinegar-baked bupleuriradix increased not only their distribution in liver, but also decreased their distribution in other tissues, also showing a liver targeting effect. Compared the sensitivity of rhein, oxymatrine together with their metabolites to the effect of vinegar-baked bupleuriradix, rhein metabolite was less sensitive than its native form, and rhein dose had marginal effect. However, the sensitivity of oxymatrine to the effect of vinegar-baked bupleuriradix was dependent on its dose, in high dose group of oxymatrine, oxymatrine was more sensitive than its metabolite, anyhow, in low dose group of oxymatrine, matrine was more sensitive than its native form.

When comparing their own distribution and the effect of vinegar-baked bupleuriradix, it is found that for the components which are sensitive to the effect of vinegar-baked bupleuriradix, their main distribution is not in liver. For rhein and oxymatrine, liver distribution was only 5% and 3.8% of the total drug in vivo respectively. However, the two components were less sensitive to the effect of vinegar-baked bupleuriradix, their distribution in liver was relatively high, AUC in liver was 17% and 17.9% for gentiopicroside and resveratrol respectively.

2.1.2 Liver targeting effect mechanism of Vinegar-baked bupleuriradix

Effect of vinegar-baked bupleuriradix on drug distribution implied that vinegar-baked bupleuriradix may affect cell uptake of the drug and this is related with membrane constituents. Therefore, the effect of vinegar-baked bupleuriradix on membrane permeability, membrane constituents, pHi and morphology of BRL cell line were investigated (unpublished data). In these studies, samples were divided into four groups according to the concentration of vinegar-baked bupleuriradix, 10 mg/mL, 2 mg/mL, 0.4 mg/mL and drug free group, respectively. In each group, samples were further divided into 3 h, 6 h, 10 h, 18 h, 24 h, 48 h and 72 h subgroups according to the culture time for permeability study (n=5), and 3, 6, 12, 24, 48 h for membrane constituents study (n=5), and 12 h sample for morphology study. Each experiment was repeated five times. Membrane permeability was determined by flow cytometry, membrane morphology of BRL was observed by electronic microscope, and constituents were determined by automatic biochemistry analysator and thin layer chromatography scanning method.

Vinegar-baked bupleuriradix increased the BRL membrane permeability significantly, and this effect was vinegar-baked bupleuriradix concentration dependent, at all the time points, high concentration vinegar-baked bupleuriradix had a stronger effect than that of low concentration, and as the culture time prolonged, the effect of vinegar-baked bupleuriradix concentration on the permeability was more obvious. Further study showed that the membrane permeability increase was not due to membrane breakage, but prompting the growth of BRL cell. Morphology study showed that compared with the control group, the cell surface was much smoother after co-cultured with medium and high dose of vinegar-baked bupleuriradix, the effect was drug dose dependent. In order to study the reason, the content of cholesterol, protein and lipids were determined. Vinegar-baked bupleuriradix had marginal effect on the content of cholesterol, and the effect of vinegar-baked bupleuriradix on the lipids and protein content was dependent on the culture time and drug dose.

Cholesterol/phospholipids reflected cell integrity and permeability, when it decreased, the increase of permeability is toxic to cells, in this study, however, compared to the control group, high and medium dose of vinegar-baked bupleuriradix increased the ratio at 3, 12, 24 h, only decreased the ratio at 6 h, low dose of vinegar-baked bupleuriradix had marginal effect on the ratio.

Proportion among lipids is related with membrane fluidity, and it is related with membrane permeability, especially phosphatidylcholine/phosphatidyl ethanolamine ratio. Like cholesterol/phospholipids ratio, when it is decreased, cells are under danger. However, vinegar-baked bupleuriradix increased the ratio before 12 h, and thereafter, it had marginal effect on it. Membrane constituents were related with transporters, and the effect of vinegar-baked bupleuriradix on the activity of P- glycoprotein in BRL cell line was also studied, and the results showed that vinegar-baked bupleuriradix inhibited the activity of P-glycoprotein, this is in accordance with the results of morphological and membrane constituents results, and indicated that liver targeting effect of vinegar-baked bupleuriradix may be related with transporters.

2.2 Study of lung meridian guide drug: platycodiradix

Platycodiradix is the root of *Platycodon grandiflorum* A. DC, and it is widely used in treating diseases of lung and respiratory system, such as laryngopharyngitis, bronchitis, asthma, pulmonary tuberculosis, and pneumonia in clinics in China. Pharmacological research showed that it is responsible for diverse effects including anti-inflammation, anti-allergy, anti-tumor, augmentation of immune response, anti-obesity, anti-oxidation, hypoglycemic activity etc (Y.Tai et al, 2009). It is described in book <Ben Cao Qiu Zhen> that platycodiradix could promote the function of lung, and guide other drugs to lung. Therefore, it is the meridian guide drug of lung.

The lung target enhancing effect of platycodiradix was studied by pharmacokinetics method. Animals were divided into two groups, drug alone group and drugs co-administration with platycodiradix. Drug concentration and the target evaluation were listed in Table 3. The studied components included levofloxadin (Y.L, Li et al., 2006), florenicol (Y.L. Li et al., 2008), and roxithromycin (Y.L. Li et al., 2005).

component	animal	Detection method	Detected components	Drug dose	Target evaluation
levofloxacin	chicken	HPLC	levofloxacin	10mg/kg	Cmax, AUC
Florfenicol	rabbit	HPLC	florfenicol	30mg/kg	Cmax, AUC
roxithromycin	chicken	Biological effect method	roxithromycin	8,10,12mg/kg	Cmax, AUC

Table 3. Experiment design of lung targeting effect of platycodiradix

Platycodiradix increased the distribution of levofloxacin, florfenicol in lung significantly and this effect is platycodiradix dose dependent and components property related. The most sensitive component was levofloxacin. When co-administered with platycodiradix, Cmax of levofloxacin in lung increased 4.4 times; and its AUC increased 470%, although platycodiradix also increased the AUC of levofloxacin in heart and kidney, the increased extent was far less than that in lung. Florfenicol was less sensitive than levofloxacin. Platycodiradix increased Cmax and AUC of florfenicol in lung. However, it also increased the distribution of florfenicol in liver. Meanwhile it decreased Cmax of florfenicol in blood and kidney with the decreased extent of 28% and 44% respectively.

Drugs	AUC Changed extent in lung	Cmax Changed extent inlung	AUC Changed extent in other tissues	Cmax Changed extent in other tissues	Drug distribution original	Distribution ratio of drug in lung
levofloxacin	440%	470%	-15% in liver, 50% in kidney, 44% in heart	-14% in liver, 72.7% in heart, 103% in kidney	Kidney>=liver >heart=lung	8.5%
Florfenicol	50%	59.7%	-26% in blood, 76.8% in liver	-28% in blood, -44% in kidney 110% in liver,	Kidney> lung≈ liver> heart	10.4%
Roxithro-mycin	No significance	36%	_	_	_	_

Table 4. Results of lung targeting effect of Platycodiradix, _ represent no data

Effect of platycodiradix on the distribution of roxithromycin was a little different from that of others. Although at 10mg/kg dose, platycodiradix increased Cmax of roxithromycin, it had marginal effect on AUC, platycodiradix enhanced drug absorption, Tmax of roxithromycin was 3 or 4 h for medium and low dose respectively, when co-administered with platycodiradix, Tmax was 0.75 h and 1.5 h respectively. In control group, drug was absorbed slowly, and there were 3 peaks, but in experimental group, there was only 1 peak. Multi-peak usually indicated liver-intestine cycle, and platycodiradix may be able to inhibit this cycle and induce a rapid elimination. Since effect of platycodiradix on drug distribution in other tissues was not studied, effect of platycodiradix on roxithromycin is not complete. This limited our knowledge.

2.3 Effect of borneol on brain targeting

Borneol, a simple bicyclic monoterpene with acrid-bitter flavor, belongs to heart, spleen and lung meridian, it has the effect of communicating holes and scattering stagnant fire, detumescencing and relieving the pain. It is frequently used in the treatment of encephalopathy, such as stroke, epilepsy and headache. Pharmacological study showed that borneol had the effect of anti-excitation of central nerve induced by picrotoxin, prolong the delitescence of hyperspasmia, prolong the survival time of mice under oxygen deficiency, and prolong the awareness of tired rats (S.R.Wu & G.Cheng et al, 2001).

In the book "Amplification on Canon of Materia Medical", it is said that "borneol is weak when used alone, it strengthens the therapeutic action of other herbs when it is used as an adjuvant and message drug", it also had the effect of "commanding other drugs". In <Plain Questions of Huangdi's Internal Classic>, it is said that "Heart, King of organs, mind efferens", "heart controls mental and emotional activities", that is to say, brain function in ancient China was listed as "Heart". Therefore it is the meridian guide drug of brain.

2.3.1 Borneol increased drug concentration in brain

Brain targeting effect of borneol was studied by determining drug concentration in brain and pharmacological method. Drugs studied using the first method included sodium ferulate (Z.Z. Lin et al, 2008), carbamazepine (H.Y. Zhou et al, 2008), tetramethylpyra (Y.

Wang et al, 2006), methotrexat (Gao et al, 2009), rifampici (S.R. Wu et al, 2004), Panax pseudo-ginsing (S.X. Wang et al, 2009), puerarin (C.Y. Gao et al, 2010), gastrodin (Cai et al, 2008), cidomycin (Q.D. Liu et al, 1994), danshensu (J. Liu et al, 2008) et al. The study design was listed in Table 5.

Drugs	Animal	Detection method	Detected components	Drug dose g/kg	Meridian guide drug dose (g/kg)	Target evaluation
Sodium ferulate	mice	HPLC-MS	Sodium ferulate	0.2	0.05,0.002	Concentration in brain and blood
Carbamazepine	mice	HPLC	Carbamazepine, 10,11- epoxide carbamazepine		0.75	Cmax, AUC
Tetramethyl-pyrazine	rat	HPLC	Tetramethyl-pyrazine	0.0034	0.034	Concentration in blood and brain
methotrexat	Rabbit	HPLC	Methotrexat	0.1	0.75	Concentration in brain
Cidomycin	rat	Enzyme immu-nization	cidomycin	0.035	1.0	Concentration in brain
rifampici	Mice	HPLC	rifampici	0.182	0.6	AUC
notoginsenoside R1	rabbit	HPLC	notoginseng R1	15.0	0.085	Concentration in tissues
Ginsenoside Rg1	rabbit	HPLC	ginsenoside Rgl	15.0	0.085	Concentrationin tisues
Ginsenoside Re	rabbit	HPLC	ginsenoside Re	15.0	0.085	Concentration in tissues
Puerarin	Rats	HPLC	puerarin	0.0625	0.3	AUC in brain
gastrodin	mice	HPLC	gastrodin	0.2	0.4, 0.6	AUC in brain and blood
danshensu	rabbit	HPLC-MS	Danshnsu	10	0.18	Concentration in tissues

Table 5. Experiment design of brain targeting effect of borneol

Among these drugs, cidomycin is aminoglycoside antibiotic, puerarin is a kind of flavonoid, notoginsenoside R1, ginsenoside Rg1 and Re are saponin, rifampici is rifomycins antibiotics, methotrexat is antifolate drug. Borneol increased their distribution in brain, and this effect is borneol dose dependnt and chemical structure related. In the study of borneol to the distribution of gastrodin, 40 and 60 mg/kg borneol increased the distribution of gastrodin in brain significantly. However, 20 mg/kg had marginal effect on the distribution of gastrodin. Among the reported study, Ginsenoside Rg1 was the most sensitive compound to the effect of borneol, and drug concentration increase in brain was 2438%. Although it also increased drug concentration in other tissues, the increased ratio was far less than that in brain. The second sensitive component was notoginsenoside R1, the increased ratio of drug concentration in brain was 523%, and borneol also increased drug concentration in other tissues in the meantime. The originally distribution of these two components in brain was very low. Borneol also had the effect of decreasing drug concentration in non-target tissues. For example, borneol decreased the concentration of tetramethylpyrazine in blood, and decreased the concentration of rifampici in liver and kidney.

Drugs	% Change of AUC in Brain	% Change of Concentration in brain	AUC Change in other tissues	Cmax Change in other tissues	Drug distribution original
Sodium ferulate	66%	47%	No significance	46% in blood	_
Carbamazepine	24.5%	129%	-9%~- 37% in lung, liver, heart and kidney	14%~29%, in liver, lung, blood, heart, muscle, 175% in spleen	Lung> brain> fat> liver> blood> kidney> spleen >heart > muscle
epoxide carbamazepine	174.5%	56%	-52~- 40% in lung, liver and heart	146% in spleen, -38%, -20.5%,-53% in lung, liver and heart respectively	Lung>heart> liver> kidney> blood> brain> fat> spleen> muscle
Tetramethylpyrazine	30%	26 %	-15% in blood	-10%	_
methotrexat	75%	56.5%	No significance	No significance	_
Cidomycin	-	142%	-	22.8	_
rifampici	99%	79%	-12%, -17%, 64%, 46% in liver, kidney lung and blood respectively	-40%,-24% 75% in liver , kidney and lung respectively	Liver> kidney> lung> blood> brain
notoginsenoside R1	--	523%	--	497% , 227% , 36% 20% in liver, lung, heart, kidney	Heart> kidney> lung> liver> brain
ginsenoside Rgl	_	2438%	_	927%, 567% and 491% in heart, kidney, liver	lung> liver >kidney >heart >brain
ginsenoside Re	_	71%	_	264%, 251%, 85% 73% in, liver, lung, heart, kidney	Kidney >heart > brain= liver > lung
Puerarin	191%		-	-	Lung>>kidney> pancreas> liver> heart> spleen> brain
gastrodin	109%	80%	No significance	No significance	
Danshensu	_	355%		-100%, 158%, 104%in heart, liver, kidney respectively	Kidney> heart> brain >liver

Table 6. Effect of borneol on drug distribution of other drugs

Among these studies, only in the study of carbamazepine, the effect of borneol on the metabolite of carbamazepine was studied. Borneol also increased the distribution of the metabolite of carbamazepine in brain, and decreased its distribuion in lung, liver and heart, also showed a brain targeting effect. However, since most of these studies only pay attention to the blood-brain barrier, effect of borneol on drug distribution in other tissues was neglected, and this limited our knowedge of borneol on the absorption, distribution, elimination and excretion of the studied drugs.

2.3.2 Brain action enhancing effect of borneol

Besides pharmacokinetics study, pharmacological method was also used to demonstrate the effect of borneol. Ischemic reperfusion usually induces brain injury. Although some drugs are effective for ischemic reperfusion, low drug concentration in brain limited their effect. Sodium ferulate is one of these drugs.

Chen Xiao-Hong et al studied the brain curative enhancing effect of borneol on sodium ferulate by ischaemia reperfused model (X. H. Chen et al, 2010). Mice were randomly divided into 6 groups (n = 6): sham-treated, which was administered 10% ethanol, treated group included sodium ferulate 100 mg/kg per day, sodium ferulate 400 mg/kg per day, borneol 10 mg/kg per day, sodium ferulate 100 mg/kg +10 mg/kg borneol per day, sodium ferulate 400 mg/kg +10 mg/kg borneol per day. Therapy was initiated 30 min before or after ischaemia reperfused. To evaluate the treatment effects, tissues of the mice were collected for brain oedema analysis after 24 h of ischaemia reperfusion, for BBB permeability detection after 48 h and for Morris water maze test after 4 days of ischaemia reperfusion. Ischemic reperfusion model was made by the bilateral common carotid artery occlusion method. The results showed that compared with sham-operated group, the ischaemia reperfused mice were associated with long-lasting spatial learning deficits in the absence of other behavioral impairments and with neurodegeneration in the hippocampal CA1 region. However, the histological injuries were significantly attenuated by oral co-administration of sodium ferulate with borneol. Furthermore, combined treatment with sodium ferulate and borneol resulted in a significant reduction in brain oedema, gliofibrillar acid protein-positive cells, and blood–brain barrier permeability, but an increase in superoxide dismutase activity, indicating a brain targeting enhancing effect.

Artherosclerosis is the patho-basis for coronary disease and stroke. Dioscin, a component from plants of dioscoreaceae, lilium and pulse family, is usually used to treat coronary disease but due to blood- brain barrier, it is seldomly used to treat stroke. Wang Guang-Jian et al investigated the cure effect of dioscin on stroke when co- administered with borneol (G.J. Wang, 2010).

Rats were divided into five groups randomly, that is control group (sham operation group), model group, dioscin group (0.2g / kg), dioscin (0.2g / kg) co-administered with borneol (0.01g/kg) and dioscin (0.2g / kg) co-administered with borneol (0.02g/kg). Animals were administered drugs or equal volume of isotonic Na chloride (for control and model group). After 7 days, besides control group, animals in other groups were made into cerebral ischemia model by block arteria cerebri media. After the animals were recovered, their neurology was given a mark. Thereafter, animals were sacrificed, brain were taken out, dyeing and calculated the ratio of cerebral infarction.

The results showed that no neurologic impairment was found in control group. Animals in model group appeared ptosis, enophothamos, the neurology mark increased significantly, and cerebral infarction ratio was 12.9%. Compared with model group, cerebral infraction ratio and neurology mark of animals in dioscin and dioscin co-administration with low dose of borneol group had a tendency of decreasing, however, dioscin co-administered with high dose of borneol decreased the cerebral infarction ratio and neurology mark significantly, indicating a very obvious synergy effect.

2.3.3 Mechanism study of borneol

The most accepted thought is that low drug concentration in brain is due to blood- brain barrier. And mechanism studies about borneol were focused on the blood- brain barrier and its tight junction. Zhao Bao-Sheng and Liu Qi-De studied the effect of borneol on blood-brain barrier, and compared its effect with the blood-brain opening under pathological condition (B.S.Zhao & Q.D. Liu, 2002). The activity of anti-induce nitric oxide synthetase antibody (iNOS) in capillary endotheliocyte of brain was determined by streptomycin-bioepiderm – oxidase linking method. Compared with normal control group, iNOS in normal animals administered with borneol did not increase, while in animals with brain injured iNOS increased significantly, indicating that the opening of blood-brain barrier induced by borneol was different from that under pathological conditions. Ultrastructure of the blood-brain barrier influenced by borneol were also studied (Ge et al, 2008). It was showed that compared with the control group, borneol loosened the tight junction and some of the tight junction was not continuous. After 24h, the ultrastructure turned to normal, also indicating a reversible effect.

Since many factors are not easily controlled in vivo, people studied the effect of borneol on tight junction of BBB using different cell models. Chen Yan-Ming & Wang Ning-Sheng et al studied effect of borneol on the BBB model constructed by MDCK cell line (Y.M. Chen and N.S. Wang, 2004). First, borneol was administrated to rabbits for 4 consective days, and blood were taken out, the concentration of borneol in serum determined by GC-MS was 133 μg/ mL. Study was carried out by comparing the BBB among MDCK cells co-cultured with serum at different time and concentration, containing or not containing borneol. After 4 h co-culture with serum containing 0.086 μmol/L borneol, the tight junction was open, after 24h co-culture with serum containing borneol at the same concentration, the number and volume of pinocytosis vesicles in the BBB cells increased significantly, thus accelerating the transport of substances by cell pinocytosis. However, 24h after removing serum contained borneol, effect of borneol disappeared and there was no difference in morphology when compared with normal cell. This is in accordance with the in vivo effect, also indicating a reversible effect.

P-glycoprotein is multidrug resistant protein. There are lots of P-glycoprotein in BBB, and some people think it is one of the reasons that BBB restrains other drugs from getting into the brain. Chen Yan-Ming & Wang Ning-Sheng studied the effect of borneol on the vinblastine toxicity in MDCK and Hela cell line, verapamil was the positive control. It was found that borneol increased the toxicity of vinblatine in both cell lines significantly, and the increased degree was similar to that of verapamil, indicating that borneol may be able to inhibit the activity of P-glycoprotein (Y.M Chen. & N.S.Wang, 2003).

Histamine and 5- hydroxytryptamine take part in the regulation of BBB, therefore, Li Wei-Rong et al studied the effect of borneol on the content of histamine and 5-hydroxytryptamine. The results showed that borneol increased the contents of histamine and 5-hydroxytryptamine in brain significantly, indicating that effect of borneol on BBB may be related with histamine and 5-hydroxytryptamine (W.R. Li et al, 2006).

2.4 Meridian guide effect of achyranthisradix

Achyranthisradix is the radix of *Achyranthes bidentata Bl*. It tastes sweet, a little bitter and sour, belongs to kidney, liver meridian. It had the effect of enforcing the function of liver and kidney, strengthening bones and muscle, inducing float fire to descend and promoting diuresis for stranguria. In clinic, it is usually used to treat gonarthritis, swelling of throat caused by flaring up of stomach fire, and gingivitis etc. A famous physician Wang Ang in Qing dynasty said in his book <Essentials of Metea Medica> that "achyranthisradix induces fire to descend". Zhang Xi-Chun said in his book <Yi Xue Zhong Zhong Can Xi Lu> that "achyranthisradix induces fire and blood to descend". In book <Han Wen Tiao Bian>, it is described that "achyranthisradix, when used without baking, its property descends quickly, it could cure emia and amenia, induce other drugs to descend". In book <Ben Cao Feng Yuan>, it was reported that "achyranthisradix induces other drugs to the lower part, arthrolithiasis of bones and muscles at the lower part should use it". It is the meridian guide of lower limb.

Pharmacological study revealed that achyranthisradix enhanced lympholeukocyte to reproduce, and increased the secretion of IL-2, decreased the Sil-2 content in old rats. It also increased the SOD activity, LPO content in old and feeble rats. Besides, it had the effect of anti-tumor, anti- inflammatory, anti- bacteria, and analgesic (Meng & Li, 2001). Its meridian guide effect was studied by pharmacokinetics combined with pharmacological method.

Rats were divided into five groups randomly, that is normal control group, model control group, achyranthisradix group (5g/kg), diclofenac sodium (10mg/kg) group, achyranthisradix (5g/kg) co-administered with diclofenac sodium group (10mg/kg for diclofenac sodium). Besides normal group, Freud's compete adjuvant (0.1mL) were injected at right voix pedis of rats in other groups, and made the inflammatory model for 28 days by measuring weights and the volume of voix pedis each week. At the 22 day, drugs were administered to rats and the drug administration continued to the 28 day. On the last day, after measuring weight and volume of voix pedis, rats were anesthetized, and blood was collected from hepatic portal vein. Afterwards rats were sacrificed, right voix pedis was cut down and the skin was removed, the soft tissues were weighed and homogenized, the content of diclofenac sodium in blood, and voix pedis was determined by high performance liquid chromatography, the content of PGE2 was determined by kit., the content of IL-1β was determined by radio-immunity kit.

Compared with normal control group, right voix pedis in model group swelled significantly (P<0.01), both PGE and IL-1β increased significantly. In the study of diclofenac sodium, compared to the model group, both diclofenac sodium and its co-administration with achyranthisradix inhibited the swell significantly, achyranthisradix alone had marginal effect on the swell. Compared with diclofenac sodium, effect of inhibited swell was more effective in the group co-administered with achyranthisradix, showing a synergistic effect. Diclofenac sodium decreased both the PGE content in blood and inflammatory tissues significantly, and there was no difference between the decreased ratio in blood and inflammatory tissues. Achyranthisradix had marginal effect on PGE content, however when co-administered with diclofenac sodium, it decreased PGE content both in blood and inflammatory tissues significantly, and the decreased ratio in inflammtory tissues was more obvious, and this is different from the effect of diclofenac sodium. Same results was obtained when comparing the content of IL-1β. Both diclofenac sodium alone and co-administration with achyranthisradix decreased the content of IL-1β significantly, the latter had no significance when compared with normal control group, all these results showed that achyranthisradix could enhance the effect of diclofenac sodium. Besides, compared with model group, diclofenac sodium decreased the weight of rats significantly, when co-administered with achyranthisradix, the weight of rats increased, indicating that achyranthisradix decreased the side effect of diclofenac sodium (Y.Q Lin, 2009).

Drug concentration in tissues gave a clue for the pharmacological results. When co-administered with achyranthisradix, concentration of diclofenac sodium in blood decreased, and drug concentration in inflammatory site increased significantly, the decreased and increased extent were 75% and 10% respectively.

3. Meridian guide drug and transporters

Above results showed that meridian guide drug enhanced the curative effect of the co-administered drugs and this effect was induced by the increased distribution of other drugs in target site or decreased distribution in non-target site. This is in accordance with modern theory, and demonstrated that meridian guide drug could be used as a target delivery method. Drug concentration in tissues is a balance of uptake and elimination. Uptake could be reflected by Cmax. Almost all the results in pharmacokinetics studies showed that meridian guide drug increased a Cmax of other drugs in target site, this indicated that increasing the uptake is one of the ways for the effect of meridian guide drug. Elimination rate could be calculated by the concentration- time profile. Meridian guide drug usually increased the elimination in non- target site in above studies. Usually, drug uptake into cells and efflux to outside through two methods, one is passive diffusion, the other is active transport. Passive diffusion mainly depends on the property of the drugs, and fewer factors could affect it. Active transport is different, since it needs the help of carriers, factors which affected the activity directly or indirectly would affect its transport efficiency. Above results indicated that the effect of meridian guide drug may be related with influx and efflux transporters.

Mechanism study also gives some clues for meridian guide drug with transporters. In cell surface, there are lots of lipid raft related with the transport of xenobiotics and endogenous metabolites. Vinegar-baked bupleuriradix increased the permeability of BRL cell line, and in high dose the cell surface changed smoothly, indicating a change at transport capability. Further study indicated that this change was due to membrane constituents change.

Transporters is a kinds of protein resides in membrane and is responsible for the across of xenobiotics and endogenous metabolites into cells. Transporters could be divided into two families according to their transport directions, and they are influx transporters and efflux transporters. Influx transporters include organic anion transport protein (OAT), organic anion transport polypeptide (OATP), organic cation transport protein (OCT) and organic cation transport polypeptide (OCTP). Efflux transporters, also named as ATP- binding cassette (ABC) transporter super-family, include P- glycoprotein (P-gp), the multi-drug resistance protein family (MRP1-9), the breast cancer resistance protein (BCRP). There are many excellent reviews about them (H. Miyazaki et al, 2004; Kusuhara & Sugiyama, 2002; Shirata et al, 2006; M. L. Elaine et al, 2005; S. Gergely, 2008). The distribution of transporters is vary with different tissue, and the results are listed in Table 8. For example, OAT1 was expressed in kidney, brain, uterus, but OCT 1 was predominantly expressed in liver, and had trace amount in kidney; OAT3 was expressed in kidney, liver, brain, and eye; MRP1 was extensively expressed in most organs, and had a high expression in lung, testicle, kidney, musculi skeleti, peripheral blood mononuclear cell etc, but had a relatively low expression in liver (B. Hagenbuch & C. Gui, 2008; M. Huls et al, 2009; M. Elaine, 2005; C. J. Endres, 2006). More and more studies showed that transporters play a major role in drug absorption, distribution, toxicity, efficacy, elimination and excretion. And it is a main reason for drug-drug interaction. Some drugs affected the activity of transporters and as a consequence affected the distribution of the substrate of transporters (S. Eberl et al, 2007; A.Y. Coban et al, 2004 ; A. Seithel, et al, 2007, Sikri et al, 2004). Most of the meridian guide drugs had the effect of inhibiting the activity of P-gp (Q. Wu, 2005), and many drugs studied above such as resveratrol (A.Lancon et al, 2004, Juan et al, 2010), rhein (Garbap, 2002), levofloxacin (T. Ito et al, 1997), danshensu (P.F.Yu et al, 2011) are the substrate of P-gp or Mrp, indicating that meridian guide drug may influence the activity of these transporters and affect drug distribution and its pharmacological action.

By analyzing the pharmacokinetics data, this hypothesis could be further elucidated. Cmax is a parameter reflecting drug absorption. The increase in Cmax suggested an uptake increase and efflux decrease in intestine. Levofloxacin is the substrate of OATP (T. Maeda et al, 2007), P-gp (T. Ito et al, 1997) and MRPs (H. Polache et al, 2010), which are located in intestine, platycodiradix inhibited the activity of P-gp and Mrps and may also increase the activity of OATP, the Cmax of levofloxacin increased 470%. Resveratrol is the substrate of MRP2 (M. E. Juan et al, 2010; Lancan A, 2004), which transported drug from the liver to blood and induced a significantly increased blood concentration. Drug distribution and elimination is the balance of drug affinity to different tissues. As shown in Table 8, different tissues had different transporters or different content of the same transporters, and the affinity with different transporters was determined by the influx and efflux rate of the drug and as a sequel, the balance in different tissues determined distribution, elimination, and excretion of the drug.

Transporters	Gene	Transporter distribution	Substrates	Inhibitors
P-gp	ABCB1	**brain**, intestine, liver, kidney, placenta, lung, stomach, colon, pancreatic gland, oesophagus	danshensu, roxithromycin, quinolone, levofloxacin, berberine, rifampicin, ofloxacin	Bupleuri Radix, cimicifugate, cortex moutan, coptis chinensis, cortex phellodendri, anemarrhenae, Tetramethylpyrazine, platycodiradix, borneol, berberine, matrine, saikosaponin, paeoniflorin, baicalin, Roxithromycin, puerarin
Mrp1	*ABCC1*	Testicle, skeletal muscle, heart, kidney, lung, Brain, intestine, liver (trace)	rhein, methotrexate	puerarin
Mrp2	*ABCC2*	liver, gut, kidney, brain, placenta	Methotrexate resveratrol diclofenac baicalein	Tetramethylpyrazine, puerarin
Mrp3	ABCC3	Adrenal gland, Intestine, Pancreas, Gallbladder	Methotrexate	Tetramethylpyrazine, puerarin,
Mrp4	*ABCC4*	Placenta, Liver,	Methotrexate	

Transporters	Gene	Transporter distribution	Substrates	Inhibitors
		Kidney, Prostate Ovary, Testis, **Kidney**, Lung, Prostate		
MRP5	ABCC5	Liver, Testis, Skeletal and Cardiac Muscle, Brain		Tetramethylpyrazine
MRP6	ABCC6	Kidney, **keratinocytes**, liver tracheal, bronchial, epithelium, intestinal mucosa, corneal epithelium, smooth muscle cell		
BCRP	ABCG2	**Placenta, colon, intestine,** liver, heart, brain, kidney, prostate, ovary	Methotrexate, resveratrol Ofloxacin	
OAT1	SLC22A6	**Kidney**, brain, eye, placenta		Cidomycin, diclofenac, Methotrexate
OAT2	SLC22A7	**Liver**, kidney		Methotrexate
OAT3	SLC22A8	Liver, intestine, liver, Blood cerebrospinal fluid barrier, placenta		Methotrexate
OAT4	SLC22A11	Liver, placenta, kidney, adrenals		Methotrexate
OAT5	SLC22A	Liver, kidney		Methotrexate
OAT10	SLC22A13	Kidney, brain, heart, colon		
OCT1	SLC22A1	**Liver**, intestine, lung, heart, placenta		
OCT2	SLC22A2	Liver, **kidney**, brain, intestine		
OCT3	SLC22A3	**Liver**, intestine, placenta, brain,heart		
OCTN1	SLC22A4	Kidney, liver, testis, muscle, heart		

Transporters	Gene	Transporter distribution	Substrates	Inhibitors
OCTN2	SlC22A5	Kidney, liver, brain, intestine, testis		
OATP1A2	SLCO1A2	**Brain**, liver, kidney, eye	Levofloxacin Methotraexate	rifampicin
OATP2B1	SLCO2B1	Brain, **liver**, kidney, placenta, **intestine**	levofloxacin	Roxithromycin, rifampicin
OATP1B1-3	SLCO1B	**Liver**	Rifampicin, methotrexate	Rifampicin cimicifugae
OATP3A1	SLCO	ubiquitous	Rifampicin, methotraexate	Rifampicin
OATP4A1	SLC	ubiquitous		Rifampicin
OATP1C1	SLC	Brain, testis, heart, lung, eye		Rifampicin
OATP1AB3	SLC	**Liver**		Rifampicin
PEPT1	SLC	Liver, kidney, **intestine**		
PEPT2	SLC	**Kidney**, brain, lung, spleen, lacteal gland		

Table 8. Distribution, substrate, and inhibitors of transporters.

The activity and expression of transporters could be affected by many factors, such as xenobiotics, diseases, stress, metabolism enzyme, microenvironment change. And as a sequence, meridian guide drug may affect drug distribution by affecting these factors directly or indirectly. Efflux transporters are usually ATP dependent, drugs affecting ATP enzyme would affect activity of transporters and then affect drug effectiveness and toxicity (MunićV. et al, 2010; Regev et al, 1999). Bupleuriradix inhibited the activity of Na-K ATP enzyme (Q.L. Zhou et al, 1996), and may indirectly affected the activity of transporters.

Different transporters may be affected by different factors, and a factor may have different effect on different transporters. MRP is affected by many factors, and even in this family, despite of a great homology in family members, factors had different effect on different MRPs. Drugs may affect transporters by affecting the factor and thereafter affected other drugs distribution. For example, MRP1 is a glutathione dependent transporter, but other transporters of MRP family are glutathione independent. Water extract of bupleuriradix increased the glutathione content (M.H. Yen et al, 2005), and enhanced the activity of MRP1. MRP1 is expressed widely in other tissues but less in liver, leading to a fast elimination rate in other tissues, while it had marginal effect on drug elimination in liver. This may be one of the reasons for its toxicity reducing effect.

In spite of above well known transporters there are some transporters such as Mate1-2, RLIP76, and aquaporin, may play a role in meridian guide effect (Tanihara 2007, Ohta et al, 2009; Singhal, 2009). For example, carbamazepine is an active drug for epilepsy, and it has drug-resistant phenomenon. P-gp was first considered as the reason, however, study showed it is not the substrate of P-gp (Maines, 2005). Further studies showed that it is also not the substrate of MRP (Luna-Tortós et al, 2010; F. Rivers, 2008), BCRP (L. Cerveny et al,

2006). Recently, Awasthi et al found that RLIP76, a multifunctional modular protein, was involved in its drug-resistance (S. Awasthi et al, 2005). Borneol increased the brain concentration of carbamazepine, probably by inhibiting the activity of RLIP76.

Besides transporters, drug metabolism enzyme had an important effect on drug absorption, distribution, elimination and excretion. Most of meridian guide drug affected the activity of metabolism enzyme, such as pueraria, cassia bark, incised notopterygium rhizome, coptis chinensis, cortex phellodendri, evodiaefructus, angelica root, forsythia suspensa, paeoniaeradix and bupleuriradix, angelica dahurica etc. And this also may be one of reasons for its meridian guide effect (Yang et al, 2002; Mao et al, 2007, X.L. Bi et al, 2010). However, there are many herbs which could affect drug transporters and metabolism enzyme and they are not the meridian guide drug. For example, ginseng is drug usually used to invigorate vital energy, the main components of it not only affected drug metabolism but inhibited P-gp as well (C.H. Choi et al, 2003; S.W. Kim et al, 2003; S. Kitagwa Et al, 2007; Y.R. Pokharel, 2010); many herbs contained flavone, such as sophoraeflos, Chinese hawthorn, soybean which also could affect drug metabolism enzyme and transporters (R.X. Zhu et al, 2011; Y.H. Liu et al, 2011) and only few of them are meridian guide drug, therefore, there must be other factors co-operating this effect and further study is required.

4. Conclusion

In summary, meridian guide drug had the effect of synery and attenuation, and this effect is based on drug concentration at target-site. Meridian guide effect had a close relationship with drug transporters and metabolism enzymes. Different components had different affinity to transporters or enzymes, and meridian guide effect is a combination of all components in meridian guide drug. Therefore, it is necessary to investigate the exact effect of main components of meridian guide drug on transporters and metabolism enzymes, establish the relationship between its dose and its effect as well as effects on different kinds of diseases. As we know more about the relationship among components in meridian guide drug, kinds of transporters and metabolism enzymes, activity in nomal and disease state, we could design target delivery system freely as desired.

5. Acknowledgements

This research was financially supported by the found of National Science Foundation of China (Grant No. 30672668, 81073063)

6. References

Awasthi S., Hallene K. L, Fazio V., Singhal S. S , Cucullo L., Awasthi Y. C , Dini G. and Janigro D. (2005). RLIP76, a non-ABC Transporter, and Drug Resistance in Epilepsy, *BMC Neuroscience*, VOL. 6, *No.* 61, doi:10.1186/1471-2202-6-61

Bi X.L., Du Q, Di L.Q., (2010). Important Application of Intestinal Transporters and Metabolism Enzymes on Gastrointestinal Disposal of Active Ingredients of Chinese Materia Medica, *Zhongguo Zhongyao Zazhi*, Vol.35, No.3, (February, 2010), ISSN 1001-5302

Cerveny L., Pavek P., Malakova J., Staud F., and Fendrich Z., (2006). Lack of Interactions between Breast Cancer Resistance Protein (BCRP/ABCG2) and Selected Antiepileptic Agents, *Epilepsia*, Vol.47, No.3, pp.461–468, ISSN 0013-9580

Chen S.M., Sato N., Yoshida M., Satoh N., Ueda S. (2008). Effects of *Bupleurum scorzoneraefolium, Bupleurum falcatum*, and Saponins on Nephrotoxic Serum Nephritis in Mice. *Journal of Ethnopharmacology*, No 116 , (November, 2008) ,pp. 397–402, ISSN 0378-8741

Chen X. H., Lin Z.Z., Liu A.M, Ye J.T., Luo Y.Y, Mao X.X., Liu P.Q. and Pi R.B., (2010). The Orally Combined Neuroprotective Effects of Sodium Ferulate and Borneol Against Transient Global Ischaemia in C57 BL/6 Mice, *Journal of Pharmacy and Pharmacology*, No.62, (July, 2010), 915–923, ISSN 0022-3573

Chen Y.M., Wang N.S., (2004). Effect of Borneol on the Intercellular Tight Junction and Pinocytosis Vesicles in vitro Blood ·Brain Barrier, *Zhongguo Zhongxiyi Jiehe Zazhi*, Vol.24, No. 7,(July, 2004), pp.632-634, ISSN 1003-5370

Chen Y.M., Wang N.S., (2003). Effect of Borneol on P-gp, *Zhongyao Xinyao Yu Linchuang Yaoli*, Vol.14, No.2, (April, 2003), pp.96-99, ISSN 1003-9783

Chiang L.C., Ng L.T., Liu L.T., Shieh D., Li C.C., (2003). Cyctoxicity and Anti-Hepatitis B Virus Activities of Saikusaponins from Bupleurum, *Planta Med*, No.69, pp. 705-709, ISSN 0032-0943

Coban A. Y., Ekinci B., Durupinar B., (2004). A Multidrug Efflux Pump Inhibitor Reduces Fluoroquinolone Resistance in *Pseudomonas aeruginosa* isolates, *Chemtherapy*, No.50, pp.22-26. ISSN 0009-3157

Eberl S., Renner B., Neubert A., Reisig M., Bachmakov I., König J., Dörje F., Thomas E. M, Ackermann A., Dormann H., Gassmann K.G., Hahn E. G., Zierhut S., Brune K. and Fromm M. F. (2007). Role of P-Glycoprotein Inhibition for Drug Interactions Evidence from In Vitro and Pharmacoepidemiological Studies, *Clin Pharmacokinet*, Vol.46, No,12, pp.1039-1049, ISSN 0312-5963

Elaine M. Leslie, Roger G. Deeley, Susan P.C. Cole, (2005). Multidrug Resistance Proteins: Role of P-glycoprotein, MRP1, MRP2, and BCRP (ABCG2) in Tissue Defense, *Toxicology and Applied Pharmacology*, No.204, pp.216– 237, ISSN 0041-008X

Endres C. J., Hsiao P., Chung F. S., Unadkat J.D., (2006). The Role of Transporters in Drug Interactions, *European journal of pharmaceutical sciences*, No. 27, pp. 501–517, ISSN 0928-0987

Fu W. K., (1990). *History of Chinese medicine* (1st), ShangHai Zhongyi Xueyuan Publishing Company, Shanghai, China. ISBN 7-81010-093-9

Gao C., Gao M., Shi W.Z., Zhao Z.G, Sun H., Zhao X.L., (2009). Experimental Study on the Effect of Borneol for Methotrexate Penetrating Across Blood Brain Barrier, *Zhongguo Linchang Yaolixue Zazhi* Vol.25, No.2, (April, 2009), pp. 134-137, ISSN 1001-6821

Gao C.Y, Li X.R., Li Y.H., Wang L.J. and Xue M., (2010). Pharmacokinetic Interaction Between Puerarin and Edaravone, and Effect of Borneol on the Brain Distribution Kinetics of Puerarin in Rats. *Journal of pharmacy and pharmacology*,No.62, (March, 2010), pp.360-367, ISSN 0022-3573

Ge C.L, Han M.F, Bai R.T., Yu C.,(2008). Effect of Borneol Oil the Ultrastructure of Promoting Blood Brain Barriar Open, *Zhongxiyi Jiehe XinNao Xueguanbing Zazhi*, Vol.6, No. 10, (October, 2008), pp. 1183-1185, ISSN 1672-1349

Gergely S., Andras V., Csilla O.L., and Balazs S. (2008). The Role of ABC Transporters in Drug Absorption, Distribution, Metabolism, Excretion and Toxicity (ADME-Tox), *Drug Discovery Today*, Vol.13, No. 9/10, pp.379-393, ISSN 1359-6446

Gorkom BAP van, Timmer-Bosscha H., Jong S de, Kolk DM van der, Kleibeuker JH and Vries EGE de (2002). Cytotoxicity of Rhein, the Active Metabolite of Sennoside

Laxatives, is Reduced by Multidrug Resistance-associated Protein 1, *British Journal of Cancer*, No. 86, pp.1494 – 1500, ISSN 0007-0920

Hagenbuch B. & Gui C., (2008). Xenobiotic Transporters of the Human Organic Anion Transporting Polypeptides (OATP) Family, *Xenobiotica*, Vol.38, No.7–8, (July–August, 2008), pp.778–801, ISSN 0049-8254

Huls M., Russel F. G. M., and Masereeuw R., (2009). The Role of ATP Binding Cassette Transporters in Tissue Defense and Organ Regeneration, *The Journal of Pharmacology and Experimental Therapeutics*, Vol. 328, No.1, (January, 2009), pp. 3-9, ISSN 0022-3565

Ito T, Yano I, Tanaka K., and Inui, (1997), Transport of Quinolone Antibacterial Drugs by Human P-glycoprotein Expressed in Kidney Epithelial Cell Line, LLC-PK, *The journal of Pharmacology and Expermental Therapeutics*, No. 282 pp. 955-960, ISSN 0022-3565

Juan M. E., Gonzalezález-Pons E., and Planas J. M., (2010). Multidrug Resistance Proteins Restrain the Intestinal Absorption of trans-Resveratrol in Rats, *The Journal of Nutrition*; Vol.140, No.3, (March, 2010), pp.489-495, ISSN 0022-3166

Kim S.W., Kwon H.Y., Chi D.W., et al, (2003). Reversal of P-glycoprotein- Mediated Multidrug Resistance by Ginsenoside Rg3, *Biochem Pharmacol*, No.65, pp.75-82, ISSN, 0006-2952

Kitagwa S., Takahshi T., Nabekura T., Tagchikawe, and Hasegawa H, (2007). Inhibitory Effects of Ginsenosides and Their Hydrolyzed Metabolites on Daunorubicin Transport in KB-C2 Cells, *Biol. Pharm. Bull.*, Vol.30. No. 10, pp.1979 – 1981, ISSN 1347-5215

Kou W-M., 2006. Effect of Radix Bupleuri Processing Method on the Drug Action and its Rule in Clinical Use, *Shizhen Guoyi Guoyao*, Vol.17, No. 10 (October, 2006), pp. 1998-1999, ISSN 1008-0805

Kusuhara H., Sugiyama Y., (2002). Role of Transporters in the Tissue-Selective Distribution and Elimination of Drugs: Transporters in the Liver, Small Intestine, Brain and Kidney, *Journal of Controlled Release* No.78, pp.43–54, ISSN 0168-3659

Lancon A., Delmas D., Osman H., J.-P. , Thenot, and Jannin B., Latruffe N., (2004). Human Hepatic Cell Uptake of Resveratrol: Involvement of Both Passive Diffusion and Carrier-mediated Process, *Biochemical and Biophysical Research Communications* No.316, (February, 2004), pp. 1132–1137, ISSN 0006-291X

Lin Y.Q.,Sun B., Yang S.Y., Lv L., Liu Y., (2009). Therapeutic Effect of Radix Achyranthis Bidentatae Guiding Function on Diclofenac Sodium Induced Adjuvant Rats Arthritis, *Zhongyao Xinyao Yu Linchuang Yaoli*, Vol.20, No.5, (October, 2009), pp. 408-411, ISSN 1003-9783

Lin Z.Z, Yao M.C., Lan M. X., Liu P.Q., Zhong G.P., Pi R. B., (2008). Effects of Borneol on Distribution of Sodium Ferulate in Plasma and in Brain Regions of Mice, *Zhong Cao Yao*, Vol.39, No.4, (April, 2008), pp.551-556, ISSN 0253-2670

Liu J., Li X., Hu S.S., Yu Q.L, Sun W.J., Zheng X.H., (2008). Studies on the Effects of Baras Camphor on the Tissue Distribution of *Salvia miltiorrhiza Bge*. in Complex Danshen Prescription in Rabbits, *Yaowu Fenxi Zazhi*, Vol.28, No.10, (October, 2008), pp.1612-1615, ISSN 0254-1793

Liu Q.D., Liang M.R, Chen Z.X., (1994). The Influence of Borneol on the Passing of Gentamycin through Blood-Brain Barrier, *Guangzhou Zhongyiyao Daxue Xuebao* Vol.11, No.1, (January, 1994), pp.87-90, ISSN 1007-3213

Liu Y.H., Mo S.L., Bi H.C., Hu B.F., Li C.G., Wang Y.T., Huang L., Huang M., Duan W., Liu J.P., Wei M.Q., Zhou S.F., (2011). Regulation of Human Pregnane X Receptor and its Target Gene Cytochrome P450 3A4 by Chinese Herbal Compounds and a Molecular Docking Study, *Xenobiotica*. Vol.41, No.4, (April, 2011), pp.259-80, ISSN 0049-8254

Li W.R., Yao L.M., Mi S.Q., Wang N.S., (2006). Relation of Openness of Blood-Brain Barrier by Borneol with Histamine and 5-Hydroxytryptamine, *Zhongguo Linchuang Kangfu*, Vol.10, No.3, pp.167-169, ISSN 1671-5926

Li X.D., (2000). Comparative Analysis of Active Composition of Radix Bupleuri Before and After Being Processed, *Zhong YI Yao Xue Bao, Vol.* 22, No.7 (July, 2000), pp.483-484, ISSN 1002-2392

Li Y. L., Cui H.M., Chen H. W., (2008). Effect of Platycodon Grandiflorum on Pharmacokinetics of Florfenico, *Zhongguo ShouYi Xuebao*, Vol. 28, No.10 (October, 2008), pp. 1203-1207, ISSN 1005-4545

Li Y. L, Jiang Z. G., He X. L. (2006). Effect of Chinese Herb Platycodon Grandiflorum Leading Action on Distribution of Levofloxacin in Chickens After Oral Administration, *Zhongguo ShouYi Xuebao* Vol.26, No.5, (May, 2006), pp.541-543, ISSN 1005-4545

Li Y. L., Lu S. M., Jian M., (2005). Effect of Chinese Herb Platycodon Grandiflorum on Roxithromycin Concentration of Lung Tissue, *Zhongguo ShouYi Xuebao*, No. 3, (March, 2005), pp.3-6 ISSN 1005-4545

Luna-Tortós C., Fedrowitz M. , Löscher W., (2010). Evaluation of Transport of Common Antiepileptic Drugs by Human Multidrug Resistance-Associated Proteins (MRP1, 2 and 5) that Are Overexpressed in Pharmacoresistant Epilepsy, *Neuropharmacology*, No. 58, (January, 2010), pp 1019-1032, ISSN 0028-3908

Maeda T., Takahashi K., Ohtsu N., Oguma T., Ohnishi T. Atsumi R., and Tamai I., (2006). Identification of Influx Transporter for the Quinolone Antibacterial Agent Levofloxacin, *Molecular Pharmaceutics*, Vol. 4, No. 1, (October, 2007), pp.85-94, ISSN 1543-8384

Maines L. W., Antonetti D. A., Wolpert E. B., Smith C.D., (2005). Evaluation of the Role of P-Glycoprotein in the Uptake of Paroxetine,Clozapine, Phenytoin and Carbamazapine by Bovine Retinal Endothelial Cells, *Neuropharmacology* No.49, pp. 610-617, ISSN 0028-3908

Mao X.Q, Xie H.T., Zhou H.H, (2007). MDR- and CYP3A4- Mediated Drug-herb Interactions, *Zhongguo Linchuang Yaolixue Yu Zhiliaoxue*, Vol 12, No 7 (July, 2007), pp 728-734, ISSN 1009-2501

Meng D.L. & Li X., (2001). The Research Development of Achyranthesbidentata B1, *Zhongguo Yaowu Huaxue Zazhi*, Vol. 40, No.2, (February, 2001): 120-124, ISSN 1005-0108

Miyazaki H., Sekine T. and Endou H., (2004). The Multispecific Organic Anion Transporter Family: Properties and Pharmacological Significance, *TRENDS in Pharmacological Sciences*, Vol.25, No. 12, pp. 654-662, ISSN 0165-6147

Nie S., Liu X.P., Chen Sh.W, Li K., (2008). Study on Fingerprint of Bupleurum Chinese and Vinegar-baked Bupleurum Chinese in Hubei Province, *Zhong Yao Cai, Vol* .31, No.5, (May, 2008), pp. 657-659，ISSN 1001-4454

Nie S.Q, Yang Q., Li L.F, Huang L.Q, (2002). Pharmacokinetics Comparisons of Bupleurum Root and Red Peony Root, Vinegar-baked Bulpeurum Root and White Reony Root between Compatibility and Single Application, *Zhongguo Shiyan Fangji Xue Zazh*, *Vol.*8, No.3, (March, 2002), pp. 11-14, ISSN 1005-9903

Ohta K.Y., Imamura Y., Okudaira N., Atsumi R., Inoue K., and Yuasa H., (2009). Functional Characterization of Multidrug and Toxin Extrusion Protein 1 as a Facilitative Transporter for Fluoroquinolones, *The Journal of Pharmacology and Experimental Therapeutics*, Vol. 328, pp.628–634, ISSN 0022-3565

Pokharel Y.R., Kim ND, Han HK, Oh WK, Kang KW, (2010). Increased Ubiquitination of Multidrug Resistance 1 by Ginsenoside Rd. *Nutr Cancer*. Vol.62, No.2, pp.252-9, ISSN 1531-7914

Choi C.H., Kang G., Min Y.D, (2003). Reversal of P-glycoprotein-mediated Multidrug Resistance by Protopanaxatriol Ginsenosides from Korean Red Ginseng.*Planta Med.*, Vol.69, No. 3 (Mar,2003), pp.235-40, ISSN 0032-0943

Regev R., Assaraf Y. G. and Eytan G. D., (1999). Membrane Fluidization by Ether, Other Anesthetics, and Certain Agents Abolishes P-glycoprotein ATPase Activity and Modulates Efflux from Multidrug-resistant cells, *Eur. J. Biochem.* 259, 18-24, ISSN 0014-2956

Rivers F., ÓBrien T. J., Callaghan R., (2008). Exploring the Possible Interaction between anti-Epilepsy Drugs and Multidrug Efflux Pumps; in vitro Observations, *European Journal of Pharmacology* No.598, (September, 2008),pp 1–8, ISSN 0014-2999

Seithel A., Eberl S., Singer K., Auge D., Heinkele G., Wolf N. B., Dorje F., Fromm M.F., and Konig J., (2007). The Influence of Macrolide Antibiotics on the Uptake of Organic Anions and Drugs Mediated by OATP1B1 and OATP1B3, *Drug Metabolism and Disposition*, No.35, (May, 2007) pp.779–786, ISSN 0090-9556

Shitara Y., Horie T., Sugiyama Y., (2006). Transporters as a Determinant of Drug Clearance and Tissue Distribution, *European Journal of Pharmaceutical Sciences*, No.27, pp. 425–446, ISSN 0928-0987

Sikri V., Pal D., Jain R., Kalyani D., and Mitra A. K., (2004). Cotransport of Macrolide and Fluoroquinolones, a Beneficial Interaction Reversing P-glycoprotein Efflux, *American Journal of Therapeutics* No. 11, pp.433–442, ISSN 1075-2765

Singhal S.S., Yadav S., Roth C., Singhal J., (2009). RLIP76: A Novel Glutathione-conjugate and Multi-drug Transporter Biochemical Pharmacology, No. 77, pp. 761– 769, ISSN 0006-2952

Tai Y., Hou J. P., Meng J.G., Xu W.W., Wang Q., (2009). Pharmacological Development of Platycodiradix, *Xiandai Zhongyiyao*, No.6, (June, 2009), pp. 74-75, ISSN 1672-0571

Tanihara Y., Masuda S., Sato T., Katsura T., Ogawa O., Inui Ken-ichi, (2007). Substrate Specificity of MATE1 and MATE2-K, Human Multidrug and Toxin Extrusions/H+-Organic Cation Antiporters, *Biochemical Pharmacology*, No.74, pp.359– 371, ISSN 0006-2952

Wang B.J., Liu C.T., Tseng C.Y., Wu C.P., Yu Z.R., (2004). Hepatoprotective and Antioxidant Effects of Bupleurum Kaoi Liu (Chao et Chuang) Extract and Its Fractions Fractionated Using Supercritical CO_2 on CCl_4-induced Liver Damage, *Food and Chemical Toxicology*, No. 42, (November, 2004) , pp. 609–617, ISSN 0278-2915

Wang G. J., Zhang B., Zhang X. S., Zhang E. H., (2010). Effect of Dioscin Co-administration with Borneol on Cerebral Ischemia Induced by MCAO, *Zhongyao Yaoli Yu Linchuang* Vol. 26, No. 5, (October, 2010), pp. 54-55, ISSN 1001-859X

Wang S. X., Miao W. L., Fang M. F., Nan Y. F., Meng X., Yu J., Zheng X. H., (2009). Effect of Borneol on the Tissue Distribution of Notoginseng R1, Ginsenoside Rgl and Re in

Rabbits, *DiSi Junyi Daxue Xuebao, Vol.* 30, No.23, (December, 2009), pp. 2750-2752, ISSN 1000-2790

Wang Y., Zhang Z.Y., Xu F., Wang B.J., Zhang S.Y., (2006). Effects of Borneol on Concentration of Tetramethylpyrazine in Blood and Distribution in Brain of Rat, *Zhongguo Yaoye*, Vol.15, No.1, (January, 2006), pp.30-31, ISSN 1006-4693

Wu J., (2008). Effect of Process on Components and Pharmacological of Radix Bupleurum, *Hubei Zhongyi Zazhi* Vol. 30, No. 9, (September, 2008), pp.60-61, ISSN 1000-0704

Wu S. R., Cheng G., He Y.X., Hao X. H., Wang L., Sun J., (2004). Studies on the Effects of Borneol on the Distribution of Rifampicin in Mice, *Zhongguo Yaoxue Zazhi* , Vol. 39, No.4 (April, 2004), pp. 289-291, ISSN 1001-2494.

Wu Q., (2005). Effect of Meridian Guide Drug on P-gp, *Xiandai Yufang Yixue*, Vol.32, No.7, (July, 2005), pp.855-856, ISSN 1003-8507

Wu S.R., Cheng G.,(2001). Pharmacological Development of Borneol, *Zhong Cao Yao*, Vol.32, No.12, (December, 2001), pp.1143-1145, ISSN 0253-2670

Yang X. F., Wang N. P., Zeng F. D., (2002) Effect of the Active Components of Some Chinese Herbs on Drug Metabolizing- Enzymes, *Zhongguo Zhongyao Zazhi*, Vol. 27, No. 5 (May, 2002), pp. 325-328, ISSN 1001-5302

Yu P.F., WangW. Y., Eerdun G., WangT., Zhang L.M., Li C., and Fu F.H,2011. The Role of P-Glycoprotein in Transport of Danshensu across the Blood-Brain Barrier, *Evidence-Based Complementary and Alternative Medicine* Vol. 2011, Article ID 713523, 5 pages doi:10.1155/2011/713523

Zhao B.S., Liu Q. D, (2002). Difference Between Borneol and Pathological on Blood-Brain Barrier, *Zhongyao Xinyao Yu Linchuang Yaoli*, Vol.13, No. 5, (October, 2002), pp. 287-288, ISSN 1003-9783

Zhao R.Z., Liu S.J, (2005). TCM Tradicinal Guide Theory and Target-tropism Administration, *Zhong Yi Za Zhi*, volume 46, No. 9, (September, 2005), pp. 643-645, ISSN 1001-1668

Zhao R.Z., Liu S.J., Mao S. R., Wang Y.J., (2009). Study on Liver Targeting Effect of Vinegar-baked Radix Bupleuri on Resveratrol in Mice, *Journal of Ethnopharmacology*, No.126, (September, 2009), pp.415-420, ISSN 0378-8741

Zhao R.Z., Yuan D, Liu S.J., Chen YJ., Liu L.J. Zhao Y. (2010). Liver Targeting Effect of Vinegar-baked Radix Bupleuri on Rhein in Rats, *Journal of Ethnopharmacology*, No. 132, (October, 2010), pp. 421-428, ISSN 0378-8741

Zheng C., Xiang H. S., Li Y. B., Zhao B. B., Yang Z. X., Xu S.G., Pu J.X., (2008). Effect of Borneol on the Distribution of Gastrodin to the Brain in Mice via Oral Administration, *Journal of Drug Targeting*, Vol.16, No.2, (February, 2008), pp178-184, ISSN 1061-186X

Zhou H. Y., Chen X. Y., Huang C. K., Jiang W. G., Hu G. X.. (2008), Effect of Borneol on Distribution of Carbamazepine in Mice, *Wenzhou Yixueyuan Xuebao*, Vol.38, No.4, (July, 2008), pp.300-305, ISSN 1000-2138

Zhou Q.L., Zhang Z.Q., Nagasawa T., and Hiai S., (1996). The Structure Activity Relationship of Saikosaponins and Glycyrrhizin Derivatives for Na+, K+ ATPase Inhibiting Action, *Yaoxue Xuebao*, Vol.31, No.7, (July, 1996), pp 496-501, ISSN 0253-3707

Zhu R.X., Hu L.W., Li H.Y., Su J.,Cao Z.W., and Zhang W.D.,(2011) Novel Natural Inhibitors of CYP1A2 Identified by *in Silico* and *in Vitro* Screening, *Int J Mol. Sci.* Vol. 12, No.5, (May, 2011), pp.3250–3262, doi: 10.3390/ijms12053250, ISSN 2306-2321

6

Knowledge-Based Discovery of Anti-Fibrotic and Pro-Fibrotic Activities from Chinese Materia Medica

Qihe Xu et al.[*]
King's College London, Department of Renal Medicine,
The Rayne Institute, London,
United Kingdom

1. Introduction

Fibrosis, also known as scarring, sclerosis or cirrhosis, is characterised by excessive accumulation of extracellular matrix (ECM) proteins leading to tissue contraction, disruption of tissue architecture and eventually chronic organ failure (Wynn, 2007; Xu et al., 2007). Research and development of anti-fibrotic drugs are generally based on two distinct but interactive strategies, with one based on mechanism studies and another based on exploring efficacy. In principle, the mechanism-based strategy begins with identification of molecular targets through mechanistic studies, and then development of inhibitors or enhancers targeting the molecules. On the other hand, efficacy-based strategy starts with screening drug candidates in disease models to identify activities and efficacy, with less reliance on analysis of mechanisms of action. There are certain limitations in both the mechanism-based strategy and the efficacy-based strategy, which largely account for the lack of success in development of anti-fibrotic drugs. The former is often associated with identification of multiple molecular targets impeding development of a single drug that tackles multiple targets, while the latter is often hampered by establishment of apt models ideal for efficacy-driven drug screens.

Efficacy-based strategy has been employed in development of both traditional and modern medicines. In the context of traditional medicine, the knowledge about efficacy of a given drug is largely derived from a trial-and-error process, namely by assessing patients' response upon treatment with natural drug candidates. However, in modern medicine, it is impossible to directly test any new drugs in patients. Solid scientific evidence on efficacy and safety of a given drug in experimental models is required prior to clinical trials. Understandably, quality of these models would determine the specificity and efficiency of the tested drug.

---

[*] Yuen Fei Wong[1], Shanshan Qu[1], Qingyang Kong[1], Xiu-Li Zhang[2], Xin-Miao Liang[2], Qin Hu[1], Mazhar Noor[1] and Bruce M. Hendry[1],
[1]*King's College London, Department of Renal Medicine, The Rayne Institute, London, United Kingdom*
[2]*Multi-Component TCM Group, Dalian Institute of Chemical Physics,*
Chinese Academy of Sciences, Dalian PR China

In vivo models are invaluable research tools but not without its limitation, especially in the development of drugs targeting fibrosis given the complex aetiologies and inflammatory processes involved in this pathological condition. In particular, drug leads displaying effectiveness in *in vivo* models of fibrosis may stem from (i) inhibition of the primary aetiological factors, (ii) inhibition of inflammation, a common inciting factor of fibrosis, (iii) inhibition of fibrosis *per se*, or (iv) a net effect of any combinations of the aforementioned. For the initial development of drugs with specific anti-fibrotic effects independent of anti-inflammatory actions and any specific aetiological factors, *in vitro* models of fibrosis appear to be more appropriate. Our laboratory recently reported transforming growth factor-β1 (TGF-β1)-induced inflammation-free *in vitro* models of fibrosis in mesenchymal cells, featuring 2-dimentional (2D) ECM protein accumulation reflecting net collagen accumulation, and 3-dimentional (3D) nodular formation following ECM protein-induced disruption of cell monolayer, which can both be objectively quantified. By coating specific matrix on 96-well plates, which determines the 2D or 3D nature of the models, we are able to quantify readouts more reliably, permitting high-throughput screening of compounds with anti-fibrotic activities (Xu et al., 2007).

In contrast to the lack of "anti-fibrotics" in Western medicine clinics, there is accumulating evidence suggesting anti-fibrotic effects of Chinese materia medicas (CMMs), i.e., medicinal materials used in traditional Chinese medicine (TCM) (Hu et al., 2007). However, most of these conclusions were drawn from animal models or patients and hence it was not clear whether the reported efficacy of those CMMs was secondary to inhibition of aetiological factors or inflammation, or whether they exerted genuine anti-fibrotic activities (Hu et al., 2009). We hypothesised that at least some of the "anti-fibrotic" herbal derivatives reported in the literature are indeed anti-fibrotic by antagonising TGF-β1-specific pro-fibrotic pathways or common pathways of fibrosis. By employing the 2D *in vitro* model (Xu et al., 2007), we tested the anti-fibrotic activity of 21 CMM-derived compounds, 11 methanolic extracts of single CMMs and 27 formulae that contained two or more CMMs as mixtures, and found that five compounds, three single CMM extracts and 16 formulae had *in vitro* anti-fibrotic activities (Hu et al., 2009). Among the five CMM-derived compounds, three flavonoids (quercetin, baicalin and baicalein) showed similar dose-dependent *in vitro* anti-fibrotic activities while two non-flavonoids (salvianolic acid B and emodin) showed varied *in vitro* anti-fibrotic activities with poor dose dependency. Among the three CMM extracts showing significant *in vitro* anti-fibrotic activities, Huangqin (root of *Scutellaria baicalensis* Georgi) is rich in baicalin and baicalein, Danshen (root of *Salvia miltiorrhiza* Bunge) is rich in salvianolic acid B and Dahuang (root of *Rheum palmatum* L.) is rich in emodin. Among the 16 herbal formulae with *in vitro* anti-fibrotic effects, eight contained neither Huangqin, Danshen nor Dahuang, while the remaining eight contained at least one of the three CMMs (Hu et al., 2009).

Following successful identification of *in vitro* anti-fibrotic activities in herbal entities, we have extended our work to focus on TCM knowledge-based discovery of novel anti-fibrotic drug leads from natural sources, especially CMMs. In TCM, fibrosis is diagnosed as a kind of "Jie Zheng" which means "lump or clot". Based on this concept, two senior TCM practitioners were invited to choose a collection of 27 CMMs, including 26 medicinal plant parts and one medicinal fungus, which they would consider using in patients with fibrotic diseases. Based on the traditional categories of CMMs, the 27 CMMs fall into three functional subgroups, namely "Huo Xue Hua Yu" ("promoting the circulation and resolving the clot"), "Hua Tan" ("resolving the sputum") and "Bu Xu" ("tonifying the deficiency"), where "clot" and "sputum" in TCM do not mean the same as the terms in Western medicine. In addition to the 27 CMMs, Chuanwutou, an unprocessed herb with well-known toxic effects, was also tested to serve as a control for cytotoxic effects, if any. In fact, owing to its strong "Qu Feng Shi" ("dispelling the wind and damp" or anti-rheumatic function) property, Chuanwutou is rather commonly prescribed to patients with diseases complicated by fibrosis, although only processed Chuanwutou is allowed for clinical use.

The aim of this project was to examine the *in vitro* anti-fibrotic and pro-fibrotic activities of these 28 CMMs (Table 1) and herein we report that eight CMMs (Baibeiyegen, Liedang, Gusuibu, Jixueteng, Lingzhi, Meiguiqie, Moyao and Shiliuhua) have *in vitro* anti-fibrotic activities while three (Chuanwutou, Dangshen and Yimucao) have pro-fibrotic activities.

2. Materials and methods

2.1 CMMs and extraction methods

Liedang was authenticated according to the criteria described in *Jilin Zhongcaoyao* (Changchun TCM College Revolutionary Committee (Ed.), (June 1970), *Jilin Chinese Herbal Medicine,* Jilin People's Press, Changchun, China) and all other CMMs were authenticated according to Chinese Pharmacopeia (2005 Edition). Voucher specimens were deposited at Dalian Institute of Chemical Physics, Chinese Academy of Sciences, Dalian, China. Individual CMM was grounded into fine powder, from which 85 g was precisely weighed out and added to 600 ml of 80% ethanol. The mixtures were boiled for 2 h and filtrated, after which the residual ethanol was evaporated. Ethanolic extracts were then concentrated and dried in an oven, and were stored at room temperature before use. For experimental purpose, ethanolic extracts were reconstituted in dimethyl sulfoxide (DMSO, Sigma-Aldrich Company Ltd., Dorset, UK) and were stored in freezer at -20 °C until use.

2.2 TGF-β1, Alk5 inhibitor and PPAR antagonists

Human TGF-β1 in lyophilised powder form (R&D Systems Europe Ltd., Abingdon, UK) was reconstituted in filter-sterilised buffer consisting of 1 mg/ml bovine serum albumin in 4 mM HCl, to a final concentration of 10 μg/ml and kept frozen at -80 °C before experiments. IN-1130, a selective inhibitor of TGF-β type I receptor (Alk5), was a kind gift from Dr Dae Kee Kim, Ewha Women's University, Korea, and was used as a positive control for *in vitro* anti-fibrotic activity (Moon et al., 2006). Peroxisome proliferator-activated receptor (PPAR) antagonists, including PPARα antagonist GW6471 (Xu et al., 2002), PPARβ/δ antagonist GSK0660 (Shearer et al., 2008) and PPARγ antagonist T0070907 (Lee et al., 2002) were purchased from Sigma-Aldrich.

2.3 Cell culture, TGF-β1-induced *in vitro* models of fibrosis and related assays

A normal rat kidney fibroblast cell line (NRK-49F) was purchased from European Collection of Cell Cultures (ECACC, Health Protection Agency, Salisbury, UK). The cells were maintained in Dulbecco's Modified Eagle Medium (DMEM, PAA Laboratories Ltd., Somerset, UK) supplemented with 100 U/ml of penicillin G (PAA), 100 μg/ml of streptomycin (PAA), 0.25 μg/ml of amphotericin B (Invitrogen Ltd., Paisley, UK) and 5% foetal calf serum (FCS, Sigma-Aldrich), in Falcon tissue culture flasks (Marathon Laboratory supplies, London, UK), and incubated at 37 °C and 5% CO_2. During routine maintenance,

Functional group	Pinyin name	Part, Latin name and authority	Authenticator	Extraction yield (%)	Voucher number
"Bu Xu"	Baibeiyegen	Dried roots of *Mallotus apelta* (Lour.) Muell.-Arg.	SJS*	21	B012081
	Liedang	Dried whole plants of *Orobanche coerulescens* Steph.	SJS	28.5	C013081
	Dangshen	Dried roots of *Codonopsis pilosula* (Franch.) Nannf.	SJS	58.7	D001081
	Gancao	Dried roots and rhizomes of *Glycyrrhiza uralensis* Fisch.	SJS	81.7	G010081
	Roucongrong	Dried fleshy stem with scales of *Cistanche deserticola* Y. C. Ma	SJS	82.2	R002081
	Yinyanghuo	Dried rootless plants of *Epimedium brevicornum* Maxim.	SJS	42.1	Y006081
"Bu Xu" & "Hua Tan"	Lingzhi	Dried mushroom of *Ganoderma lucidum* (Leyss. Ex Fr.) Karst.	SJS	8.33	L003081
"Hua Tan"	Baiguo	Dried ripe seeds of *Ginkgo biloba* L.	HXR**	7.9	B013041
	Jiegeng	Dried roots of *Platycodon grandiflorum (Jacq.)* A. DC.	SJS	12.3	J009081
	Meiguiqie	Dried flowers of *Hibiseus sabdariffa* L.	SJS	37.6	M004081
	Tiannanxing	Dried tuberous roots of *Arisaema erubescens* (Wall.) Schott.	SJS	2.34	T001081
"Hua Tan" and "Huo Xue Hua Yu"	Yinxingye	Dried leaves of *Ginkgo bilobla* L.	SJS	65	Y009081
"Huo Xue Hua Yu" & "Qing Re Jie Du"***	Baihuasheshecao	Dried plants of *Oldenlandia diffusa* (Willd.) Roxb.	HXR	18	B010041
"Huo Xue Hua Yu"	Ezhu	Dried rhizomes of *Curcuma kwangsiensis* S. G. Lee et C. F. Liang	HXR	60.1	E001041
	Gusuibu	Dried rhizomes of *Drynaria fortunei* (Kunze) J. Sm.	SJS	27	G007081
	Jixueteng	Dried stem of *Spatholobus suberectus* Dunn	SJS	33.9	J001081
	Maqianzi	Dried ripe seeds of *Strychnos nux-vomica* L.	SJS	7.7	M003081
	Moyao	Dried resin of *Commiphora myrrha* Engl.	SJS	33.7	M002081
	Niuxi	Dried roots of *Achyranthes bidentata* Bl.	SJS	9.9	N002081

Functional group	Pinyin name	Part, Latin name and authority	Authenticator	Extraction yield (%)	Voucher number
	Ruxiang	Dried oleogum resin of *Boswellia carterii* Birdw.	SJS	60.6	R001081
	Sanleng	Dried tuberous roots of *Sparganium stoloniferum* Buch.–Ham.	SJS	25.1	S003081
	Sheputaogen	Dried roots of *Ampelopsis (Miq.)* W. T. Wang	SJS	14	S011081
	Shiliuhua	Dried flowers of *Punica granatum* L.	SJS	88	S012081
	Taoren	Dried ripe seeds of *Prunus persica (L.)* Batsch.	SJS	35.6	T004081
	Yanhusuo	Dried tuberous roots of *Corydalis yanhusuo* W. T. Wang	HXR	69.5	Y010041
	Yimucao	Dried rootless plants of *Leonurus japonicus* Houtt.	SJS	12.8	Y005081
	Zhenzhumei	Dried bark of the stems of *Sorbaria sorbifolia (L.)* A. Brown.	SJS	33.1	Z004081
"Qu Feng Shi"	Chuanwutou	Dried main roots of *Aconitum carmichaeli* Debx.	SJS	18.2	C005081

Table 1. Functional groups, species names and parts, authenticators, extraction yield and voucher numbers of the 28 test materials. * SJS: Shi Jian Sa, Tong De Chinese Materia Medica Co. Ltd., Anguo, Hebei, China; ** HXR: He Xi Rong, Institute of Chinese Materia Medica, China Academy of Chinese Medical Sciences, Beijing, China; *** "Qing Re Jie Du" means "clearing heat and detoxifying".

NRK-49F cells were sub-cultured before they became confluent to prevent transformation. The 2D model was employed for experiments in this project. Cells were seeded in collagen type I-coated 96-well plates (BD Biosciences, Oxford, UK) at a density of 1×10^4 cells per well in 200 µl DMEM supplemented with 2.5% FCS and 2.5% Nu-Serum™ V serum replacements (NU, BD Biosciences). After three days, the medium was changed to serum-free DMEM supplemented with 1% insulin-transferrin-selenium liquid media supplement (ITS, Sigma-Aldrich) for four days, and then changed to fresh ITS-supplemented serum-free medium containing 5 ng/ml TGF-β1 in the presence of different concentrations of herbal extracts or a vehicle control (an equal volume of DMSO) for 48 h. In all the experiments, 1 µM IN-1130 was used as a positive control for anti-fibrotic activities. For initial screening, the concentrations of CMM extracts tested were 10, 20, 40, 80, 160 and 200 µg/ml, 3-6 wells per group, and the screening was repeated at least twice. For follow-up confirmation studies, four herbal extracts were selected based on the results from initial screening studies, and their effects were further confirmed using three different concentrations, 3-6 wells per group. Each follow-up experiment was performed four times.

2.4 Cell detachment index (CDI) and lactate dehydrogenase (LDH) release assay

For the screening studies, *in vitro* cytotoxicity at the end of 48 h treatment was assessed by phase-contrast microscopy using the same CDI criteria that we reported before (Hu et al.,

2009). In brief, CDI reflects cell monolayer disruption, including cell detachment from the adherent surface and disorganisation of cell monolayer. Scores of 0, 0.5, 1, 1.5, 2, 2.5, 3, 3.5 and 4 represented an area of 0, 5%, 10%, 20%, 30%, 40%, 60%, 80% and 100%, respectively, of the total adherent surface not covered by cells. This method was used to approximate cytotoxicity, as well as to ensure the reliability of subsequent picro-Sirius red (PSR) staining results, which required minimum cell (and matrix) detachment and disruption of cell monolayer. For follow-up studies, LDH release assay was used to assess *in vitro* cytotoxicity at the end of 48 h treatment. Fifty microlitre of supernatant from each well was collected and tested for LDH release according to the manufacturer's instructions (Promega, Southampton, UK). LDH release was measured using a Dynex Technologies MRX spectrophotometer (Prior Laboratory Supplies Ltd., East Sussex, UK), at optical density (OD) value of 490 nm.

2.5 Microscopic examination
Microscopic examination was performed on a Nikon Eclipse TE2000-S microscope (Nikon Instruments Europe B.V., The Netherlands). Bright-field and phase-contrast images were captured with a DXM1200F Nikon digital camera (Nikon UK Limited, Surrey, UK) and processed with Adobe Photoshop (Adobe System Europe Ltd., London, UK).

2.6 PSR staining and spectrophotometric analysis
Total collagen accumulation was assessed qualitatively by microscopic examination of PSR-stained cells and quantitatively by spectrophotometric analysis of PSR staining. After CDI determination and conditioned medium collected for LDH release assay, cell monolayer in 96-well plates were fixed in ice-cold methanol (200 µl per well) overnight at –20 °C. Cells were carefully washed twice (5 min each) with 1x phosphate buffered saline (PBS, 200 µl per well) and then stained with 0.1% w/v PSR solution (200 µl per well, Sigma-Aldrich) at room temperature for 4–6 h. The staining solution was then removed and excessive PSR stain was carefully washed off with 0.1% v/v acetic acid (200 µl per well, VWR International Ltd, Lutterworth, UK) three times (5 min each). The stained wells were left to air dried for 24–48 h. PSR stain was then observed under bright-field microscopy and microscopic pictures were taken. Finally, PSR stain was eluted in 0.1 N NaOH (200 µl per well) on a rocking platform at room temperature for 1 h. The plate was then subjected to spectrophotometric analysis of OD at 540 nm on a Dynex Technologies MRX spectrophotometer (Hu et al., 2009).

2.7 PPARα, PPARβ/δ and PPARγ agonistic activities of Shiliuhua extract and effect of Shiliuhua extract in the presence of PPAR antagonists
We commissioned Tebu-bio Laboratories, Le Perray en Yvelines, France, to perform a pilot test on Shiliuhua extract for its isotype-specific PPAR activation. In brief, the assay was carried out *in vitro* in three HeLa cell lines stably expressing a chimeric protein containing the yeast transactivator GAL4 DNA binding domain fused to ligand binding domain regions of human PPARα, PPARβ/δ or PPARγ, and a luciferase reporter gene driven by a pentamer of the GAL4 recognition sequence in front of the β-globin promoter (Seimandi et al., 2005). The PPAR reporter cell lines were seeded in a 96-well plate in triplicates, and treated with 40 µg/ml Shiliuhua extract, or an equal volume of DMSO as negative control, for 24 h. Luciferase activity was determined with a luminometer and relative light units (RLU) were recorded. Three independent experiments were performed and the fold changes of RLU were normalised to the mean of negative control.

The effect of PPAR antagonism on Shiliuhua extract treatment was assessed following the protocol as described in sections 2.3-2.6. Cells were treated with 40 μg/ml Shiliuhua extract with and without PPARα antagonist, GW6471 (0.01-10 μM), PPARβ/δ antagonist, GSK0660 (0.001-1 μM), or PPARγ antagonist, T0070907 (0.1-25 μM). Three independent biological experiments were performed, 3-6 wells per group.

2.8 Statistical analysis
Results of PSR and LDH OD values were expressed as mean ± SEM unless stated otherwise. Statistical differences were computed with Prism 4.0 (GraphPad Software, San Diego, CA, USA), by one-way analysis of variance and Dunnett post test for comparison between a control group and all other groups; for PPAR reporter activity, one-tail paired t test was performed on log-transformed fold changes. $p < 0.05$ was regarded as statistically significant.

3. Results

3.1 Initial screening
The screening results of CMM extracts were summarised in Table 2. Anti-fibrotic and pro-fibrotic effects were defined as PSR OD values significantly lower and higher than that of TGF-β1-treated group, respectively; cytotoxicity was defined as CDI significantly higher than that of TGF-β1-treated group. Doses at which extracts exhibited reproducible effects were indicated in the table. The CMMs were categorised into four groups, i.e., eight in Group A showed *in vitro* anti-fibrotic activities; three in Group B showed pro-fibrotic activities; six in Group C showed prominent cytotoxicity; 11 in Group D did not have profound effects on total collagen accumulation nor integrity of cell monolayer. In Group A, Liedang, Meiguiqie and Gusuibu extracts were well-tolerated agents with anti-fibrotic activities noted within the range of 80-200 μg/ml; extracts of Shiliuhua, Baibeiyegen, Jixueteng, Moyao and Lingzhi showed anti-fibrotic effects at concentrations ranging from 10–80 μg/ml, beyond which cytotoxicity was noted. In Group B, Chuanwutou showed a pro-fibrotic effect at concentrations as low as 20 μg/ml whereas pro-fibrotic effect of Dangshen and Yimucao were observed only at higher concentrations (160–200 μg/ml).

3.2 Follow-up studies
Based on the initial screening results, Shiliuhua (SLH), Liedang (LD), Meiguiqie (MGQ) and Chuanwutou (CWT) extracts were selected for follow-up studies in view of their minimum CDI changes indicating low cytotoxicity, and the results are shown in Fig. 1. In contrast to SLH, LD and MGQ extracts, which showed varying degrees of *in vitro* anti-fibrotic effects, CWT extract exhibited a marked pro-fibrotic effect. Representative effects of SLH, LD, MGQ and CWT extracts on PSR staining, relative PSR OD values and LDH release are shown in Fig. 2 and Fig. 3.

3.3 Activation of PPARs by SLH extract
As SLH extract is one of the CMM extracts with the most potent *in vitro* anti-fibrotic activity and it was previously reported to interfere with the PPAR signalling pathway (Li et al., 2008), we hypothesised that the anti-fibrotic effect of SLH extract was at least in part mediated by activation of one or more PPAR receptors. Indeed, SLH extract induced PPARα- and PPARγ-mediated reporter activity; it also marginally activates PPARβ/δ but the induction of reporter activity was just above the threshold of significance ($p=0.066$) (Fig. 4a). In order to

determine if the agonistic effect of SLH extract has an impact on TGF-β1-induced fibrogenesis, cells were treated with SLH extract and individual PPAR antagonists. PPARβ/δ antagonist, GSK0660 (IC$_{50}$ 160 nM) (Shearer et al., 2008), did not affect the anti-fibrotic activity of SLH extract at all concentrations tested (up to 6.25-fold higher than its IC$_{50}$); PPARα antagonist, GW6471 (IC$_{50}$ 240 nM) (Xu et al., 2002), also did not show any significant effect at concentrations up to 4.2-fold of its IC$_{50}$, but at 10 μM (42-fold higher than its IC$_{50}$), it did moderately suppress the anti-fibrotic activity of SLH extract; PPARγ antagonist, T0070907 (IC$_{50}$ 1 nM in inhibiting rosiglitazone binding to PPARγ and 3.2-24.3 μM in inhibiting proliferation of different cancer cell lines) (Lee et al., 2002; Burton et al., 2007), did not show any significant effect at concentrations of 0.1, 1 and 10 μM, but further increased the anti-fibrotic effect of SLH extract at 25 μM (Fig. 4b).

Group	Pinyin name	Anti-fibrotic or pro-fibrotic doses (μg/ml)	Changes at optimum doses compared to TGF-β1 treated group	Cytotoxic doses (μg/ml)
A. Anti-fibrotic	Baibeiyegen	20-40	-81.4% (40 μg/ml) -63.3% (20 μg/ml)	≥80
	Liedang	80-160	-61.2% (160 μg/ml) -59.3% (80 μg/ml)	200
	Gusuibu	160-200	-36.8% (200 μg/ml) -30.0% (160 μg/ml)	–
	Jixueteng	10-40	-75.0% (20 μg/ml) -63.0% (10 μg/ml)	≥80
	Lingzhi	10-80	-34.9% (80 μg/ml) -47.4% (40 μg/ml)	≥160
	Meiguiqie	160-200	-28.0% (200 μg/ml) -21.0% (160 μg/ml)	–
	Moyao	10-40	-57.2% (40 μg/ml) -67.9% (20 μg/ml)	≥80
	Shiliuhua	10-40	-78.0% (40 μg/ml) -61.2% (20 μg/ml)	≥80
B. Pro-fibrotic	Chuanwutou	≥20	+90.2% (40 μg/ml) +68.5% (20 μg/ml)	–
	Dangshen	200	+32.4% (200 μg/ml)	–
	Yimucao	160-200	+65.7% (200 μg/ml) +53.9% (160 μg/ml)	–
C. Cytotoxic	Baihuasheshecao (≥80 μg/ml), Ruxiang (≥10 μg/ml), Sheputaogen (≥80 μg/ml), Tiannanxing (≥80 μg/ml), Yinxingye (≥20 μg/ml), Zhenzhumei (≥40 μg/ml).			
D. Inert	Baiguo, Ezhu, Gancao, Jiegeng, Maqianzi, Niuxi, Roucongrong, Sanleng, Taoren, Yanhusuo, Yinyanghuo.			

Table 2. Initial screening results of CMMs in TGF-β1-induced *in vitro* fibrogenesis. Minus (-) and plus (+) percentages represent relative reduction and increase in TGF-β1-induced PSR OD values, respectively. " – ": Cytotoxicity, assessed from CDI, was not significantly different from TGF-β1-treated group at all concentrations tested (10-200 μg/ml).

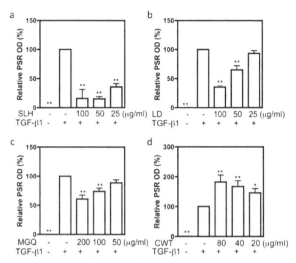

Fig. 1. *In vitro* anti-fibrotic and pro-fibrotic effects of four selected extracts, Shiliuhua (SLH) (a), Liedang (LD) (b), Meiguiqie (MGQ) (c) and Chuanwutou (CWT) (d) at three selected concentrations. Shown here are relative PSR OD changes of four independent experiments. The CDI changes were minimum and not shown. The average PSR OD values of negative control group and TGF-β1-treated group were normalised to 0 and 100%, respectively, and changes in percentage of herbal extract-treated groups were relative to the TGF-β1 only group. *, **: p<0.05 and p<0.01 vs TGF-β1 only group.

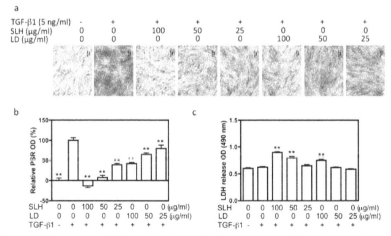

Fig. 2. Effects of Shiliuhua (SLH) and Liedang (LD) extracts on PSR staining (a), relative PSR OD values (b) and LDH release (c). Results in (b) and (c) shown here are in Mean ± SEM from one representative experiment, ** p<0.01 vs TGF-β1 only group, n=6 wells. The average PSR OD values of negative control group and TGF-β1 only group were normalised to 0 and 100%, respectively, and changes in percentage of herbal extract-treated groups were relative to the TGF-β1 only group.

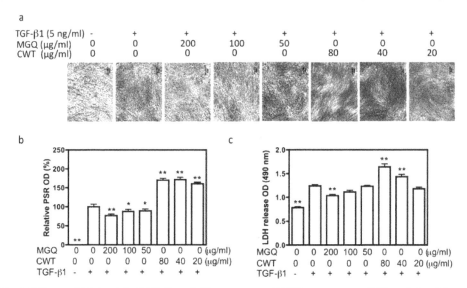

Fig. 3. Effects of Meiguiqie (MGQ) and Chuanwutou (CWT) extracts on PSR staining (a), relative PSR OD values (b) and LDH release (c). Results in (b) and (c) shown here are in Mean ± SEM from one representative experiment, *, ** $p<0.05$, $p<0.01$ vs TGF-β1 only group, n=6 wells. The average PSR OD values of negative control group and TGF-β1 only group were normalised to 0 and 100%, respectively, and changes in percentage of herbal extract-treated groups were relative to the TGF-β1 only group.

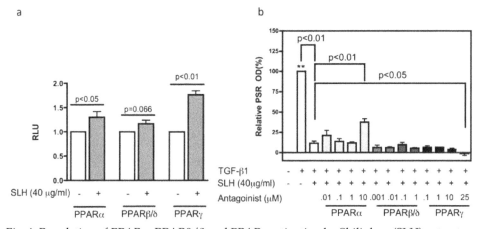

Fig. 4. Regulation of PPARα, PPARβ/δ and PPARγ activation by Shiliuhua (SLH) extract and effects of PPARα, PPARβ/δ and PPARγ antagonists on the anti-fibrotic effect of SLH extract. a. Effects of SLH extract on PPARα, PPARβ/δ and PPARγ activation, n=3 independent biological experiments; b. effects of increasing doses of PPARα, PPARβ/δ and PPARγ antagonists on the anti-fibrotic effect of SLH extract. ** $p<0.01$ vs control group, n=3 independent biological experiments. Other statistical results are as indicated in the figures.

4. Discussion

4.1 Knowledge-based discovery of anti-fibrotic activities from CMMs

Further to the evidence-based approach that we used in our earlier screens (Hu et al., 2009), in which we selected CMMs that had been reported to reduce fibrotic lesions *in vivo*, we used a knowledge-based approach in this study, namely, to screen candidate CMMs that were believed to be beneficial in treating fibrotic diseases based on the theory and practice of TCM. Of the 28 CMM extracts examined, eight (28.5%) showed reproducible *in vitro* anti-fibrotic activities, *i.e.*, Baibeiyegen, Liedang, Gusuibu, Jixueteng, Lingzhi, Meiguiqie, Moyao and Shiliuhua. Identification of these CMMs with anti-fibrotic activities *in vitro* underscores their inflammation-independent activities to inhibit TGF-β1-induced total collagen accumulation, perhaps through inhibiting TGF-β1-specific signalling or common pathways of fibrogenesis.

Among the eight CMM extracts with anti-fibrotic activities, Baibeiyegen (Zhao et al., 2002), Lingzhi (Lin et al., 2006; Wang et al., 2009; Wu et al., 2010), Meiguiqie (Liu et al., 2006), Moyao (Massoud et al., 2004) and Shiliuhua (Huang et al., 2005) have been reported anti-fibrotic in animal models of liver fibrosis or in hepatic stellate cells; Gusuibu was one of the weakest and its effect on fibrosis has never been previously reported either *in vivo* or *in vitro*; Liedang has not been reported on its effect on fibrosis either, but the ethanolic extract of its closely related family member *Boschniakia rossica* (Cham. & Schltdl.) B. Fedtsch. has been reported to mitigate liver fibrosis in a rat model of dimethylnitrosamine-induced liver fibrosis (Piao et al., 2005); Jixueteng is used in some herbal formulae, such as Huangqijixuetengtang (Li et al., 2006; Li et al., 2007) and Herbal Compound 861 (also known as Fufangdanshenheji) (Wang 2000; Wang et al., 2008), which were reported to be anti-fibrotic in patients and *in vitro*, but has never been reported as an individual anti-fibrotic herb.

Although only a quarter of the selected CMMs showed anti-fibrotic activities in our model, we do not exclude the possibilities that some of these CMMs might have a favourable effect in treating fibrotic diseases by interfering with other factors *e.g.* inflammation, TGF-β1 production and activation, molecules upstream of TGF-β1 signalling and TGF-β1-independent pro-fibrotic signalling pathways. Of note, CMMs which were identified as cytotoxic in the NRK-49F renal fibroblast model might be of therapeutic value in fibrotic diseases since loss of fibroblasts, the main producers of pathological matrices, may result in reduced ECM accumulation hence promoting regression of fibrosis. It is also worth reiterating that the results presented here were derived from extracts of CMMs in boiling 80% ethanol. Different extraction methods, including extraction solutions and efficiency, might have different impact on *in vitro* activities of the materials. Nevertheless, it would be of particular interest to isolate compounds contained in the eight ethanolic CMM extracts with *in vitro* anti-fibrotic activities, and further test individual compounds for their *in vitro* anti-fibrotic activities.

4.2 *In vitro* anti-fibrotic activities and TCM categorisation of the CMMs

CMMs are traditionally characterised based on their function, nature, taste and channel tropism. By focusing on functional groups of the selected CMMs, we found that four out of 15 (27%) CMMs of "Huo Xue Hua Yu" group, two out of six (33%) CMMs of "Hua Tan" group and three out of seven (43%) CMMs of "Bu Xu" group, had *in vitro* anti-fibrotic activities. In view that "Hua Tan" and "Bu Xu"groups had rarely been the focus of previous evidence-based studies of anti-fibrotic CMMs, we consider our findings significant in guiding future studies of anti-fibrotic herbal medicines and in selecting therapeutic options in the clinic. However, due to the small sample numbers involved in this study, we do not intend to conclude that CMMs of certain functional groups have a higher chance of being anti-fibrotic than another. For example, results of Danshen, a drug in the "Huo Xue Hua Yu" group, was excluded from this project as it has been tested and reported elsewhere (Hu et al., 2009). In fact, Danshen is the most used herb in the 16 herbal formulae that showed *in vitro* anti-fibrotic activities (Hu et al., 2009). On the other hand, our results do not negate the fact that other functional groups of CMMs may possess anti-fibrotic activities. For example, Dahuang (root of *Rheum palmatum* L.) and Huangqin (root of *Scutellaria baicalensis* Georgi), both not in these three functional groups, had been previously reported to be anti-fibrotic and their activities had been confirmed in our earlier studies (Hu et al., 2009).

4.3 Shiliuhua and PPAR

In this study, Shiliuhua extract was one of the most potent CMMs in reducing TGF-β1-induced matrix accumulation. Extracts of Shiliuhua had been previously reported to activate PPARα and induce PPARγ expression. We found that ethanolic extract of Shiliuhua significantly activated both PPARα and PPARγ, which might account for its anti-fibrotic activity since agonists of PPARα (Toyama et al., 2004; Iglarz et al., 2003) and PPARγ (Milam et al., 2008; Kawai et al., 2008; Iglarz et al., 2003) were previously reported to suppress fibrosis of liver, lung, heart and kidney. Contrary to our hypothesis, we found that the anti-fibrotic activities of Shiliuhua extract can only be partially blocked by GW6471, a PPARα antagonist, at a dose 42-fold of its reported IC_{50}. Since the dose of PPAR antagonists were selected based on their IC_{50} reported in other cell types, it is possible that the doses we employed were sub-optimal in blocking PPARs in NRK-49F renal fibroblast cells. More interestingly, T0070907, a PPARγ antagonist, further increased the anti-fibrotic effect of shiliuhua extract when used at high dose (25 μM). Thus, it appears that Shiliuhua extract can activate both PPARα and PPARγ, but this property could not explain the anti-fibrotic activity of Shiliuhua in full. Further studies are required to elucidate the involvement of PPAR signalling pathway in anti-fibrotic activities of shiliuhua, for example to establish if these two PPAR isotypes have opposing functions in regulating fibrogenesis in renal fibroblasts in view that they did have opposing effects on monocyte chemotaxis in endometriosis (Hornung et al., 2001).

4.4 *In vitro* pro-fibrotic activities observed in this project

The *in vitro* pro-fibrotic activities of Chuanwutou, Dangshen and Yimucao deserve special attention. It rationalises pharmacovigilant studies to establish clinical relevance of these effects. Before clinical conclusions are drawn, it might be wise to avoid un-necessary, large-dose and long-term use of these herbs, especially in patients prone to fibrotic diseases. This issue is important because Dangshen and Yimucao are commonly used in formulae for fibrotic diseases (Yao et al., 2003) and Chuanwutou is indicated for conditions such as osteoarthritis, muscular diseases and stroke that often are complicated by fibrosis as well. As CMMs are rarely used individually, it is important to explore if their pro-fibrotic activities could be antagonised or eliminated when used in formulae. Of note, Yimucao had been reported in animal models to induce nephrotoxicity, including renal fibrosis, but its toxicity was reduced when used in formulae (Sun et al., 2005a, 2005b).

Among the three pro-fibrotic herbs, Chuanwutou appeared to be the most potent. Chuanwutou has well-known toxic effects that are believed to be reduced through a special processing procedure known as "Paozhi" (Chan et al., 1994; Singhuber et al., 2009), but as far as we know, this is the first report linking Chuanwutou to potent pro-fibrotic activities. The Chuanwutou we examined in this project was a raw material that had not undergone any "Paozhi" before ethanolic extraction. It is important to establish if the potent pro-fibrotic effect of this toxic herb could be reduced or even eliminated through traditional "Paozhi" and if this newly identified adverse effect contributes to any known clinical toxicity and adverse effects, in view that only processed Chuanwutou is allowed to be used in TCM practice according to the Chinese Pharmacopeia.

Interestingly, while extract of Dangshen, the root of *Codonopsis pilosula* (Franch.) Nannf. was found pro-fibrotic in this study, pollen of the same plant had been previously reported to be effective in preventing carbon tetrachloride-induced liver damage including fibrosis (Xiao et al., 1989). Furthermore, Fuzi, the daughter roots of the same plant as Chuanwutou, is a CMM categorised into a different functional group. We examined Fuzi in our *in vitro* model but it did not show any pro-fibrotic, anti-fibrotic or apparent cytotoxicity (data not shown). Thus, different parts of the same plant might have different and even opposite effects in regulating fibrogenesis.

5. Conclusion

Among the 28 herbal and fungal materials tested, eight showed *in vitro* anti-fibrotic activities while another three, especially Chuanwutou, showed pro-fibrotic activities. These results warrant further prudent investigations of their potential translation into clinical efficacy and their adverse effects.

6. Acknowledgements

We thank Ms. Dan Jiang (Acu-herb Clinic Sheffield, Sheffield, UK) and Professor Dunxu Wu (Shanghai University of Traditional Chinese Medicine) for recommending CMMs screened in this project. We are grateful to Dr Dae Kee Kim (Ewha Women's University Korea) for his kind gift of IN-1130, a selective inhibitor of TGF-β type I receptor (Alk5). The project was funded by Innovation China UK, Kidney Research UK, as well as European Union's Framework Programme 7 Coordination Action grant, Good Practice in Traditional Chinese Medicine Research in the Post-genomic Era.

7. References

Burton, J.D.; Castillo, M.E.; Goldenberg, D.M. & Blumenthal, R.D. (2007). Peroxisome proliferator-activated receptor-γ antagonists exhibit potent antiproliferative effects versus many hematopoietic and epithelial cancer cell lines. *Anticancer Drugs*, Vol. 18, No. 5, (June 2007), pp. 525-34, ISSN 0959-4973

Chan, T.Y.; Tomlinson, B.; Tse, L.K.; Chan, J.C.; Chan, W.W. & Critchley, J.A. (1994). Aconitine poisoning due to Chinese herbal medicines: a review. *Veterinary and Human Toxicology*, Vol. 36, No. 5, (October 1994), pp. 452-455, ISSN 0145-6296

Hornung, D.; Waite, L.L.; Ricke, E.A.; Bentzien, F.; Wallwiener, D. & Taylor, R.N. (2001). Nuclear peroxisome proliferator-activated receptors a and g have opposing effects on monocyte chemotaxis in endometriosis. *The Journal of Clinical Endocrinology & Metabolism*, Vol. 86, No. 7, (July 2001), pp. 3108-3114, ISSN 0021-972X

Hu, Q.; Jiang, D. & Xu, Q. (2007). In vitro models of fibrosis: Anti-fibrotic herbal medicines revisited. In: *Elements of fibrosis and the prevention and treatment of fibrosis in traditional Chinese medicine*, J. Niu, (Ed.), pp678-pp682, People's Health Press, ISBN 978-7-117-09337-8, Beijing, China

Hu, Q.; Noor, M.; Wong, Y.F.; Hylands, P.; Simmonds, M.S.J.; Xu, Q.; Jiang, D.; Hendry, B.M. & Xu, Q. (2009). *In vitro* anti-fibrotic activities of herbal compounds and herbs. *Nephrology Dialysis & Transplantation*, Vol. 24, No. 10, (October 2009), pp. 3033-3041, ISSN 0931-0509

Huang, T.H.; Yang, Q.; Harada, M.; Li, G.Q.; Yamahara, J.; Roufogalis, B.D. & Li Y. (2005). Pomegranate flower extract diminishes cardiac fibrosis in Zucker diabetic fatty rats: modulation of cardiac endothelin-1 and nuclear factor-κB pathways. *Journal of Cardiovascular Pharmacology*, Vol. 46, No. 6, (December 2005), pp. 856-862, ISSN 0160-2446

Huang, W. & Sun, R. (2010). Pathological damage mechanism of rats' nephrotoxicity caused by alcohol extracted components of Herba Leonuri. *Chinese Journal of Experimental Traditional Medical Formulae*, Vol. 16, No. 9, pp. 111-114, ISSN 1005-9903

Iglarz, M.; Touyz, R.M.; Viel, E.C.; Paradis, P.; Amiri, F.; Diep, Q.N. & Schiffrin, E.L. (2003). Peroxisome proliferator-activated receptor-alpha and receptor-gamma activators prevent cardiac fibrosis in mineralocorticoid-dependent hypertension. *Hypertension*. Vol. 42, No. 4, (October 2003), pp. 737-43, ISSN 0914-91IX

Kawai, T.; Masaki, T.; Doi, S.; Arakawa, T.; Yokoyama, Y.; Doi, T.; Kohno, N. & Yorioka, N. (2009). PPAR-γ agonist attenuates renal interstitial fibrosis and inflammation through reduction of TGF-beta. *Laboratory Investigation*, Vol. 89, No. 1, (January 2009), pp. 47-58, ISSN 0023-6837

Lee, G.; Elwood, F.; McNally, J.; Weiszmann, J.; Lindstrom, M.; Amaral, K.; Nakamura, M.; Miao, S.; Cao, P.; Learned, R.M.; Chen, J.L. & Li, Y. (2002). T0070907, a selective ligand for peroxisome proliferator-activated receptor γ, functions as an antagonist of biochemical and cellular activities. *Journal of Biological Chemistry*, Vol. 277, No. 22, (May 2002), pp. 19649-19657, ISSN 0021-9258

Li, R. & Zhao, M.Y. (2006). Effects of Huangqijixueteng decoction on TGF-β1, CTGF and PDGF-BB expression in experimental rat liver fibrosis. *Proceeding of Clinical Medicine*, Vol. 15, No. 9, (2006), pp. 659-661, ISSN 1671- 8631

Li, R.; Lu W. & Zhao, M.Y. (2007). Preventive effect and mechanism of Huangqijixueteng decoction on hepatic fibrosis in rats. *Chinese Journal of Integrated Traditional and Western Medicine on Digestion*, Vol. 15, No. 2, (2007), pp. 99-103, ISSN 1671-038X

Li, Y.; Qi, Y.; Huang, T.H.; Yamahara, J. & Roufogalis, B.D. (2008). Pomegranate flower: a unique traditional antidiabetic medicine with dual PPAR-α/-γ activator properties. *Diabetes, Obesity and Metabolism* Vol. 10, No. 1, (January 2008), pp. 10-17, ISSN 1463-1326

Lin, W.C. & Lin, W.L. (2006). Ameliorative effect of Ganoderma lucidum on carbon tetrachloride-induced liver fibrosis in rats. *World Journal of Gastroenterology*, Vol. 12, No. 2, (January 2006), pp. 265-270, ISSN 1007-9327

Liu, J.Y.; Chen, C.C.; Wang, W.H.; Hsu, J.D.; Yang, M.Y. & Wang, C.J. (2006). The protective effects of Hibiscus sabdariffa extract on CCl4-induced liver fibrosis in rats. *Food and Chemical Toxicology*, Vol. 44, No. 3, (March 2006), pp. 336-343, ISSN 0278-6915

Massoud, A.M.; El Ebiary, F.H. & Abd El Salam, N.F. (2004). Effect of myrrh extract on the liver of normal and bilharzially infected mice. An ultrastructural study. *Journal of the Egyptian Society of Parasitology*, Vol. 34, No. 1, (April 2004), pp. 1-21, ISSN 1110-0583

Milam, J.E., Keshamouni, V.G.; Phan, S.H.; Hu, B.; Gangireddy, S.R.; Hogaboam, C.M.; Standiford, T.J.; Thannickal, V.J. & Reddy, R.C. (2008). PPAR-γ agonists inhibit profibrotic phenotypes in human lung fibroblasts and bleomycin-induced pulmonary fibrosis. *American Journal of Physiology - Lung Cellullar and Molecular Physiology*, Vol. 294, No. 5, (May 2008), pp. L891-901, ISSN 1040-0605

Moon, J.A.; Kim, H.T., Cho, I.S.; Sheen, Y.Y. & Kim, D.K. (2006). IN-1130, a novel transforming growth factor-β type I receptor kinase (ALK5) inhibitor, suppresses renal fibrosis in obstructive nephropathy. *Kidney International*, Vol. 70, No. 7, (October 2006), pp. 1234-1243, ISSN 0085-2538

Piao, X.-X.; Huang, H.-G. & Piao, D.M. (2005). Therapeutic role of ethanolic extract of Boschniakia Rossica in dimethylnitrosamine-induced liver fibrosis in rats. *World Chinese Journal of Digestology*, Vol. 13, No. 18, (September 2005), pp. 2205-2209, ISSN 1009-3079

Seimandi, M.; Lemaire, G.; Pillon, A.; Perrin, A.; Carlavan, I.; Voegel, J.J.; Vignon, F.; Nicolas, J.C. & Balaguer, P. (2005). Differential responses of PPARα, PPARδ, and PPARγ reporter cell lines to selective PPAR synthetic ligands. *Analytical Biochemistry*, Vol. 344, No. 1, (September 2005), pp. 8-15, ISSN 0003-2697

Shearer, B.G.; Steger, D.J.; Way, J.M.; Stanley, T.B.; Lobe, D.C.; Grillot, D.A.; Iannone, M.A.; Lazar, M.A.; Willson, T.M. & Billin, A.N. (2008). Identification and characterization of a selective peroxisome proliferator-activated receptor β/δ (NR1C2) antagonist. *Molecular Endocrinology*, Vol. 22, No. 2, (February 2008), pp. 523-529, ISSN 0888-8809

Singhuber, J.; Zhu, M.; Prinz, S. & Kopp B. Aconitum in traditional Chinese medicine: a valuable drug or an unpredictable risk? *Journal of Ethnopharmacology*, Vol. 126, No. 1, (October 2009), pp. 18-30, ISSN 0378-8741

Sun, R.; Wu, X.; Liu, J.; Sun, L. & Lv, L. (2005a). Experimental study of the rat renal toxicity of Tripterygium wilfordii, Caulis aristolochiae and Leonurus. *Pharmacology and Clinics of Chinese Materia Medica*, No. 2, 2005, pp. 26-28, ISSN 1001-859X

Sun, R.; Sun, L.; Wu, X. & Lv, L. (2005b). Formulation reduces the renal toxicity of Yimucao. *Chinese Journal of Pharmacovigilance*, No. 3, (June 2005), pp. 144-147, ISSN 1672−8629

Toyama, T.; Nakamura, H.; Harano, Y.; Yamauchi, N.; Morita, A.; Kirishima, T.; Minami, M.; Itoh, Y. & Okanoue, T. (2004). PPARα ligands activate antioxidant enzymes and suppress hepatic fibrosis in rats. *Biochemical and Biophysical Research Communications. Vol. 324, No. 2*, (November 2004), pp. 697-704, ISSN 0006-291X

Wang, B.E. (2000). Treatment of chronic liver diseases with traditional Chinese medicine. *Journal of Gastroenterology & Hepatology*, No. 15 Suppl, (May 2000), pp. E67-70, ISSN 0815-9319

Wang, L.; Wang, B.E.; Wang, J.; Xiao, P.G. & Tan, X.H. (2008). Herbal compound 861 regulates mRNA expression of collagen synthesis- and degradation-related genes in human hepatic stellate cells. *World Journal of Gastroenterology*, Vol. 14, No. 11, (March 2008), pp. 1790-1794, ISSN 1007-9327

Wang, G.J.; Huang, Y.J.; Chen, D.H.; Lin, Y.L. (2009). Ganoderma lucidum extract attenuates the proliferation of hepatic stellate cells by blocking the PDGF receptor. *Phytotherapy Research*, Vol. 23, No. 6, (June 2009), pp. 833-939, ISSN 0951-418X

Wu, Y.W.; Fang, H.L. & Lin, W.C. (2010). Post-treatment of Ganoderma lucidum reduced liver fibrosis induced by thioacetamide in mice. *Phytotherapy Research*, Vol. 24, No. 4, (April 2010), pp. 494-499, ISSN 0951-418X

Wynn, T.A. (2007). Common and unique mechanisms regulate fibrosis in various fibroproliferative diseases. *Journal of Clinical Investigation*, Vol. 117, No. 3, (March 2007), pp. 524-529, ISSN 0021-9738

Xiao, J.C.; Liu, H.J.; Han, D.; Li, Z.; Jiang, J.X. & Qing, C. (1989). Protective effects of the pollen of Codonopsis pilosula (Franch.) Nannf. on liver lesions at the ultrastructural level. *Zhongguo Zhong Yao Za Zhi*. Vol. 14, No. 3, (March 1989), pp. 42-44, ISSN 1001-5302

Xu, H.E.; Stanley, T.B.; Montana, V.G.; Lambert, M.H.; Shearer, B.G.; Cobb, J.E.; McKee, D.D.; Galardi, C.M.; Plunket, K.D.; Nolte, R.T.; Parks, D.J.; Moore, J.T.; Kliewer, S.A.; Willson, T.M. & Stimmel, J.B. (2002). Structural basis for antagonist-mediated recruitment of nuclear co-repressors by PPARα. *Nature* Vol. 415, No. 6873, (February 2002), pp. 813-817, ISSN 0028-0836

Xu, Q.; Norman, J.T.; Shrivastav, S.; Lucio-Cazana, J. & Kopp, J.B. (2007). *In vitro* models of TGF-β-induced fibrosis suitable for high-throughput screening of antifibrotic agents. *Am J Physiol Renal Physiol* Vol. 293, No. 2, (August 2007), pp. F631-40, ISSN 0363-6127

Yao, C.F. & Jiang, S.L. (2003). Prevention and treatment of pulmonary-fibrosis by traditional Chinese medicine. *Zhong Xi Yi Jie He Xue Bao*. Vol. 1, No. 3, (September 2003), pp. 234-238, ISSN 1672-1977

Zhao, J.; Lü, Z.; Wang, X. & Zhang, X. (2002). The study on the anti-oxidation effect of root of Mallotus apelta in the rat model of liver fibrosis. *Zhong Yao Cai*. Vol. 25, No. 3, (March 2002), pp. 185-187, ISSN 1001-4454

7

Traditional Chinese Medical Criteria About the Use of Yongquan as a Life Support Maneuver

Adrián Angel Inchauspe
La Plata National University,
Argentina

1. Introduction

Although I consider the beginning of my formal Dim Mak education since 1993 –when Master Erle Montaigue spread out this theory in the western world *("Dim Mak –Death Point Striking")*, my first contact with K-1 Yongquan was in 1976, when I had the opportunity to explore some "almost secret" scripts about this subject.

I waited until 1987, during my surgical residence, to apply this knowledge in my first case – a cardiac arrest derived from a pulseless activity with no response of the life support therapy, but with great success using the K-1 maneuver.

Since then, my researches are continuous about the acupuncture-point Yongquan manipulation results after both basic and advanced Cardio-Pulmonar Resuscitation (CPR) protocol failure. It surprising results guide me to call this phenomenon the "Lazarus Effect". It's necessary to describe briefly the principles that give sense to the K-1 Yongquan maneuver, in order to integrate them to western medical concepts.

2. *Jing:* Our energetic inheritance

The ancestral u original energy represents the value of our energetic inheritance, or *Jing*.

The *Innate Jing*, received from our parents is hidden in the Kidneys (Yin) and in the Mingmen (Yang) to generate the initial Qi for our vital processes *(Jing Yue Quan Shu – Zhang Jie Bin)*.

The *Adquired Jing* gives the substrate of the anterior one. It is contained into the five *zhang* and the six *fu*, nurturing our vital substance.

The *Yin or Nurture Qi* enters in our energy system from the Earth through K-1 Yongquan; and it will be selected in its "pure form" by the Spleen before reaching the Lungs and Heart. In that way, the last organs will be able to elaborate *Zheng Qi* or Central (thoracic) energy for its vital priority of his active cardio-respiratory function.

3. Kidney and traditional Chinese medicine

In acupuncture, the Kidneys (Shen) represents Water, so that is the Yin organ "par excellence". Their main function, similar to the allopathic medical knowledge, is" *to control the body Water distribution*" (*Su Wen*, chap. 34). In the same way, it will be responsible of filtering wastes, eliminate toxins, the water intake excess and the mineral salts incorporated by diet, in order to regulate the blood Ph.

For the Chinese Medicine, the Kidney develops the following functions:

1.   *"to store the Jing and dominate reproduction, growth and development"*

This includes the mastering of derived functions as birth, growing, development and reproduction, for   Kidneys are our natural ancestral energy depot - the purified and condensed modality of Qi *(Jing)* - that will aid us to get each of the human development stages *(Su Wen ,chap.1)*.

2.   *"to produce the bone marrow" (Su Wen , chap.5)*.

This statement involves the following properties:

-     The control of the bones and their marrow *(Su Wen, chap.23)*.
-     To elaborate the blood –Xue-(were the Chinese intuitive about erythropoietin's existence?).
-     To nurture the brain (for Chinese people, the brain represents the "Sea of Marrow").

We can see that the "Medullae concept" in TCM results very much transcendental than their western significance. Not only involves the bone marrow, but the matrix of the fundamental components of the Central Nervous System.

3.   *"to dominate Water" (Su Wen, chap.34)*

This function has been analyzed before in this chapter. Is obvious to understand this meaning in the regulation of the methabolism of water and corporal fluids *("Jin ye")*.

4.   *"to control the reception of Qi"*

In the sense that Shen is the depot of the Ancestral energy or *Yuan Qi (Ling Shu.chap.5)*, Kidneys are capable to captivate the Qi for recycle it energetically, taking influence over the following *zhang*:

•   Over the Spleen and its "couple in Earth" Stomach, allowing the correct digestives procedures
•   Over the Heart, getting the equilibrium in the Water. Fire harmony *(Kan Li)*
•   Over the Lungs, helping to gather and descend the Qi during inspiration
•   Over the Liver, ensuring a soft and harmonious Qi flux all around the body
•   Over the Triple Heater, promoting the "Water transformation" through its energetic methabolism

5.   *"It manifests in the hair"*.

As indicated in *Su Wen (chap.5)*, hair's characteristics show the internal sufficiency of the Qi of Shen.

6.   *"to open the ears" (Ling Shu, chap.17)*.

It was written in this chapter " *The Qi of the Kidneys go to the ears; when the Kidneys are in harmony, the ears can hear the Five Sounds"…* _ thus referring not only to the five notes from the pentathonic Chinese music, but the effect of the Kidneys (Shen) over the other organs or *zhang*.

We must remember the hearing disorders as a consequence of treating patients with nephrotoxic drug (ej. antibiotics) to understand how advanced was the Chinese medical wisdom.

Among this, and searching for motives of the spectacular reaction through Yongquan in resuscitation, again in *Ling Shu* (chap. 10) appears the link between Kidney and Heart(by its internal vessel) and with the Lungs (by a secondary vessel),that justifying this powerful influence.

4. Specific analysis about the K-1 Yongquan acupuncture point

Its name means "Gushing spring" or "Bubbling well".The ancient book I-Ching instructs us about the Water ("Kan") trigram:"...*its correspondence is to Water; is the Water in movement, the spring that falls into deepness...*"

4.1 K1-Resuscitation maneuver: Chinese fundamentals

Located in the sole of the foot, in a depression where the sole makes its plantar flexion. Tracing a line from the base of the second toe up to the heel, and dividing it in three equal parts, the point is found at the junction between the anterior and the middle third.

Anatomically speaking, Yongquan´s precise ubication is between the second and third metatarsal bones, at the level of the plantar fascia. Medial to it are the longus and brevis flexor digitorum pedis tendons and the second lumbricalis pedis muscles.

In its deepest position, the point lay in the interossei plantaris muscles. It is innervated by the second common plantar digital nerve, and irrigated by the lateral plantar and the anterior tibial arteries anastomose in the plantar arch.

In the major acupuncture classical texts, K-1 Yongquan is considered the first and Jing (Tsing)-well point of the Kidney meridian. But through the *Ling Shu* analysis (chap.5),

K-1 is also hierarched as the "root" point of the *Shao Yin* .This energetical level, formed by the Kidneys and the Heart, is the most profound among all others, giving us a special reason why K-1 Yongquan can act as an effective cardiac pacemaker.

Moreover, Yongquan is the main place for the ascending Yin Qi from the Earth into our body. Therefore, this kind of energy will nurture the *zhang*, especially those placed in the most Yang part of the torso, in order to interact and compensate the Heavenly energy, essential for organs with a non-interruptable function to maintain our life, like the heart and the lungs. It can be read in *Ling Shu, chap 9:"Yin rules the organs, while Yang rules the viscus. Yin absorbs the Heavenly energy, while Yang absorbs the energy from the Five Organs"*. Thus, the Celestial Yang Qi provides them with continous motility in the Upper Jiao of our body, for a perfect vital equilibrium.

4.2 Main applications for K-1 Yongquan in TCM

Traditional Chinese Medicine "officially" recognizes the following as the main applications of K-1 Yongquan:

-	Respiratory diseases	-	Nasal obstruction - Epistaxis (nosebleed).
-	O.R.L diseases	-	Dry tongue – Amigdalitis – Swollen throat – Odinophagia –Vertigo
-	Digestive diseases	-	Abdominal colics -Vomits – Diarrhea – Difficult defecation
-	Urinary conditions	-	Difficult urination – Dysuria
-	Genital conditions	-	Functional sterility
-	Psychiatric conditions	-	Insomnia – Psychosis
-	Cardiovascular diseases	-	Arterial hypertension – Syncope
-	Neurological conditions	-	Blurred vision – Vertex headaches – Peripheral neuropathy – Infantile convulsions – Epilepsy – Lower limbs paralysis (Zheng Li)-Stroke – Loss of consciousness (Coma)

Among this indications, in relative recent times (2006), Chinese doctors added a case of subdural hematoma.

Since.1987, my specific and new use is as a rescue point against both basic and advanced CPR failure. Currently, a new paper has been sent to the World Journal of Critical Care Medicine in order to present a complete protocolization about K-1 uses during life- support maneuvers.

5. Bioenergetic survival axis

5.1 Valorative comparison between Oriental and Occidental axioms
In "Impending Death situation" patients, both Oriental and Western Medicines explain some biological reactions that make organs and viscus to take a peculiar concatenation that could be followed by a logical sequence. In this manner, we can understand this mutual cooperation as a result of K-1 stimulation in a dynamic way.

5.2 A common embryological origin
It is well known in Occident that both the skin and the Central nervous System recognize a common embryological origin.

In the beginning of the 3th week, a trilaminar embrion enhance its cranial extreme, and an axial depression appears in its ectoderm. This fissure is the Neural fold ;a structure that few days later will make the Neural tube ,and the first draught of raquis.

Over this, alternative medicines found arguments that support their action vehicled by the skin.This represents, in current neurological physiology ,the visceral-cutaneous reflex.

5.3 Survival axis components
Among the Kidneys, there are another organs to be integrated under the structure of what is presented as the "Survival Axis".

Integrated diagrams will configure this notions in a dynamic way.

SURVIVAL AXIS -   Dr. Inchauspe

6. Suprarenal glands

Not only an anatomical relationship – for there are positioned over- entail them with the Kidneys, but also represent the Yang function of the mentioned channels (remember that Kidneys themselves maintain the Yin part of this balance).

In the mid 20th century, german investigator Hans Seyle described the "Stress reaction", while in North America, Cannon menctioned it as the "Fright, fight or flight" behaviour. Both were clearly coincident about the suprarenal response to an emergency state, producing glucocorticoids (the main one in primates is cortisol), mineralocorticoids (aldosteron) and androgens. The final release of catecholamines (L-dopa, ephynefrine, norephynefrine) will prepare our body to stress. All the last derive from phenylalanine´s molecule; so that it injection can enhance our alarm reaction.

This hypothesis is another evidence of the "Mother and son" rule from the Five Element´s theory in TCM.

K1-Yongquan hypothalamus-adrenal bio-feedbak

7. Brain

Above all emotions, **FEAR** is the natural response against any situation that put life into risk (is the emblematic emotion of the Water element). The sensorial perceptions are interpreted as a menace in the limbic system. From this site of the temporal lobe, signals will run down from the hypothalamus to hypofisis to stimulate suprarenal glands, preparing us to face **DANGER**.

Among all the cutaneous reflexes, the Babinski one is the best known and of utmost importance, because this plantar stimulation ,after the age of 2 ,can diagnose a pyramidal lesion with a patognomonic hallux extension –casualty scratching near the K-1 Yongquan!.

This evidence even more the axiom "*Kidney masters the Sea of Marrow*".

Interaction of the Water Element (Tai Yang Level)

8. Heart

Chinese related it with the Kidney by internal passways. Moreover, TCM considered this two organs conform the most profound energetic level in a human being: *The Shao Yin*.

Heart could be conceived in a Yin and a Yang phase: the "right heart" includes the right auricule and ventricle; same consideration can be made with the left side.

The right side acts as an "admission pump" the blood *(Xue)* follows a centripetal route towards the heart, so it can be understood with a Yin nature.

The left auricle and ventricle transport oxygenated blood to the body, reaching them in a centrifugal travel impulsed by the systolic ejection. So this "propulsive part" of the Heart behaves as the Yang side.

In the right auricle, Keith & Flack´s sinoauricular node normally functions as our cardiac pacemaker. Because its same Yin polarity line of Kidney –and connected by profound collaterals -, it could be very influenced by it.

9. Kidneys and the Ancestral Energy

For the Chinese, they are the "Ancestral Energy Depot", and they also considered it as the "Prenatal Emperor" for their activity during pregnancy (perhaps they already knew that Kidneys are directly involved in the amniotic fluid production).

During the 3th week –in the vitelin sack, very near from the alantoid process -,a group of haploid cells travel through the inguinal stretch to testicles (or to ovaries) where will rest the cromosomic potential for our species perpetuation.

This essential energy, or *Yuan* is a kind to be convoked into emergency states, so that stimulating the route of our "Survival Axis".

In Traditional Chinese Medicine (TCM), it is generally accepted that, if the principal property from the Curious Vessels is to conduct the *Yuan* or ancestral energy into themselves, the reason is that all of this Particular Meridians have their origin in the Kidneys (Shen).

In chapter 9, *Ling Shu* tells us: "*Curious Vessels as Chong Mai and Ren Mai are connected to the Chao (Shao) Yin level*". So through the Chong Mai –the "*Mother of the Twelve Meridians*" – it can be understood in what way Kidney influences over the other body channels.

More specifically talking, those Curious Vessels of Yin nature (Yin Wei – Yin Qiao –Chong Mai) recognize their initial point in K-1 Yongquan, while the rest of them endowed with

Yang polarity (Yang Qiao – Yang Wei – Dai Mai) are born in the final point of the Yang descendent (centrifugal) channels in the inferior limbs. If you pay attention to the names of this points – ex.Gb 44: Zu Qiao Yin ("Passage to the Yin"); or B 67: Zhi Yin ("That who meets the Yin"), make us evident how close are they to contact the major Yin source ever known _ the terrestrial energy_ and their main entrance: the K-1 acupuncture point.
Yuan Considerations.

10. The *Shao Yin* level

The *Shao Yin* commands the vital functions, although the brain´s energy had been impaired.
Up to the 60´s, cardiac activity´s suspension was evident by a fail in both breathing and pulse perception. Only this allowed the doctor to declare a clinical death.
With the development of the organ –transplantation therapy,death was not more the absence of vital signs,but a non – reactive EEG.So with the brain activity in suspension ,we are able to define a legally death patient, turning it into a "living donor".
In the *Shao Yin level* resides the last quantum of energy before life abandon us. For its connection with Earth –the most powerful Yin source available, K-1 Yongquan - the "root" point of the *Shao Yin* that enables the Terrestrial energy to rush up towards the cranial Yang pole – deserves the possibility of rescuing us with a simple maneuver, pressing the most dark and retired place of the body: in the sole of the foot!

11. Results

Since 1987, of a current statistic of 44 cases, 39 patients were admitted in hospital, while 5 external cases in "impending death situation" received life-support attention with failure of both basic and advanced CPR protocol.
The next table summarizes the demography and outcome of this people assisted with the "Lazarus Effect".

- Stroke	7 cases	1 death
- Severe hypertension	8 cases	no death
- Electrocution	1 case	1 death
- Chest crush	3 cases	1 death
- Chest trauma with skull and bilateral femur fractures	1 case	1 death
- Post-operative shock	4 cases	1 death
- Intraoperative heart stoppage	6 cases	1 death
- Pulseless activity	3 cases	1 death
- Ventricular fibrillation	5 cases	1 death
- Gas embolism	1 case	no death
- Renal failure post-sepsis	2 cases	1 death
- Anaphylactic shock (post oncology drugs)	3 cases	no death

12. Conclusions

Comparison between my first 30 patients against the best results of Emergency Services and Rescue Teams (around 19 % survival in CPR), justified its publication in the Resuscitation Journal (j.resus. 4183. JAN-2010; DOI information: 10.1016).

In October, 2010 I was invited to participate as speaker in the 8th International Congress of Drug Development, Science and Technology in the Convention Center of Beijing. There I exposed about the theoretical effect of phenylalanine inyection over K-1 Yongquan, based in its convertion into catecholamines and its action over the glomic micro-structure of the acupuncture point (Dr. Sergio Gutierrez Morales, Canarias). Hipothetically speaking, this allows the cardiac arrest victims to "respond" more effectively to the Yongquan maneuver, thus improving to higher survival rates.

Actuarial statistics show a mortality percentage in heart stoppage in aprox. 1,5/1000 healthy individuals. Translating this proportion to the current world population, nearly 8.000.000 deaths occur per year for this cause, a very much lethal situation that any epidemic or pandemic danger actually known. From them, only a limited 19% -it means, 1.520.000 persons – can be rescued.

The K-1 Yongquan resuscitation maneuver could raise up this rate to, at least, 38%.This signifies that more than 3.500.000 people could be potentially saved each year –as was informed in FILASMA Congress in Sevilla, in November 2010, where Dr.Enrique Ruffa summed another new 3 cases to the Yongquan resuscitation statistics. This number is comparable with the actual population of our neighbough country, Uruguay –aprox. 4.000.000 people.

Once the World Resuscitation Committee accepts this therapeutic maneuver, this whole theory will open the possibility of converting cardiac arrests victims into responders, allowing the K-1 Yongquan maneuver inclusion in the life-support protocols, upgrading the survival rates even much more.

13. References

Borison, R.L. et al: "Metabolism of amino acid with antidepressant properties". Res Commun Chem Pathol & Pharmacol, 1978; 21 (2):363-6.

Chamorro, C. et al: "Can heart donation exclusion factors be overcome?" Rev.Esp. Cardiol., 2006; 59:232-7.

Chamorro, C.: "Mantenimiento especifico del posible donante cardíaco". Conferencia como Coordinador de Transplantes – Servicio de Medicina Intensiva". Clinica "Puerta de Hierro", Madrid.

Gutierrez Morales, A.R.; Smith Agreda, V.: "Mecanismos de acción de la analgesia acupuntural: Biomedicina, practica clinica e investigación". Edit. Mandala, Madrid, 2001

Gray, B.: "The Advanced Iron Palm. Unique Publications, Burbank, California, 1995; (2), 11.

Huang Di: "Ling Shu, Yellow Emperor´s Canon of Acupuncture" 1° Edition, Madrid, 2002.

Huang Di: "Su Wen, Nan Jing"7° Edition, Ed. Plaza, Madrid, 2002.

Hsieh, D.: "Advanced Dim Mak". Meadea Enterprise Co., Inc. Republic of China, 1995; (7).87.

Inchauspe, A.: "Phenylalanine injection over K-1 Yongquan: a theoretical way of upgrading survival rates in CPR".speaker of the 8th IDDST Congress. Beijing, China. October 23-26th, 2010

Inchauspe, A.: "Traditional Chinese Medicine K-1 Yongquan and resuscitation: another Kind of "Lazarus phenomenon". Resuscitation (2010), doi: 10.1016/j. resuscitation. 2009.12.009.

Kitade, T.; Odahara, Y.; Shinohara, S. et al:"Studies on the enhanced effect of acupunture analgesia and acupuncture anesthesia by D-phenylalanine (2nd report) — schedule and administration and clinical effects in low back pain and tooth extraction". Acupunct. Electrother rev., 1990; 15 (2):121-35.

Len Kevin, MD.: ".DL-fenilalanina(DLPA):el agente analgesico y terapeutico natural". Conferencia como miembro de la Chemical Royal Society.

Long, H: "Advanced Dragon´s Touch – Anatomical targets and techniques. Paladin Press, Boulder, Colorado, 1995

Montaigue, E.: "Dim Mak –Death Point Striking", chap.4."The points and what they do". Paladin Press, Boulder, Colorado, 1993; 85.

Montaigue, E: "Advanced Dim Mak – The finer points of Death-Point Striking" chap. 8:"Point Power". Paladin Press, Boulder, Colorado, 1994, 198, fig.263 -264.

Poewe, W.: "Treatment for Parkinson disease---past achievements and current clinical Needs. Neurology, 2009.Feb.17; 72 (7 Suppl):s65-73.

Russell, A.L.; Mc Carthy, M.F.: "DL-phenylalanine markedly potentiates opiate analgesia - an example of nutrient/pharmaceutical up-regulation of the endogenous analgesic system.Med. Hypothesses.2000; 55 (4):283-8.

Sabelli, H.C.; Fawcett, J.; Gusovsky, F. et al.: "Clinical Studies on the phenylalanine hipótesis of affective disorders: urine and blood phenylacetic acid and phenylalanine dietary supplements".J. Clin Psychiatry, 1986; 47 :66-70.

Steven, D.; Ehrlich, NMD: "Solution Acupuncture, a private practice specializing in Complementary and Alternative Medicine". Verified Health Network.

Solorzano del Rio, H.."Funciones de la Fenilalanina".Conferencia como coordinador del Departamento de Medicinas Complementarias. Univ. Guadalajara, Mexico.

Szabo, G.: "Physiologic changes alter brain death".J. Heart Lung Transplant 2004; S223-6.

Walsh, N.E.; Ramamurthy, S.; Schoenfeld, L.; Hoffman, J."Analgesic effectiveness of D-phenylalanine in cronic pain patients".Arch. Phys. Med. Redhabil., 1986; 67(7):436-9.

8

Chinese Medicine and Integrative Approaches in the Prevention of Breast Cancer – Acupuncture Meridian, Pulsed Eletromagnetic Field Test and Chinese Food Therapy

Lulu Fu and Hong Xu
Victoria University,
Endeavour College of Natural Health,
Australia

1. Introduction

A series of studies conducted demonstrate the integrative abilities of hormone regulation and subsequent preventative strategies with the use of Chinese Medicine (CM) in the prevention of breast cancer and balancing hormones.

These investigations studied the patterns of disharmony for groups of middle aged women and explored the relationship between the CM patterns of disharmony and specific bio-markers (Xu, 2004; Fu & Xu, 2011).

Chinese medicine assessment in Fu and Xu's study (2011) indicated that the participants felt correspondingly weaker and their health conditions also had adverse trends in their middle age. They commonly had mood swings which relates to *Liver Qi stagnation*. Peri-menopausal symptoms also affected their daily life. Data collected from these participants indicated that the adverse symptoms and relative signs changed after the treatment resulting in the levels of disharmony being reduced. The changes of patterns of disharmony indicated in the Chinese medicine assessment are relevant to the change of biomedical markers, which may be useful in western-medical assessment of hormones fluctuation and pre-clinical breast diseases. If Chinese medicine diagnostic methods indicate that *Liver Qi stagnation* and *Liver-Kidney Yin deficiency* are the main patterns of middle aged women hormone fluctuation or pre-clinical breast diseases, it is reasonable to argue that the treatment principle should be based on regulating *Qi* and nourishing *Yin*. This study has provided a repeatable evidence of using the Chinese kiwi fruit extract for the regulation of hormonal disorder and Chinese medicine patterns of disharmony.

The bio-markers used in these studies are the 2-hydroxyestrone and 16α-hydroxyestrone (2-OHE: 16α-OHE), they are both reliable and sensitive in order to investigate the hormone imbalance. These can be easily applied as early preventative strategies that integrate both CM and Western diagnostic methods. The selected Chinese kiwi fruit (*Actinidia chinensis var. deliciosa*) extract could benefit women with hormone imbalance or hormone related diseases (Xu & Xu, 2006). In another clinical trial, 16 participants, who were diagnosed with breast cancer and had just completed chemotherapy, were given this Chinese kiwi fruit drink (equal to 20g) daily over a seven day period. The results indicated that the rate of binucleate lymphocyte cells with micronuclei in these participants had significantly decreased. This may indicate the recovery of chromosome change in the breast tissue (Xu, 1999). Appropriate choice of nutritional products on the scientific basis is an important aspect in cancer patients' recovery (Xu & Xu, 2006).

This study focused on the relationships between the acupuncture meridian, Chinese food therapy and pulsed electromagnetic field test in the same population group, using a double-blind, placebo-controlled clinical trial.

1.1 Acupuncture meridian

In Chinese Medicine, all the primary 12 meridians passed the trunk area and over spread to peripheral extremities. The *Yang* meridians traverse the outer surface of the arm or leg and travel to the head and the back, in spite of the *Stomach Meridian* that are running the lateral side of the *Kidney Meridian*, at the anterior of the trunk. All *Yin* meridians traverse or bypass the breast area and the special superior lateral side of the breast. These meridians each correspond to different organ (*Zang Fu*) systems. Meridians harmonise the whole body's function if *Qi* and *Blood* could circulate well, they can also reflect the direct trauma and the *Zang Fu* function. Pathogens and diseases can make visible changes on the related meridians (Tang et al., 1999). The acupuncture meridians are important transportation channels, any blockage of the meridians will cause disease and disharmony in the body.

During the fourteenth century, Dr Dan-Xi Zhu summarized the etiology of breast cancer that a woman, who was worried and depressed, could suffer from an accumulation of stagnation. The stagnation could be the cause of *Liver Qi* rebels horizontally and the stagnation finally turns into nodules (Niu, 1996). Female hormonal related diseases and breast diseases are related to the *Liver* and *Kidney Meridians* (Fu & Xu, 2011).

1.2 Pulsed Electromagnetic Field (PEMF) test

Electromagnetic fields are present everywhere in our environment but are invisible to the human eye. One of the main characteristics which define an electromagnetic field is its frequency or its corresponding wavelength. Fields of different frequencies interact with the body in different ways (WHO, 2011). The equipment selected for the PEMF test is safe according to the WHO guideline. The magnetic field changes were measured by a noninvasive medical device, which has been supplied on the market for over 10 years. This magnetic test, using a polarized light can detect a defect at the cellular level (Gianni & Liberti, 2006).

Humans have an electromagnetic energy field, the human body is an aerial that can transmit and receive energy (William, 2002). When there is a disorder, the magnetic field could be alternated by the *Qi and Blood* stagnation in CM theory. Magnetic therapy has been used in CM practices from 200 BC according to CM history.

In the early stage study of electromagnetic models, the magnetic network was recognized similar to the acupuncture meridian (Omura, 1986). Later study indicated that the acupuncture meridians were related to the electromagnetic model of transmission lines (Yung, 2005). In this study, the polarized light was used to detect the magnetic field change near and along the acupuncture meridian.

Chinese Medicine and Integrative Approaches in the Prevention of Breast Cancer – Acupuncture Meridian, Pulsed Eletromagnetic Field Test and Chinese Food Therapy

127

1.3 Chinese Kiwi Fruit Extract

Chinese herbal formulae, food therapy and acupuncture have long been used to effectively regulate endocrinal disorders in Chinese clinical practice. One Chinese food therapy of interest is the Chinese food formula - Kiwi Fruit Extract (KFE), which has been used in practice for many years and related safety tests have also been conducted. Kiwi fruit extract is rich in vitamin C, vitamin E, vitamin K, folate, antithetic acid, niacin, lutein, zeaxanthin, arytenoids, falconoid, calcium, iron, manganese, selenium, zinc, copper, potassium, magnesium, fibre and amino acids (Collins et al., 2001).

Xu (2004) in his book *The Progress of Resource, Environment and Health* indicated that: Some varieties of kiwi fruit found in China have a strong anti-mutagenesis effect. When somatic cells change into cancer cells they will go through mutation, apoptosis of cells and loss of control of proliferation. Mutagenesis can be examined by gene mutation, chromosome aberration and DNA damage in laboratory experiments. High mutagenic rates can indicate the risk of cancer. There are many mutagens in the environment, e.g., coal, petroleum, tobacco, uncompleted burning of products benzo(a)pyrene etc. Polycyclic Aromatic Hydrocarbons (PAHs); over stir fried meat PhIP; peanuts, corn etc. produce aflatoxin in the damp heat environment polluted by mould; farm chemicals that pollute food like nitrous amine compound (nitrosamine), organic chlorine, toxic algae's toxins, organic pollutions in water e.g., methyl mercury; benzene, formaldehyde which are chemical pollutants in workshops and living room air; as well as overdoses of irradiation of ultraviolet ray and electromagnetic waves. The greater concern for cancer patients is some chemotherapy drugs e.g., cyclophosphamide, radiotherapy's radiation is also a mutagen.

To reduce the effects of the mutagen and the side effects of chemotherapy and radiotherapy it is beneficial to use therapeutic fruits, i.e., kiwi fruit and hawthorn fruit, which have broad anti-mutagenesis effects. Moreover, these fruits have the effect of increasing immune function. Of course, use of expansion agents to increase the size of the kiwi fruit can damage the quality of the kiwi fruit. To enhance kiwi fruit's health care effects, withdrawing the effective components, e.g., anti-cancer isoflavones, organic acids, polysaccharide and trace element, by formulation and scientific experiments to produce functional health care products, can enhance the whole anti-cancer defensive system, e.g., Hong En Health Drink (Xu & Xu, 2006).

KFE is used to improve the quality of life of women suffering from endocrine disorders (Xu, 2004; Fu & Xu, 2011). In this study, the effects of KFE on regulating the function of acupuncture meridians and unblocking the stagnation in these meridians were evaluated.

2. Research methodologies

Thirty-six middle aged peri-menopausal women living in Melbourne Australia were recruited and randomly assigned (using numbered order as they became available) into two groups, treatment group taking KFE and control group taking placebo. The group assignments were kept blind from the participants and data collectors. All the participants were in the age range from 40 to 55 year-old. They were not taking either contraceptive pills or hormone replacement therapy. None of them suffered from either breast cancer or liver and or kidney disease according to western medicine and they did not have any food allergies.

Participants took 10g of powder, either KFE or placebo each time, twice a day, mixed with 100ml of warm water. The powder was administered one hour before each breakfast and dinner meal, over an eight week period. The selected Chinese therapeutic food is a wild resourced Chinese kiwi fruit extract, Hong En No. 1 (also known as Hong En Health Drink) in powder form, provided by Professor Houen Xu of Peking University.

Pulsed electromagnetic field changes at pre and post trial were tested, at the trunk area, where the pass way of acupuncture meridians distributed. Each test lasted about 10 minutes to go through all the meridians on both the left and right side of the body, this short time exposure to the PEMF is not expected to cause any change to the body. No adverse events were reported by any of the participants in this study.

The Ultra-long Electromagnetic Wave technique, a pulsed electromagnetic field (TW-1) was selected, supplied by Health Link Food & Equipment Pty. A polarized light was used for detecting changes in the magnetic flux, the light turns off when the magnetic flux is blocked. The results were recorded on a map where there is an anatomical drawing of the human trunk. These include the depiction of any defective areas found in the two dimensions (length and width). A 0-10 scale is used to measure the portion of the blockage, "0" represents unblocked and "10" represents fully blocked. The tested area on the body was restricted between the mid-clavicular line and mid-axillary line, from the iliac crease to the clavicula and the axillary line at the trunk area, which matches the CM *Liver Meridian* area (See Figure 1).

The detailed steps of magnetic test were to:

- Obtain consents from participants to record the dots on their bodies and to take photographs as records for the first measurement and the last measurement.
- Explain the test purposes and procedure to the participant individually. Place the patient in supine position with the arm at 90 degree abduction.
- Measure the area of the magnetic test.
- Record the magnetic flux changes on the surface of the skin with a marker. The marks will show any defective areas found along the *Liver Meridian*.
- Use a tape measure to measure the magnetic flux changes area (width and length).
- Record the dots formed on a body map, which include the trunk area of the anatomy.
- Remove the marks on the skin, cleaning with ethanol swabs or wet cotton ball.

The study was approved by the related committees and the ethics approval was gained from the Human Research Ethics Committee of Victoria University, Australia. All participants received an explanation document and a consent form for completion.

3. Results and discussion

All the 36 participants (aged 48.38 ± 3.97 in the treatment group and 48.50 ± 5.15 in the control, $p > 0.05$) completed the tests (See Table 1), the magnetic test results were positive which indicated that blockage existed in the tested areas. The *Liver* and *Kidney* meridians in breast and flank areas are mostly affected. The average of the test results of both the left and right sides of the *Liver* and *Kidney* meridians, in both the treatment and the control group were analyzed using *t-test* by SPSS 19.

The pre-trial PEMF test results indicated that both the meridians of KFE and control groups were blocked at similar levels, there were no significant differences between the pre-trial comparisons in the two groups ($p > 0.05$) (Table 1).

Chinese Medicine and Integrative Approaches in the Prevention of Breast Cancer – Acupuncture Meridian,
Pulsed Eletromagnetic Field Test and Chinese Food Therapy

129

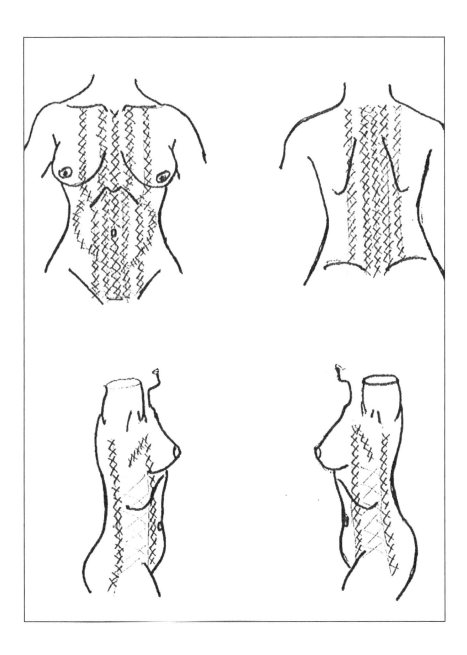

Fig. 1. PEMF test transmission lines

Groups	n	Age (years)	*Liver Meridian* PEMF test	*Kidney Meridian* PEMF test
Treatment	18	48.38 ± 3.97	7.64 ± 4.18	5.61 ± 4.99
Control	18	48.50 ± 5.15	6.11 ± 4.94	4.89 ± 4.86

Notes: *Participants in treatment group take Chinese kiwi fruit extract (Hong En No. 1) 10g X 2/days X 8 weeks; **Participants in control group take placebo
$p > 0.05$ between groups.

Table 1. Pre - trial base-line comparison of the age and PEMF test results (mean ± SD) between the treatment* and control** group of peri-menopausal women

After eight week's treatment, the results of the PEMF tests were significantly different between the two groups and between the pre and post treatment on the *Liver Meridian* (See Table 2). This indicates that KFE can improve *Liver Meridian*'s function. The results of the pre and post treatment comparison on the *Kidney Meridian* indicated a reduction of the meridian blockage while there was no change observed in the control group. However, this comparison did not achieve statistical significance (Table 3). According to common CM theory and practise, it could take much longer time to recover *Kidney* disorders, especially if the disorder is related to the pattern of deficiency. In the previous study (Fu & Xu, 2011), *Kidney* function can be improved by KFE indicated by the biomarker 2-OHE:16α-OHE change. It is therefore suggested that an integrative approach that incorporates different diagnostic methods may be a more effective way to identify and prevent breast diseases.

Groups	n	Pre-trial *Liver Meridian* PEMF test	Post-trial *Liver Meridian* PEMF test
Treatment*	18	7.64 ± 4.18	1.33 ± 2.68**
Control	18	6.11 ± 4.94	4.67 ± 4.95***

Notes: *Participants take Chinese kiwi fruit extract (Hong En No. 1) 10g X 2/days X 8 weeks. **Pre and post comparison in treatment group, $p = 0.000$, $t = 8.864$;
***Post-trial comparison between treatment and control groups, $p = 0.003$, $t = 3.252$¶

Table 2. Comparison of *Liver Meridian* PEMF test results (mean ± SD) of peri-menopausal women

Groups	n	Pre-trial *Kidney Meridian* PEMF test	Post-trial *Kidney Meridian* PEMF test
Treatment*	18	5.61 ± 4.99	4.58 ± 4.88
Control	18	4.89 ± 4.86	4.89 ± 5.00

Note: $p > 0.05$.

Table 3. Comparison of *Kidney Meridian* PEMF test results (mean ± SD) of peri-menopausal women

Most participants in the KFE group reported the improvement of general well-being after taking KFE, the details included: the decrease of hot flushes, mood swing, tiredness, abdominal distension and anger. However, these changes were not reported by the control group. There were no adverse events reported.

4. Conclusion

In this study, the pulsed electromagnetic field test is an effective diagnostic tool for the detection of acupuncture meridian disorder. The stagnation of the meridian is related to the magnetic field change. Chinese kiwi fruit extract could regulate the function of the acupuncture meridians which have been proved by the pulsed electromagnetic tests. These approaches can be easily applied as early preventative and diagnostic strategies that integrate both Chinese Medicine and contemporary therapies.

5. References

Xu, H.E. (2004). Chinese Kiwi Fruit and Health, In: *The Progress of Resource, Environment and Health in China - SCOPE China Publication Series III*, H.E. Xu, (Ed.), 113-133, Peking University Medical Press, ISBN 7-81071-559-3, Beijing, China

Fu, L.L. & Xu, H. (2011). A Preliminary Study of the Effectiveness of Chinese Therapeutic Food on Regulating Female Reproductive Hormones. *Integrative Medicine Insight*, Vol 6, (March 2011), pp. 7-12, ISSN 1177-3936

Xu, H. & Xu, H.E. (2006). Chinese Food and Cancer Healing. *Integrative Medicine Insights*, Vol 1, (Febuary 2007), pp. 1-5, ISSN 1177-3936

Xu, H.E. (1999). *Hong-En Health Drink – Development and Research*, Beijing Medical University Publishing House, pp. 11-21, ISBN 7-81034-975-9, Beijing, China

Tang, Y.X; Dang, Y. & Geng, E.G. (1999). *Acupuncture and Moxibustion*, Academy Press, pp. 462–480, ISBN 7-5077-1269-9, Beijing, China

Niu, J.Z. (1996). *Modern Gynecology of Traditional Chinese & Western Medicine*, China Science and Technology Publishing House, pp. 39-46. ISBN 9787504619402, Beijing, China

WHO, (2011). Electromagnetic Fields, Available from http://www.who.int/peh-emf/about/WhatisEMF/en

Gianni, M. & Liberti, M. (2006). Modeling Electromagnetic Fields Detectability in a HH-like Neuronal System: Stochastic Resonance and Window Behavior. *Biological Cybernetics*, Vol.94, No.2, pp. 118-127, ISSN 0340-1200

William, S. (2002). The Human Electromagnetic Energy Field: Its Relationship to Interpersonal Communication. *Journal of Theoretics*, Vol.4, No.2, ISSN 1529-3548

Omura, Y. (1986). Re-evaluation of the Classical Acupuncture Concept of Meridians in Oriental Medicine by the New Method of Detecting Meridian-like Network Connected to Internal Organs Using "Bi-Digital O-Ring Test". *Acupuncture & Electro-Therapeutic Research*, Vol.11, No.3-4, pp. 219-31, ISSN 0360-1293

Yung, K.T. (2005). A Birdcage Model for the Chinese Meridian System: Part III. Possible Mechanism of Magnetic Therapy. *The American Journal of Chinese Medicine*, Vol.33, No.4, pp. 589-597, ISSN 1793-6853

Collins, B.H.; Horská, A.; Hotten, P.; Riddoch, C. & Collins, AR. (2001). A Kiwifruit Protects
    Against Oxidative DNA Damage in Human Cells and in Vitro. *Nutrition and Cancer.*
    Vol.39, pp. 148-153, ISSN 1532-7914

Part 2

Pharmacodynamic Material Base Research

9

The MALDI-TOF Analysis of Aconitum Alkaloids in Proprietary Chinese Medicine and in the Concoction of Fuzi

Yong Wang and Chunhui Luo

College of Bioscience, Shenzhen University, Shenzhen
China

1. Introduction

In theory, the kinds and relative amounts of aconitum alkaloids in proprietary Chinese medicines should be consistent with those in Fuzi. However, this feature has not been noted enough and no direct experimental evidence to prove it. In this work MALDI-TOF-MS was used to analysis 19 kinds of proprietary Chinese medicines, benzoylmesaconine and hypaconitine have been proved to be the predominant monoester and diester alkaloids respectively. In addition, the MALDI-TOF analysis of the concoction of seven kinds of Chinese medicine has confirmed that the acidity of concoction will improve the aconitines contents and the toxicity of concoction, but this rule was not suited for Lonicera nitida, Rhizoma Chuanxiong or Chaenomeles sinensis.

The Aconitum plants are widely used in China as an analgesic, a cardiotonic, and an anti rheumatism treatment. Among all the species Aconitum, the lateral roots of Aconite (Aconitum Camicheali Debx, Fuzi), main roots of Aconite (Chuanwu) and roots of Aconitum kusnezoffii Reichb (Caowu) are the three kinds of plant medicines that are collected in Chinese Pharmacopoeia, and some of other Aconitum plants have been used as folk medicine. It is well known that diester diterpenoid aconitine (DDA) and its analogues isolated from Aconitum plants contribute to the bioactivity and the high toxicity for the heart and the central nervous system. Fortunately, aconitines are heat-unstable and will be conversed into less toxic monoester diterpenoid alkaloids (MDA) or lipo-alkaloids after processing [1], therefore, the amounts of highly toxic aconitine are lower than those of monoester diterpenoid alkaloids in processed aconite and proprietary Chinese medicines (PCMs).

For monitoring the possible toxicity of Chinese medicines, high-performance liquid chromatography (HPLC) has been frequently used for quantification analysis of aconitines. Generally, only aconitine, mesaconitine and hypaconitine three standards could be purchased and most of research was limited in these 3 alkaloids [2]. Therefore, qualitative analysis is also essential for PCM besides quantitative analysis. In contrast to chromatographic methods, matrix-assisted laser desorption time-of-flight mass spectrometry (MALDI-TOF-MS) determines the molecular mass of alkaloids, which represents an inherent physical property and is feasible for high-throughput analysis of different samples containing aconitines.

In this work, we have analyzed aconitum alkaloids in 19 kinds PCMs and found that hypaconitine is the dominant DDA in the 12 oral PCMs, which is somewhat different from previous quantitative results of aconitines in PCM reported by using HPLC method [3]. These PCMs include Guifudihuangwan (GFDHW), Fuzilizhongwan (FZLZW), Jinkuishenqiwan(JKSQW), Xiaohuoluowan (XHLW), Sanhanhuoluowan (SHHLW), Zuifengtouguwan (ZFTGW), Narusanwewan (NRSWW), Muguawan (MGW), Xiaojinwan (XJW), Haimabushenwan (HMBSW, Dahuoluowan (DHLW), Panlongqipian (PLQP), Fufangxuelianjiaonang (FFXLJN), Diedazhentonggao (DDZTG), Tiebangcuizhitonggao (TBCZTG), Guzengshengzhentonggao (GZSZTG), Shexiangzuifenggao (SXZFG), Zhentonglingding (ZTLD) and Shangtongding (STD).

On the other hand, the detoxification mechanism of aconite in concoction is far away from clear. For example, acidity is one of the factors to influence the hydrolysis of aconitines [4]. Here we have concocted Fuzi with 7 others herbal Medicines and analyzed the alkaloids in the concoction by MALDI-TOF-MS. We have found that acidity is not the only factor that affects the hydrolysis reaction of DDAs as well as the amounts of aconitines because of the complexity of Chinese medicine.

1.1 Experimental

Prepared root of aconite and all proprietary Chinese medicine (PCM) were purchased from drug store; 5g dried and powered aconite root or PCM were soaked with 60 mL ethanol for 48 h at room temperature, and the resulting solution of alkaloids was diluted with 50% ethanol for further analysis of MALDI-TOF.

1.2 Mass spectrometry

All experiments were performed using a Voyager DE-STR MALDI-TOF mass spectrometer (Applied Biosystems) The Voyager DE STR was operated in a positive reflector mode with the following parameters: acquisition mass range, 400-1000 Da; accelerating voltage, 20,000 V; grid voltage, 73%; mirror voltage ratio, 1.14; guide wire, 0.01%; low mass gate set at 300; extraction delay time, 150 ns; and the laser power attenuator set at 2700, total 100 shots/spectrum. Matrix solution was prepared by dissolving 8mg of α-cyano-4-hydroxycinnamic acid (CHCA) in 1 ml of 1:1 mixture of acetonitrile and 0.1% trifluoroacetic acid.

2. Results and discussions

2.1 The MALDI-TOF analysis of nineteen kinds of PCM

For aconitum alkaloids, protonated molecules (M+H) $^+$ were observed by MALDI-MS in positive ion mode. The structures of aconitum alkaloids are very similar and it is reasonable to assume that they have similar ionization efficiencies [5]. The alkaloids of 13 oral administration pills or tablets that using prepared aconite roots have been analyzed firstly. As shown in Fig.1-Fig.13, benzoylhypaconine (BHA, m/z 574), benzoylmesaconine (BMA, m/z 590) and benzoylaconine (BAC, m/z 604) were the major components, hypaconitine (HA, m/z 616) is the most main diester alkaloids, additionally, deoxyaconitine (DA, m/z 630), mesaconitine (MA, mz/ 632) and aconitine (AC, m/z 646) can also be observed. In all 13 PCMs, HMBSW exhibit the most high relative abundance of the highly toxic diester aconitines (Fig.12), however, different with some previous report that obtained by high performance liquid chromatography [3], it is HA other than MA is the dominant aconitine, in addition, 10-OH-MA (m/z 648) and 10-OH-AC (m/z 662) have been detected also. We believe our result is reasonable because MA is more prone to be hydrolyzed to BMA after boiling [1] and HA is the main aconitine in prepared aconite roots [5]. An exception is Daguoluowan, only BMA was detected with a weak signal. According to the ancient Chinese concept of Yin-Yang, Aconite is one of the most important herbal medicines that related Yang deficiency and relieving pain, so a certain amount of monoester aconitum alkaloids and diester alkaloids is essential for the treatment. Generally, in the mass region of m/z 400-500, talatizidine, talatisamine, neoline, fuziline and 14-acetyl- talatisamine can be detected at m/z 408, m/z422, m/z 438, m/z 545 and m/z 464 respectively owing to they also exist in prepared Fuzi [6]. Secondly, for the vitro dosage form such as plaster or tincture, some obvious changes have been observed. Aconitine at m/z 646 has been detected as the main alkaloids in DDZTG (Fig.14), TBCZTG (Fig.15), GZSZTG (Fig.16), and STD (Fig.17); thirdly, mesaconitine is the most high content alkaloids in SXZFG (Fig.18); fourthly, high abundance of HA, DA, MA and AC have been detected in ZTLD.

In sum, because of the high ionization efficiency of alkaloids, aconitines and their hydrolysis products can be easily analyzed by MALDI-TOF after extracted by chloroform, thus, MALDI-TOF mass spectrometry provides a rapid, sensitive, simple and specific method for the qualitative analysis of alkaloids mixtures in complex systems such as proprietary Chinese. By comparing the relative abundance of DDA and MDA, we can further acquire relatively quantitative information of aconitum alkaloids. Actually, as an analysis method that based on mass isolation, mass spectrometry method is especially suit for the well-known research system such as aconitum alkaloids.

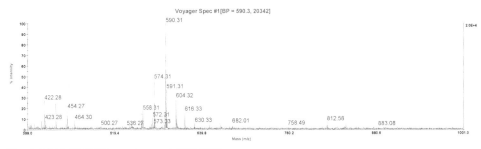

Fig. 1. MALDI-TOF spectrum of GFDHW

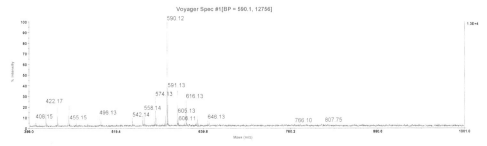

Fig. 2. MALDI-TOF spectrum of FZLZW

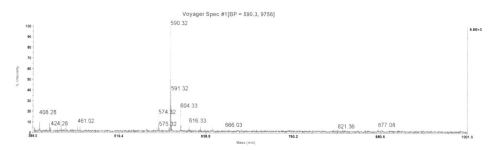

Fig. 3. MALDI-TOF spectrum of JKSQW

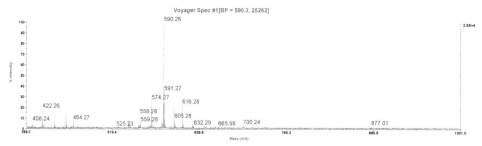

Fig. 4. MALDI-TOF spectrum of XHLW

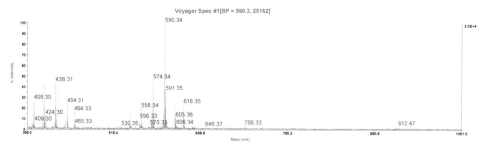

Fig. 5. MALDI-TOF spectrum of SHLLW

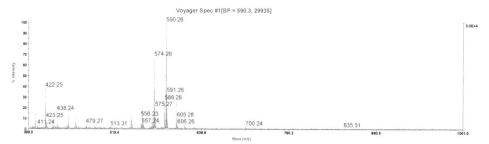

Fig. 6. MALDI-TOF spectrum of ZFTGW

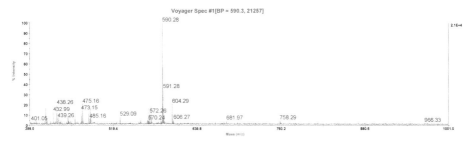

Fig. 7. MALDI-TOF spectrum of NRSWW

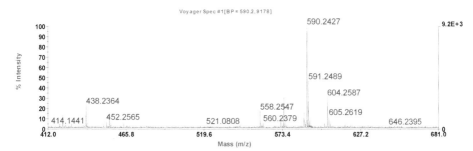

Fig. 8. MALDI-TOF spectrum of MGW

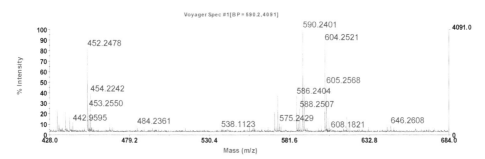

Fig. 9. MALDI-TOF spectrum of PLQP

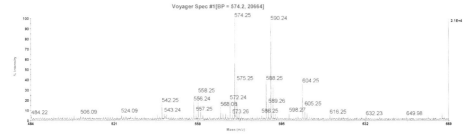

Fig. 10. MALDI-TOF spectrum of XJW

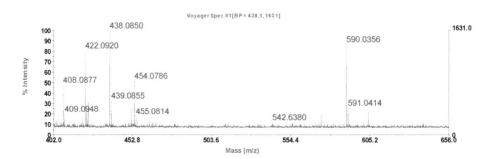

Fig. 11. MALDI-TOF spectrum of FFXLJN

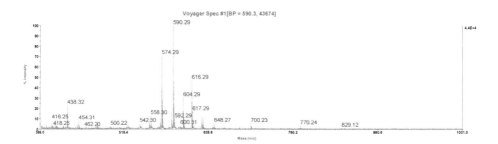

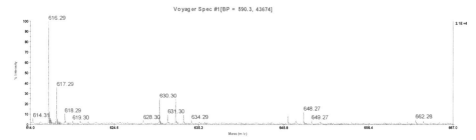

Fig. 12. MALDI-TOF spectrum of HMBSW

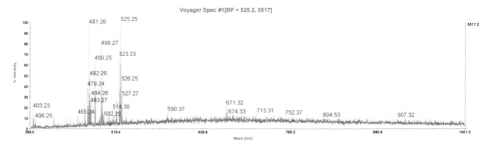

Fig. 13. MALDI-TOF spectrum of DHLW

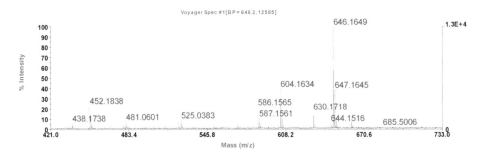

Fig. 14. MALDI-TOF spectrum of DDZTG

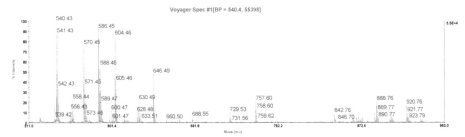

Fig. 15. MALDI-TOF spectrum of TBCZTG

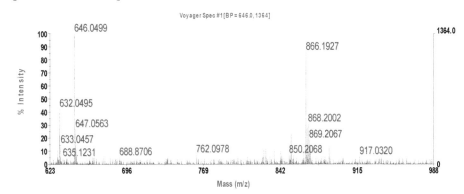

Fig. 16. MALDI-TOF spectrum of GZSZTG

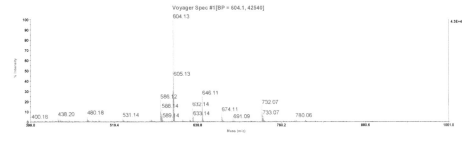

Fig. 17. MALDI-TOF spectrum of STD

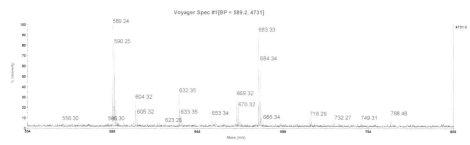

Fig. 18. MALDI-TOF spectrum of SXZFG

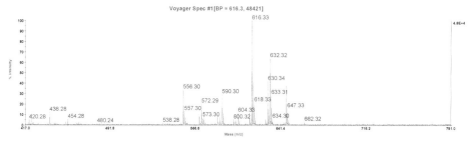

Fig. 19. MALDI-TOF spectrum of ZTLD

2.2 The MALDI-TOF analysis of alkaloids in the concoction of aconite roots with other Chinese medicine

To some extent, the combinational principles of Fuzi can be explained by the chemical reactions in the concoction, namely, DDA will be changed to MDA and lipo-alkaloids in boiling water [1]. In addition, the acidity of solution has played an important role for these chemical reactions and high acidity will inhibit the hydrolysis of aconitines [4]. However, it is still not clear that whether the acidity is the only factor for the amounts of aconitines in concoction. In this study, we have selected 7 kinds of Chinese medicines of which decoction are acidic to answer this question.

As shown in Table 1, the pH value of the Fuzi decoction is 4.73; the pH value of the decoction of Radix Glycyrrhizae is 5.54, the pH value of other 6 kinds of herbal medicine ranged from 3 to 4. The pH value of the concoction of aconite with others is similar with those of decoction.

2.3 The MALDI-TOF analysis of alkaloids in prepared Fuzi and the decoction of Fuzi

The MALDI-TOF spectrum of the ethanolic extract of prepared Fuzi provides a profile of the alkaloids. BHA, BMA and BAC are the main alkaloids in Prepared Fuzi, HA, DA, MA and 10-OH-AC has been observed as the main aconitines (Fig.20). After decocting, the relative amounts of highly toxic aconitines have been reduced because they are heat-unstable [5,6].

2.4 The MALDI-TOF analysis of alksloids in the concoction of Fuzi with Radix Glycyrrhizae, Lonicera nitida and Rhizoma Chuanxiong

It is well known that Radix Glycyrrhiza has the detoxify effect, so it is reasonable that almost no aconitines has been detected in the concoction of Fuzi with it except for low abundant

HA at m/z 616 (Fig.22). However, to our surprise, in the concoction of Fuzi with Lonicera nitida or Rhizoma Chuanxiong (Fig.23 and Fig.24), the relative intensity of aconitines is also low and other aconitines have been detected at noice lowel. Since the pH value of the concoction of Fuzi with Lonicera nitida and Rhizoma Chuanxiong is respective 3.54 and 3,75, these results have suggest that the acidity of concoction is not the only factor that effect the hydrolysis reactions of aconitines.

Aconite roots	4.73
Radix Glycyrrhizae (甘草)	5.54
Lonicera nitida (金银花)	3.54
Crateagus pinnatifida (山楂)	3.32
Chaenomeles sinensis (木瓜)	3.95
Rhizoma Chuanxiong (川穹)	3.75
Herba Potulacae Oleraceae (马齿苋)	3.84
Galla Chinensis (五倍子)	3.63
Aconite roots+ Radix Glycyrrhizae (A+RG)	5.12
Aconite roots+ Lonicera nitida (A+LN)	3.22
Aconite roots+ Crateagus pinnatifida (A+CP)	3.26
Aconite roots+ Chaenomeles sinensis (A+CS)	3.69
Aconite roots+ Rhizoma Chuanxiong (A+RC)	4.10
Aconite roots+ Herba Potulacae Oleraceae (A+HPO)	3.87
Aconite roots+ Galla Chinensis (A+GC)	3.65

Table 1. The pH value of the decoction of eight kinds of Chinese Medicine

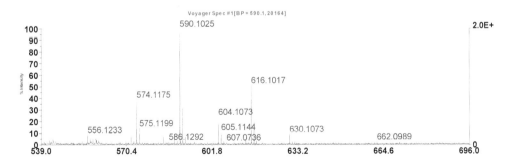

Fig. 20. MALDI-TOF spectrum of the ethanol extract of prepared Fuzi

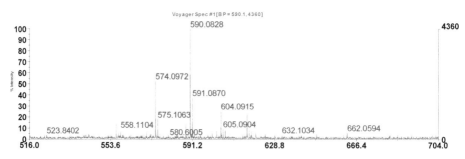

Fig. 21. MALDI-TOF spectrum of the decoction of prepared Fuzi

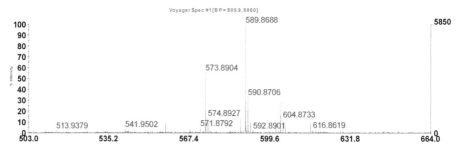

Fig. 22. MALDI-TOF spectrum of the concoction of prepared Fuzi with Radix Glycyrrhizae

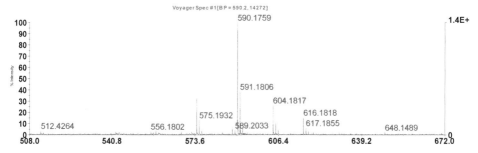

Fig. 23. MALDI-TOF spectrum of the concoction of prepared Fuzi with Lonicera nitida

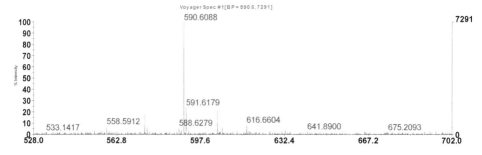

Fig. 24. MALDI-TOF spectrum of the concoction of prepared Fuzi with Rhizoma Chuanxiong

2.5 The MALDI-TOF analysis of alkaloids in the concoction of Fuzi with other 4 kinds of acidic herbal medicines

As shown in Fig.25-Fig.28, when Fuzi was concocted with Crateagus pinnatifida, Galla Chinensis, Chaenomeles sinensis or Herba Potulacae Oleraceae respectively, the relative amounts of DDA were higher that those in decoction, which suggested that these four herbal medicines should not be concocted with Fuzi. However, owing to the point-to-point difference of MALDI source, a statistical analysis is necessary. All the results have been shown in Table 3-Table 11 and summarized in Table 12.

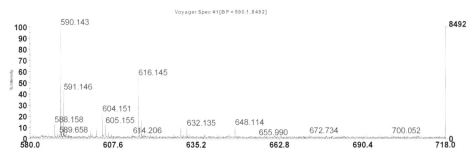

Fig. 25. MALDI-TOF spectrum of the concoction of prepared Fuzi with Crateagus pinnatifida

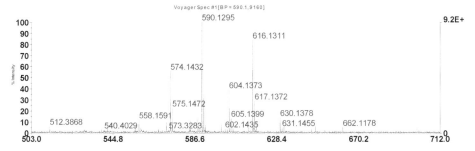

Fig. 26. MALDI-TOF spectrum of the concoction of prepared Fuzi with Galla Chinensis

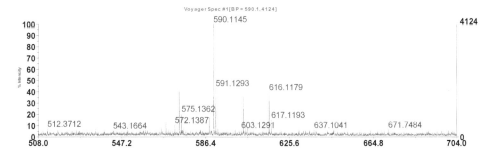

Fig. 27. MALDI-TOF spectrum of the concoction of prepared Fuzi with Chaenomeles sinensis

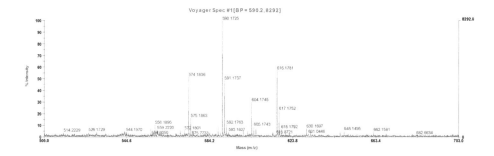

Fig. 28. MALDI-TOF spectrum of the concoction of prepared Fuzi with Herba Potulacae Oleraceae

Aconitum alkaloids	Relative intensities							Average value	RSD
	1	2	3	4	5	6	7		
Benzoylhypaconine (m/z574)	25.19	36.56	38.83	37.19	30.25	28.09	36.77	33.27	5.33
Benzoylmesaconine (m/z590)	100	100	100	100	100	100	100	100	0.00
Benzoylaconine (m/z604)	23.65	39.82	24.04	32.98	39.86	15.10	17.85	27.61	10.07
Hypaconitine (m/z616)	22.16	21.88	51.37	30.43	41.87	50.18	45.13	37.57	12.65
Deoxyaconitine (m/z630)	3.16	5.69	9.14	8.97	10.82	9.43	5.91	7.59	2.71
Mesaconitine (m/z632)	2.63	3.78	3.58	3.24	4.94	8.27	6.22	4.67	1.98
Aconitine (m/z646)	0.00	4.78	2.27	2.98	11.76	6.99	2.74	4.50	3.86
10-OH-mesaconitine (m/z648)	1.43	4.77	1.08	2.48	11.40	7.15	2.93	4.46	3.71
10-OH-aconitine (m/z662)	0.00	3.98	2.67	4.57	4.37	10.39	4.18	4.31	3.12

Table 3. The average value of relative intestines of the detected peaks from prepared Fuzi for seven times

Aconitum alkaloids	Relative intestines							Average value	RSD
	1	2	3	4	5	6	7		
Benzoylhypaconine (m/z574)	65.08	54.99	52.73	56.36	61.57	60.03	74.30	60.72	7.31
Benzoylmesaconine (m/z590)	100	100	100	100	100	100	100	100	0.00
Benzoylaconine (m/z604)	28.22	29.91	25.67	21.63	25.71	28.18	23.78	26.16	2.86
Hypaconitine (m/z616)	38.76	31.93	22.43	22.25	30.74	38.88	22.85	29.69	7.39
Deoxyaconitine (m/z630)	4.12	5.00	3.00	11.71	4.14	3.98	6.82	5.54	2.97
Mesaconitine (m/z632)	2.44	3.20	4.06	6.51	2.26	2.80	6.68	3.99	1.87
Aconitine (m/z646)	0.00	3.45	2.87	4.57	2.66	0.00	6.21	2.82	2.27
10-OH-mesaconitine (m/z648)	0.00	3.65	4.52	7.91	2.11	1.71	7.20	3.87	2.90
10-OH-aconitine (m/z662)	0.00	0.00	5.87	3.41	0.00	2.85	7.43	2.79	3.02

Table 4. The average value of relative intetie of the detected peaks from the detection of Fuzi for seven times

Aconitum alkaloids	Relative intestines							Average value	RSD
	1	2	3	4	5	6	7		
Benzoylhypaconine (m/z574)	57.73	40.16	40.63	51.59	55.97	53.19	52.16	50.20	7.04
Benzoylmesaconine (m/z590)	100	100	100	100	100	100	100	100	0
Benzoylaconine (m/z604)	23.91	24.03	21.44	38.33	28.22	28.27	36.77	28.71	6.53
Hypaconitine (m/z616)	31.67	5.56	11.75	28.82	9.85	17.67	23.82	18.45	9.97
Deoxyaconitine (m/z630)	9.91	0	0	8.33	0	0	2.62	2.98	4.33
Mesaconitine (m/z632)	8.08	0	0	3.7	0	0	6.08	2.55	3.42
Aconitine (m/z646)	5.51	1.91	2.13	2.21	0	0	4.13	2.27	2.02
10-OH-mesaconitine (m/z648)	6.71	0	1.63	2.21	0	0	5.65	2.31	2.80
10-OH-aconitine (m/z662)	4.4	0	2.2	2.5	0	0	10.13	2.75	3.66

Table 5. The average value of relative intestines of the detected peaks from the concoction of Fuzi with Radix Glycyrrhiza for seven times

Aconitum alkaloids	Relative intestines						Average value	RSD
	1	2	3	4	5	6		
Benzoylhypaconine (m/z574)	32.81	44.01	24.66	32.52	30.84	38.10	33.82	6.60
Benzoylmesaconine (m/z590)	100	100	100	100	100	100	100	0.00
Benzoylaconine (m/z604)	26.40	23.12	25.97	21.72	26.86	26.06	25.02	2.09
Hypaconitine (m/z616)	15.43	11.11	12.24	23.16	12.01	13.42	14.56	4.47
Deoxyaconitine (m/z630)	2.59	1.74	0.00	3.67	0.00	2.40	1.73	1.48
Mesaconitine (m/z632)	0.00	4.72	2.68	3.75	0.00	2.90	2.34	1.95
Aconitine (m/z646)	0.00	3.97	0.00	2.95	0.00	0.00	1.15	1.82
10-OH-mesaconitine (m/z648)	2.33	9.11	0.00	3.49	0.00	2.71	2.94	3.35
10-OH-aconitine (m/z662)	0.00	5.40	0.00	2.66	0.00	0.00	1.34	2.25

Table 6. The average value of relative intestines of the detected peaks from the concocction of Fuzi with Lonicera nitida for six times

Aconitum alkaloids	Relative intestines			Average value	RSD
	1	2	3		
Benzoylhypaconine (m/z574)	37.02	17.91	21.42	25.45	10.17
Benzoylmesaconine (m/z590)	100.00	100.00	100.00	100.00	0.00
Benzoylaconine (m/z604)	22.79	21.14	15.60	19.84	3.77
Hypaconitine (m/z616)	19.69	8.84	15.17	14.57	5.45
Deoxyaconitine (m/z630)	0.00	0.00	0.00	0.00	0.00
Mesaconitine (m/z632)	2.98	5.20	3.90	4.03	1.12
Aconitine (m/z646)	0.00	0.00	0.00	0.00	0.00
10-OH-mesaconitine (m/z648)	3.61	1.76	0.00	1.79	1.81
10-OH-aconitine (m/z662)	0.00	0.00	1.76	0.59	1.02

Table 7. The average value of relative intestines of the detected peaks from the concocction of Fuzi with Rhizoma Chuanxiong for three times

Aconitum alkaloids	Relative intestines						Average value	RSD
	1	2	3	4	5	6		
Benzoylhypaconine (m/z574)	35.39	38.94	21.33	40.68	40.24	28.24	34.14	7.79
Benzoylmesaconine (m/z590)	100.00	100.00	100.00	100.00	100.00	100.00	100.00	0.00
Benzoylaconine (m/z604)	22.79	18.42	21.20	22.46	21.01	24.09	21.66	1.95
Hypaconitine (m/z616)	54.98	56.09	38.57	80.39	51.51	53.42	55.83	13.61
Deoxyaconitine (m/z630)	9.86	5.56	8.57	7.49	13.16	12.54	9.53	2.94
Mesaconitine (m/z632)	9.92	8.74	11.58	10.90	6.60	9.80	9.59	1.76
Aconitine (m/z646)	3.86	3.56	2.42	4.54	3.85	4.56	3.80	0.79
10-OH-mesaconitine (m/z648)	10.46	6.37	5.08	6.64	6.01	7.20	6.96	1.85
10-OH-aconitine (m/z662)	3.71	4.33	0.00	3.62	4.71	3.06	3.24	1.69

Table 8. The average value of relative intestines of the detected peaks from the concocction of Fuzi with Crateagus pinnatifida for six times

Aconitum alkaloids	Relative intestines							Average value	RSD
	1	2	3	4	5	6	7		
Benzoylhypaconine (m/z574)	54.45	77.33	50.76	64.26	55.34	51.57	75.68	61.34	11.26
Benzoylmesaconine (m/z590)	89.18	98.06	84.35	84.77	100	100	81.59	91.14	8.03
Benzoylaconine (m/z604)	41.47	36.27	25.70	59.23	38.73	44.37	39.13	40.70	10.07
Hypaconitine (m/z616)	100	100	100	100	83.70	71.44	100	93.59	11.50
Deoxyaconitine (m/z630)	11.65	13.77	12.18	27.91	13.89	7.47	11.48	14.05	6.47
Mesaconitine (m/z632)	13.28	8.18	8.29	5.87	6.38	3.81	8.90	7.82	2.98
Aconitine (m/z646)	3.11	4.25	9.76	10.47	3.46	0.00	8.90	5.71	4.00
10-OH-mesaconitine (m/z648)	3.96	4.78	10.82	13.53	6.57	6.87	10.06	8.08	3.48
10-OH-aconitine (m/z662)	6.98	7.57	11.76	11.32	4.93	4.54	8.15	7.89	2.82

Table 9. The average value of relative intestines of the detected peaks from the concocction of Fuzi with Galla Chinensis for seven times

Aconitum alkaloids	Relative intestines							Average value	RSD
	1	2	3	4	5	6	7		
Benzoylhypaconine (m/z574)	41.22	33.60	25.68	29.67	48.78	44.39	33.30	36.66	8.34
Benzoylmesaconine (m/z590)	1000	100	100	100	1000	100	100	100	0.00
Benzoylaconine (m/z604)	37.32	23.85	39.65	27.92	27.20	18.33	33.73	29.71	7.60
Hypaconitine (m/z616)	39.79	15.07	24.40	26.92	24.88	15.75	19.98	23.83	8.39
Deoxyaconitine (m/z630)	7.76	2.94	9.67	6.85	4.92	6.86	8.78	6.83	2.29
Mesaconitine (m/z632)	5.29	2.26	5.82	6.61	4.02	3.64	2.73	4.34	1.62
Aconitine (m/z646)	6.28	2.90	7.55	9.68	4.84	3.85	2.00	5.30	2.71
10-OH-mesaconitine (m/z648)	4.97	2.61	6.57	7.25	6.26	5.04	3.95	5.24	1.61
10-OH-aconitine (m/z662)	3.59	2.84	5.97	8.17	5.83	2.78	4.09	4.75	1.99

Table 10. The average value of relative intestines of the detected peaks from the concocction of Fuzi with Chaenomeles sinensis for seven times

Aconitum alkaloids	Relative intestines					Average value	RSD
	1	2	3	4	5		
Benzoylhypaconine (m/z574)	30.49	51.63	20.61	43.12	30.06	35.18	12.19
Benzoylmesaconine (m/z590)	100	100	100	100	100	100	0.00
Benzoylaconine (m/z604)	15.28	30.10	18.81	19.65	18.81	20.53	5.61
Hypaconitine (m/z616)	33.70	57.20	34.36	92.86	46.45	52.91	24.34
Deoxyaconitine (m/z630)	5.85	7.59	9.45	8.27	14.36	9.10	3.21
Mesaconitine (m/z632)	5.56	5.71	4.61	7.46	10.20	6.71	2.21
Aconitine (m/z646)	0.00	4.29	5.57	4.02	4.30	3.64	2.12
10-OH-mesaconitine (m/z648)	3.21	5.45	5.76	4.79	3.32	4.51	1.19
10-OH-aconitine (m/z662)	2.95	4.55	6.10	5.93	4.16	4.74	1.31

Table 11. The average value of relative intestines of the detected peaks from the concoction of Fuzi with Herbal Potulacae Oleraceae for five times

Concoction	Relative Intensities								
	BHA	BMA	BAC	HA	DA	MA	AC	10-OH-MA	10-OH-AC
Fuzi	33.27±5.33	100	27.6±10.07	37.57±12.65	7.59±12.65	4.76±1.98	4.50±3.86	4.46±3.71	4.31±3.12
Fuzi decoction	60.72±7.31	100	26.16±2.86	29.69±2.86	5.54±2.97	3.99±1.87	2.82±2.90	3.87±2.90	2.79±3.02
Concoction of A+RG	50.20±7.04	100	28.71±6.53	18.45±9.97	2.98±4.33	2.55±3.42	2.27±2.02	2.31±2.80	2.75±3.66
Concoction of A+LN	33.82±6.60	100	25.02±2.09	14.56±4.47	1.73±1.48	2.34±1.95	1.15±1.82	2.94±3.35	1.34±2.25
Concoction of A+RC	25.4±10.17	100	19.84±3.77	14.57±5.45	0	4.03±1.12	0	1.79±1.81	0.59±1.02
Concoction of A+CS	36.66±8.34	100	29.71±7.60	23.83±8.39	6.83±2.29	4.34±1.62	5.30±2.71	5.24±1.61	4.75±1.99
Concoction of A+GC	61.3±11.26	91.1±8.03	40.7±10.07	93.56±11.50	14.05±6.47	7.82±2.98	5.71±4.00	8.08±3.48	7.89±2.82
Concoction of A+CP	34.14±7.79	100	21.66±1.95	55.83±13.61	9.53±2.94	9.59±1.76	3.80±0.79	3.69±1.85	3.24±1.69
Concoction of A+HPO	35.1±12.19	100	20.53±5.61	52.91±24.34	9.10±3.21	6.71±2.21	3.64±2.12	4.51±1.19	4.74±1.31

Table 12. The average value of relative intestines of the detected peaks from the concocction and decoction of Fuzi

Taken the ethanol extract of Fuzi as a standard, we will find that the DDAs have been reduced after decocting or concocting with Radix Glycyrrhizae, Lonicera nitida, Rhizoma Chuanxiong or Chaenomeles sinensis, respectively. Coincidentally, both Radix Glycyrrhizae and Lonicera nitida is the most popular medicine for detoxification. However, when Fuzi has been concocted with Crateagus pinnatifida, Galla Chinensis or Herba Potulacae Oleraceae, the relative amounts of all DDAs, especially of hypaconitine, have been increased significantly despite that the pH value of Lonicera nitida is smaller than that of Galla Chinensis and Herba Potulacae Oleraceae. The results have indicated that the detoxification mechanism of traditional Chinese medicine such as Fuzi is very complex and can not be explained by a simple reason such as pH value. In addition, our studies have suggested that although Crateagus pinnatifida, Galla Chinensis and Herba Potulacae Oleraceae is beyond the list that should not be combined with aconite according to traditional Chinese theory or experience, but they do increase the toxicity of Fuzi.

3. References

[1] Yong Wang, Lei Shi, Fengrui Song, Zhiqiang Liu and Shuying Li. Exploring the reaction of ester exchange for diester-diterpenoid alkaloids in the process of decocting aconite by electrospray ionization tandem mass spectrometry. Rapid Commun. Mass Spectrom, 2003, 17(4), 279-284

[2] Judith Singhuber, Ming Zhua, Sonja Prinz and Brigitte Kopp. Aconitum in Traditional Chinese Medicine—A valuable drug or an unpredictable risk? Journal of Ethnopharmacology, 2009, 126 , 18–30

[3] Ying Xie, Zhi Hong Jiang , Hua Zhoua, Hong Xi Xu, Liang Liu. Simultaneous determination of six Aconitum alkaloids in proprietary Chinese medicines by high-performance liquid chromatography. Journal of Chromatography A, 2005, 1093, 195–203

[4] Yong Wang, Fengrui Song, Zhiqiang Liu and Shuying Li. Study on the combination principles about aconite roots by electrospray ionization mass spectrometry. Acta Pharmaceutica Sinica (in Chinese).2003, 38(6): 451 - 454

[5] Yong Wang, Lei Shi, Dongming Jin, Fengrui Song, Zhiqiang Liu and Shuying Li. Stripping and hydrolyzing balance of aconitic alkaloids in processing of Sini Decoction. Chinese Traditional and Herbal Drugs. (in Chinese), 2003, 34(4): 311-314

[6] JiangshanWang, Rob van der Heijden, Gerwin Spijksma, Theo Reijmers, MeiWang, Guowang Xua, Thomas Hankemeier and Jan van der Greef. Alkaloid profiling of the Chinese herbal medicine Fuzi by combination of matrix-assisted laser desorption ionization mass spectrometry with liquid chromatography–mass spectrometry. Journal of Chromatography A, 2009, 1216 2169–2178

10

Study on Metabolism of Natural Medical Components *In Vivo*: Metabolism Study in Rat After Oral Administration of Rhubarb Decoction and Characterization, Identification of the Rat Metabolite of *Scutellaria baicalensis*

Chenggang Huang et al.[*]

Shanghai Institute of Materia Medica, Chinese Academy of Sciences, Shanghai, China

1. Introduction

Rheum palmatum L., one of the commonly used Traditional Chinese Medicines (TCMs), which is called Dahuang in Chinese, has been successfully used in China for thousands of years. The crude material of *R. palmatum* called rhubarb was widely used as laxative to treat constipation. Furthermore, it has various other pharmacological actions, such as antibacterial [1, 2], anti-inflammatory [3, 4], antiviral [5], anti-angiogenic [6], antioxidative [7], immunomodulatory [8], protecting effects in rat with chronic renal failure [9] and anti-diabetic effects on diabetic mice [10]. Although many investigations have been conducted in the fields of pharmacology, clinical trials, and phytochemistry about rhubarb, researchers still do not know what its effective constituents are, how many compounds are absorbed into blood after intragastric administration of the decoction, and what the fate of the decoction in the body is. The limited knowledge about the metabolism of rhubarb decoction restricts the deeper pharmacological mechanism study and wider clinical use of rhubarb.

It was well accepted that TCMs expressed its effects through multi-components and multi-targets. Rapid, sensitive and selective analytical method is needed to simultaneous determine of multiple components of TCMs in biological matrix with low concentrations. In recent years, HPLC/ESI/MS[n] has been proved to be a modern and powerful method for the identification of compounds in biosamples or TCM extracts [11, 12]. Metabolism of rhubarb has been reported [13], but data on pharmacokinetics are scanty. So, our interest was to utilize a solid phase extraction (SPE) and HPLC/ESI/MS[n] techniques for the detection of potentially active compounds in urine, plasma and tissue samples and for the

[*] Bin Wu[1], Shuyun Liu[1,2], Shuang Liu[3], Zhixiong Li[1], Longhai Jian[4], Yihong Tang[1], Zhaolin Sun[1] and Ke Wang[4]

[1]*Shanghai Institute of Materia Medica, Chinese Academy of Sciences, Shanghai, China*
[2]*Shuguang Hospital, Shanghai University of Traditional Chinese Medicine, Shanghai, China*
[3]*Haerbin University of Commerce, Haerbin, China*
[4]*Shanghai Institute for Food and Drug Control, Shanghai, China*

pharmacokinetic study of rhubarb. Total of 39 compounds were identified as absorbed bioactive constituents. The excretion of M22 and M39 reached more than 1000 μg in urine samples after intragastric administration of the decoction.

2. Experiments

2.1 Chemicals and materials

Standards of the rhapontin, aloe-emodin, chrysophanol, emodin, rheochrysidin and rhein were obtained from the National Institute for the Control of Pharmaceutical and Biological Products (NICPBP) (Beijing, China). The plasma, urine and tissue samples were extracted using Supelco™ LC-18 solid-phase extraction (SPE) tubes (1ml/100mg, USA). Acetonitrile (HPLC grade) was purchased from the Dikma Company (Dikma, USA). Water was deionized and double distilled. All other chemicals were of analytical grade. Blank rat plasma (drug free) was prepared in our laboratory.

2.2 Equipment

An HPLC-MS system (Agilent 1100, Agilent Technologies, Wilmington, DE, USA) with an electrospray ionization (ESI) ion source was used. The LC/MSD Trap software (version 5.3) was used for data acquisition and processing. An API 4000 triple quadrapole instrument (Applied Biosystems, Toronto, Canada) was used for the mass spectrometric detection using an electrospray ionization (ESI) source in the negative mode. A high-speed bench-top centrifuge (Sorvall ST16, Thermo Fisher Scientific, Germany) was used for centrifuge biological samples.

2.3 Preparation of rhubarb decoction

200 g rhubarb was immersed in 2000 mL distilled water and then refluxed for 1 h at 100°C. The aqueous extract was filtered and the residue was refluxed for 30 min with another 2000 mL of distilled water under the same conditions. The two water extracts were combined and condensed to 200 mL and stored at 4°C until use.

2.4 Standard preparation

The standard of rhapontin, aloe-emodin, chrysophanol, emodin, rheochrysidin and rhein were dissolved in methanol at a concentration of 100 μg/ml to obtain the standard stock solutions.

2.5 Animals

30 male Sprague-Dawley rats (200±20 g) were obtained from the Animal Center of Shanghai Institute of Materia Medica, Shanghai, China. They were kept under standard laboratory conditions (12/12 h light/darkness, 22±2°C room temperature, 50-60% humidity) for one week prior to the experiments. All animal experiments were carried out according to the Guidelines for the Care and Use of Laboratory Animals, and were approved by the Animal Ethics Committee of Shanghai Institute of Materia Medica.

Six male rats were orally administered a single dose of rhubarb decoction at 10 g/kg. After dosing, the rats were housed in separate glass metabolic cages with free access to water. Urine was collected at -8 to 0 h predose and during 0-2, 2-4, 4-6, 6-8, 8-24, 24-36, 36-48 h postdose.

Other 24 male rats were divided into four groups at random. They were used in determining the concentration of rhubarb in blood and tissues. One group of rats was killed predose to provide control blood and tissues for analysis. Other three groups of rats were orally administrated of rhubarb decoction at a dosage of 17.6 g/kg. Six rats each were anesthetized with ether and blood samples were collected from abdominal aorta of the rats at 1.0, 2.0, and 3.0 h after dosing, respectively. The following tissues and organs were collected and weighed at the time of killing for determination of rhubarb concentration: heart (HE), liver (LV), spleen (SP), lung (LU), kidney (KI), brain (BR), small intestine (SI), large intestine (LI), stomach (ST), and testis (TE). The whole tissues were homogenized with PBS to yield final concentration of 20% w/v. All the homogenates were stored at -80°C.

2.6 Extraction of rat biological samples
All samples were centrifuged at 3000×g for 10 min. The supernatants were loaded onto a C18 SPE cartridge. Before use, an SPE column was conditioned and washed with 2 ml of methanol and then 2 ml of deionized water. Then 600 µl of the selected supernatant sample was applied to the SPE well. The SPE well was washed with 1 ml of water, and then the analytes were eluted with 1 ml of methanol. The eluent was evaporated at 37°C under a gentle stream of nitrogen. The dry residue was then reconstituted with 200 µl methanol and vortex-mixed for 20 s. The solution was then centrifuged at 14000×g for 10 min, and an aliquot of 10 µl supernatant was injected into the HPLC/ESI/MS system for analysis.

2.7 HPLC condition
The metabolites of rhubarb decoction were separated on a Grace Apollo C18 reversed-phase column (250 mm×4.6 mm, 5 µm) equipped with an EasyGuard Kit C18 (4×2 mm) guard column. The column was maintained at 25°C. The mobile phase consisted of 0.5% formic acid-water (A) and acetonitrile (B) and was delivered at a flow rate of 1.0 ml/min. The detection wavelengths were set at 190-400 nm. Gradient elution was used as follows: a linear gradient from 35% to 100% B in the first 30 min, followed by 100% B for 10 min, and finally a linear gradient to 35% B at 45 min that was held for 5 min. The total run time was 50 min.

2.8 Mass spectrometry analysis for qualitation
The HPLC system used was an Agilent 1100 series LC/MSD Trap mass spectrometer (Agilent Technologies, Wilmington, DE, USA), connected to an Agilent 1100 HPLC instrument via an electrospray ionization (ESI) source. The LC/MSD Trap software (version 5.3) was used for system operation and data collection. The operating parameters in the negative ion mode were as follows: collision gas, ultra-high purity helium (He); nebulizing gas, high purity nitrogen (N_2); capillary voltage, 3.5 kV; end plate offset, 500 V; nebulizer, 30 psi; drying gas flow rate, 10 l/min; drying gas temp., 350°C. Trap: ICC, target, 30000, max accu. time, 300.00ms, averages, 5. Auto Ms. 4; MS/MS frag. ampl., 1.00V; auto MS (n>2): frag. ampl., 0.77V. Smart frag: start ampl., 30.0%; end ampl., 200%. For full-scan MS analysis, the spectra were recorded in the range of m/z 50-1500.

2.9 Mass spectrometry analysis for quantitation
An API 4000 Qtrap mass spectrometer (Applied Biosystems, Toronto, Canada) equipped with a pneumatically assisted ESI interface was linked with the HPLC system. Initially optimization of the parameters for the ESI/MS and ESI/MS/MS analyses of the standards

and the samples was performed by direct infusion into the ES ionization source. The operating parameters were as follows: negative ion scan mode, curtain gas (CUR) 30 psi, collision gas (CAD) medium, ion source gas 1 (GC1) 45 psi, ion source gas 2 (GC2) 45 psi, ion spray voltage (IS) 5000 V, entrance potential (EP) 10 V, declustering potential (DP) 160 V, collision energy 60 V, collision cell exit potential (CXP) 3 V and temperature (TEM) 350°C.

3. Results

3.1 Optimization of HPLC and MS conditions

To obtain HPLC chromatograms with good separation and peak shape, different mobile phase compositions were screened. Given the acidity of phenolic compounds, it was found that acetonitrile and 0.5% aqueous formic acid were the most suitable eluting solvent system. The proposed method was acceptable as well as adequate for further MS/MS analysis. To acquire maximum sensitivity for most compounds, MS parameters such as spray voltage, capillary temperature, sheath gas and auxiliary gas pressure, source CID, collision gas pressure and collision energy were optimized using methanol extraction of rhubarb decoction by flow injection analysis (FIA). It was found that the negative ion mode was more sensitive than positive ion mode for most of the compounds.

3.2 System suitability

The system suitability test is performed to assure that the analytical method can be executed with the existing HPLC system. A system suitability test of the chromatographic system was performed before each validation run. Five replicate injections of a system suitability/calibration standard (at concentration of 10 µg/ml) were made. Area and retention time relative standard deviation, asymmetry factor t_a and efficiency (as plate number N) for the five injections was determined. For all samples analyses, the asymmetry factor t_a was≤1.4, efficiency≥3000 and area % R.S.D.≤1.0%.

3.3 Optimization of sample preparation

Solid-phase extraction was used as an important step of the sample preparation. Quantitative elution of standard samples from SPE cartridge are apparent after 1.0 ml of methanol. The reproducibility and recovery of solid-phase extraction was determined from five repetitions. The reproducibility expressed as R.S.D. was 0.6-0.9% and recovery was 84.8-97.2% for concentration of 10 µg/ml of standard samples.

3.4 Limits of detection (LOD)/ linearity/accuracy/precision for related substances

The limit of detection of the six standard components (based on a detector signal-to-noise ratio 3:1) was 0.1 µg/ml. The method was found to be linear with correlation coefficients (R^2) of 0.986-0.997 for the six standard components, with slops near unity and y-intercepts near zero for these low-level determinations. Accuracy and precision for the standard components were satisfactory at three concentrations studied. Accuracy and intra-day and inter-day precision of the six standard components were less than 10%.

3.5 Stability of standard and sample solutions

Prepared samples and standards have been shown to be stable for at least 2 weeks when stored refrigerated. Additionally, the standard solutions have been shown to be stable while in use for assays for at least 72 h. The stability of the six standard sample solutions was evaluated after 1 and 2 weeks under refrigerated condition. The results obtained for refrigerated standard solution were 100.1 to 101.2% of the initial concentration for 1 and 2 week time points, respectively. The result for the refrigerated sample solution were 102.1 to 96.8% of its initial concentration after 1 and 2 week's storage, respectively. No degradation products were observed for any of the solutions tested. The standard solutions that had been held at room temperature for 72 h were stable with responses of 98.7-100.9%.

3.6 Fragmentation behavior of the parent compounds

To interpret the mass spectra of the metabolites using the LC/MS^n technique, it is necessary to fully understand the fragmentation behavior of the parent compound. Rhapontin, aloe-emodin, chrysophanol, emodin, rheochrysidin and rhein were selected as representative parent compounds in this study. It was found that the negative ion mode was more sensitive than positive ion mode for most of the compounds with triple quadrupole mass spectrometer, so negative ion mode was chosen. The $HPLC/ESI/MS^n$ spectra of $[M-H]^-$ ion of the six parent compounds were shown in Fig.1. As most of these metabolites remained the structural features of the parent compounds, the analysis of the fragmentation pathways greatly facilitated the identification of metabolites from rhubarb decoction.

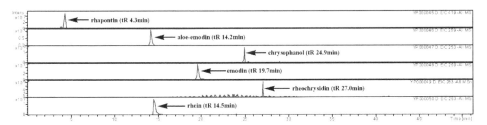

Fig. 1. The HPLC/ESI/MS spectra of the parent compounds

3.7 Identification of metabolites

Possible metabolite structures were considered based on the parent structure and the known metabolic pathways. As for MS detection, the potential metabolites were detected by comparison of the chromatograms of the drug-containing samples with those of blank samples. The retention time of each potential metabolite was ascertained by employing its mass to generate its extracted ion chromatogram (EIC) of the drug-containing sample Compared with blank samples, a total of 39 compounds were detected in extracted ion chromatograms from the drug-containing urine, plasma and tissue samples (Table 1).

The identification of the metabolites and elucidation of their structures were performed mainly based on their MS^n fragmentations. Possible metabolite structures were considered based on the parent structure and the known metabolic pathways. Then, rat urine, plasma and tissue samples after i.g. administration of rhubarb decoction were analyzed and compared with blank samples by $HPLC/ESI/MS^n$ in negative mode. Typical chromatograms resulting from the analysis of various biological samples are shown in Fig.2. Ultimately, the 39 metabolites could be generally divided into three groups: glucoside, glucuronidation and sulfation metabolites. The MS^2 spectra of the 39 compounds were shown in Fig. 3. Metabolite M4, M10 and M20 were selected as examples and the structural elucidations of the other metabolites were carried out similarly. The postulated fragmentation pathways of M4, M10 and M20 were shown in Fig.4.

Metabolites	t_R (min)	[M-H]-	UR	PL	HE	LV	SP	LU	KI	BR	SB	LB	ST	TE	ESI-MS data (% base peak) (m/z)
M1	3.3	591	+	-	-	-	-	-	-	-	-	-	-	-	MS²[591]:253(100),175(14.4) MS³[253]:253(100)
M2	3.3	383	+	-	-	-	-	-	-	-	-	-	-	-	MS²[383]:303(34.7).207(100),113(52.1) MS³[207]:207(52.8),163(100),122(10.8)
M3	3.3	445	-	-	-	-	-	-	-	-	-	-	+	-	MS²[445]:427(8.0),283(100),175(4.5) MS³[283]:283(100),239(17.4)
M4	3.4	479	+	-	-	-	-	-	-	-	-	-	-	-	MS²[479]:303(100),174(20.9) MS³[303]:303(100),259(9.8)
M5	3.4	417	+	-	-	-	+	-	-	-	-	-	-	-	MS²[417]:373(100),330(12.5),241(41.0),175(3.7) MS³[373]:373(9.1),330(100)
M6	3.5	313	+	-	-	-	-	-	-	-	-	-	-	-	MS²[313]:313(12.8),233(100),175(3.6) MS³[233]:233(100),189(11.2)
M7	3.5	459	+	+	-	-	-	-	+	-	-	-	-	-	MS²[459]:283(100),175(3.6) MS³[283]:283(100),239(9.1)
M8	3.7	475	-	-	-	-	-	-	-	-	-	-	+	-	MS²[475]:431(7.2),311(57.0),269(100) MS³[269]:269(100)
M9	3.8	287	+	-	-	-	-	-	-	-	-	-	-	-	MS²[287]:287(8.3),207(100) MS³[207]:207(85.5),163(100)
M10	4.1	621	-	+	-	-	-	-	-	-	-	-	-	-	MS²[621]:575(3.5),445(100),269(21.3) MS³[445]:311(7.8),269(100)
M11	4.1	375	-	-	+	-	-	-	-	-	-	-	-	-	MS²[375]:332(18.8),243(100) MS³[243]:243(100)
M12	4.2	445	+	-	-	-	-	-	-	-	-	-	-	-	MS²[445]:269(100),175(2.1) MS³[269]:269(100)
M13	4.2	268	+	-	+	-	-	-	+	-	-	-	-	-	MS²[269]:189(100)
M14	4.3	417	+	+	-	-	-	-	-	-	-	-	-	-	MS²[417]:399(8.1),241(5.1),175 (100) MS³[175]:113(100)
M15	4.5	435	-	-	-	-	-	-	-	-	-	-	+	-	MS²[435]:273(100),167(4.3) MS³[273]:273(100),167(53.0)
M16	4.6	431	-	-	-	-	-	-	-	-	-	-	+	-	MS²[431]:269(100) MS³[269]:269(100)
M17	4.6	459	+	-	-	-	-	-	-	-	-	-	+	-	MS²[459]:283(100) MS³[283]:283(100),257(1.9)
M18	4.7	297	+	+	+	-	-	-	+	+	-	-	-	-	MS²[297]:175(83.7),113(100) MS³[113]:95(80.0),85(100)
M19	4.9	401	-	+	-	+	-	+	+	-	+	-	-	-	MS²[401]:358(100),296(4.2),225(32.4),174(60.5) MS³[358]:313(13.5),174(100)
M20	5.2	525	-	+	-	-	-	-	-	-	-	-	-	-	MS²[525]:445(100),349(20.3),269(73.5) MS³[445]:269(100)
M21	5.3	349	+	-	-	-	-	-	-	-	-	-	-	-	MS²[349]:269(100) MS³[269]:269(100),240(5.8)
M22	5.3	363	+	-	-	-	-	-	-	-	-	-	-	-	MS²[363]:283(100) MS³[283]:283(100),239(7.0)
M23	5.4	433	-	+	-	-	-	-	-	-	-	-	-	-	MS²[433]:415(7.4),257(100),175(60.5) MS³[257]:257(100)
M24	5.6	321	-	+	+	+	-	-	-	-	-	-	+	-	MS²[321]:241(100),121(87.7) MS³[241]:241(12.3),121(100)
M25	6.0	473	-	+	-	-	-	-	-	-	-	-	-	-	MS²[473]:426(6.2),335(9.5),297(87.7),253(100) MS³[253]:253(100)

ID	tR	[M-H]													MS^n data
M26	6.0	363	+	+	+	-	-	-	+	-	-	-	-	-	MS^2[363]:283(100) MS^3[283]:283(100),239(4.7)
M27	6.3	407	-	-	-	-	-	-	-	-	-	-	+	-	MS^2[407]:369(18.7),245(100) MS^3[245]:245(100),230(50.4)
M28	6.6	431	-	-	-	-	-	-	-	-	-	-	+	-	MS^2[431]:340(3.3),269(100) MS^3[269]:269(100)
M29	6.6	429	+	+	-	-	-	-	+	-	-	-	-	-	MS^2[429]:253(100),175(6.8) MS^3[253]:253(100)
M30	6.8	415	-	-	-	-	-	-	-	-	-	-	+	-	MS^2[415]:253(100) MS^3[253]:253(100)
M31	7.0	429	+	+	+	+	-	+	+	-	-	-	-	-	MS^2[429]:253(100),175(6.8) MS^3[253]:253(100)
M32	8.2	313	-	-	-	-	-	-	-	-	-	-	+	-	MS^2[313]:269(100),201(5.4) MS^3[269]:269(100)
M33	8.4	445	+	+	+	+	-	-	+	-	-	-	-	-	MS^2[445]:269(100) MS^3[269]:269(100)
M34	8.4	459	+	-	-	-	-	-	-	-	-	-	-	-	MS^2[459]:283(100),175(7.0) MS^3[283]:283(100)
M35	10.2	443	-	-	-	-	-	-	-	-	-	-	-	-	MS^2[443]:411(100),267(87.5),253(91.5),157(10.9) MS^3[411]:335(30.2),267(100),253(88.9)
M36	11.5	297	+	+	+	+	-	-	+	-	+	-	+	-	MS^2[297]:253(100) MS^3[253]:253(100)
M37	12.9	349	+	-	-	-	-	-	-	-	-	-	+	-	MS^2[349]:269(100) MS^3[269]:269(100)
M38	14.3	561	+	-	-	-	-	-	-	-	-	-	-	-	MS^2[561]:269(100),240(9.5) MS^3[269]:269(100)
M39	14.6	283	+	+	+	+	-	+	+	-	+	-	+	+	MS^2[283]:257(100),239(66.9) MS^3[257]:257(100),239(41.0)

tR: retention time; +:found; -:not found; [M-H]: negatively charged molecular ion

Table 1. The metabolites detected in rat urine, plasma and tissues after intragastric administration of rhubarb decoction

M4, which was only detected in plasma samples produced a [M-H]$^-$ at m/z 479 with a retention time of 3.4 min. It was found that the [M-H-176]$^-$ ion plus the ion at m/z 303 were observed in its MS^2 spectrum. So, M4 was identified as the metabolite that conjugated with one molecule of glucuronic acid (GlcA). The ion at m/z 303 could produce fragment ion at m/z 259. The spectroscope (MS^n) data of M4 was different from those reported in the published literature before [14]. According to the data above, M4 was conjectured to be glucuronide conjugate of methyl catechin.

M10 gave a [M-H]$^-$ signal at m/z 621 in the mass spectrum and fragmentation of the ion with the peak at m/z 621 gave the ion peak at m/z 445 (-176 Da), involving the loss of glucuronic acid. Then, the MS^3 fragmentation yielded the ion peak at m/z 269 (-176 Da), involving another loss of glucuronic acid. The quasi-molecular ion of m/z 621 lost a 46 Da and a 30 Da fragmentation sequentially forming the product ions at m/z 575 and 591, suggesting that the mother nucleus was aloe-emodin, and the hydroxymethyl was not conjugated. Therefore, the compound M10 was identified as bisdesmoside conjugate of aloe-emodin.

The mass spectrum of the compound M20 displayed a signal at m/z 525 ([M-H]$^-$). A product ion spectrum of M20 displayed fragment ion at m/z 445, 400, 349 and 269. Fragmentation of the ion at m/z 525 gave the ion peak at m/z 349 (-176 Da), suggesting the loss of glucuronic acid. Meanwhile, fragmentation of the quasi-molecular ion yielded an ion peak at m/z 445 (-80 Da), involving the presence of sulfate. Glucuronic acid group and sulfate were not conjuncted with hydroxymethyl of the parent compound, which was judged by sequential loss of 44 Da and 46 Da. Therefore, the structure of M20 was conjectured to be glucuronide and sulfate conjugate of aloe-emodin, glucuronic acid group and sulfate occurred at the 1 and 8-hydroxy, respectively.

Based on the discussions above, the proposed metabolic pathways of rhubarb in rats are shown in Fig.5. The parent compound rhein was found in urine, plasma and most of the tissue samples.

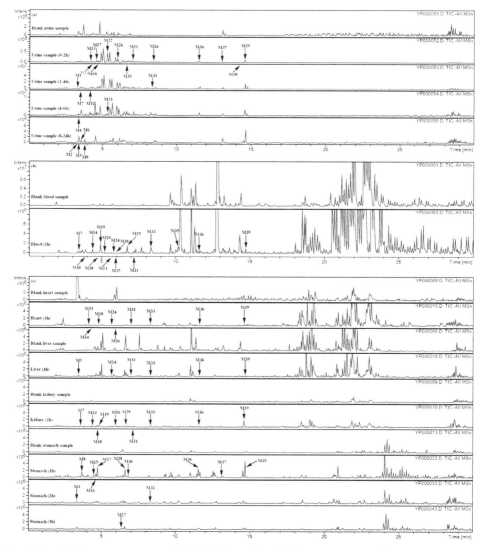

Fig. 2. Typical chromatograms of biological samples (a) chromatograms of urine samples after i.g. administration of 10 g/kg rhubarb decoction; (b) chromatograms of plasma samples after i.g. administration of 17.6 g/kg rhubarb decoction; (c) chromatograms of some tissue samples after i.g. administration of 17.6 g/kg rhubarb decoction

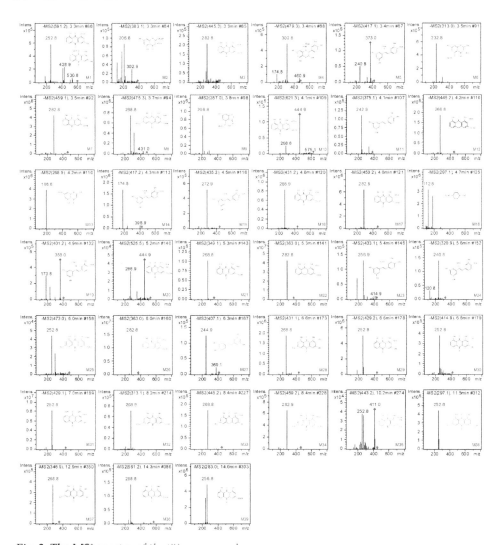

Fig. 3. The MS² spectra of the 39 compounds

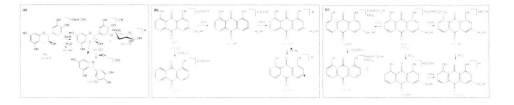

Fig. 4. Postulated fragmentation pathways of the selected metabolites (a) M4; (b) M10; (c) M20

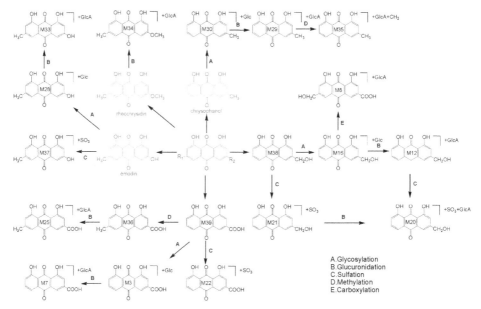

Fig. 5. The proposed transformation pathway of rhubarb in rats

3.8 Urinary excretion of rhubarb

The urinary excretion of rhubarb following a single intragastric administration of rhubarb decoction to rats is summarized in Fig.6. Among the 21 compounds detected in urine samples, the excretion of M22 and M39 were the largest, reaching more than 1000 µg in 48 h, the excretion of M5 and M26 has reached more than 500 µg.

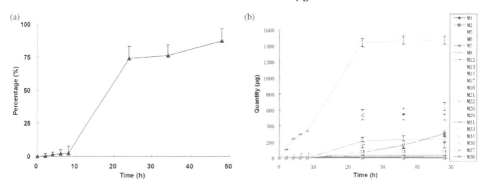

Fig. 6. Cumulative excretion curves of rhein (M39) and the metabolites of rhubarb following the intragastric administration of 10 g/kg rhubarb decoction to SD rats (a) the prototype component M39; (b) metabolites detected in urine samples

3.9 Plasma concentration of rhubarb and the metabolites

Among the 16 constituents detected in plasma, only rhein (M39) was the parent compound. The peak rhein concentration (Cmax) in plasma was 7.23 µg/ml. The peak concentration of

M19, a metabolite of emodin, reached 8.05 µg/ml at 2 h after i.g. administration of rhubarb decoction. The concentrations of the 16 compounds were shown in Table 2.

Time (h)	M7	M10	M14	M18	M19	M20	M23	M24	M25	M26	M29	M31	M33	M35	M36	M39
1	2.55	0.72	1.76	6.53	4.14	0.33	1.02	1.11	0	4.01	3.40	1.34	3.90	0.80	3.56	7.23
2	1.46	3.57	2.93	0	8.05	0.89	0.19	0.40	0.30	0	5.33	1.48	5.44	0	2.79	3.19
3	0	4.07	1.40	1.18	5.53	0.65	0.11	0	0.35	0	3.89	1.64	0	0	0.62	1.27

Table 2. The concentration of the 16 compounds detected in plasma (µg/ml)

3.10 Tissue distribution of rhubarb

Tissue distribution of the metabolites at 1.0, 2.0 and 3.0 h after a single intragastric administration of 10 g/kg rhubarb decoction to SD rats are also studied. Among the 24 metabolites found, M36 and M39 were distributed in most of the tissues, tissue concentrations of M36 and M39 are shown in Fig.7. At 1.0 h after intragastric dosing, tissue concentrations in most tissues were higher than the corresponding concentrations at 2.0 and 3.0 h. M7, M13, M18, M26, M29 and M33 reached the highest amount of concentration in kidney, M3, M8, M15, M16, M17, M27, M28, M30 and M37 reached the highest amount in stomach at 1.0 h after intragastric dosing. A total of nine compounds were detected in heart samples, seven in liver samples, four in lung samples, ten in kidney samples, thirteen in stomach samples, one in large intestine samples, three in small intestine samples and one in testis samples. The metabolites detected were shown in Table 1. The highest level of most of the metabolites was observed in the stomach, while none of the metabolites was found in spleen and brain.

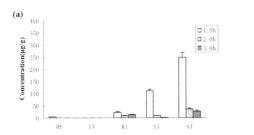
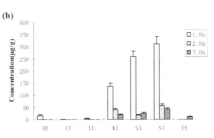

Fig. 7. Distribution of (a) M36, (b) M39 at 1.0h, 2.0h and 3.0h following intragastric administration of 10 g/kg rhubarb decoction to SD rats. Each value represents mean and SD of six animals.

4. Discussion

Many medicinal herbs have a long history of clinical use. However, the safety and efficacy of most of these herbs in relation to their pharmacological activities are poorly understood. Furthermore, knowledge of the pharmacokinetics of the main bioactive ingredients of these herbs is extremely limited. Dahuang is one of the most commonly prescribed Chinese medicinal herbs for the treatment of constipation. However, pharmacokinetics of the main bioactive ingredients in this herb is largely unknown.

In this paper, we developed a triple quadruple MS method for analysis and identification the main bioactive components and their possible metabolites in urine, plasma and tissues. Following a single intragastric administration of rhubarb decoction to rats, 21 constituents in urine samples and 16 compounds in plasma samples were identified. Some constituents of rhubarb were rapidly absorbed into blood and tissues, indicating that the compounds might be responsible for curative effects of rhubarb decoction. Ten compounds were detected in kidney samples, it may elucidate that rhubarb decoction has the effects of anti-diabetic and protecting chronic renal failure in rats. [9, 10].Their conjugations of glucosides, glucuronide and sulfates were also detected and two of the parent compound aloe-emodin and rhein. The developed method was simple, reliable and sensitive, which revealed that it will be appropriate for rapid analysis and identification the characterization of main bioactive components and their metabolites in biosamples. However, the present study still demonstrated the analytical potential of this approach for identification of metabolites. This identification and structure elucidation of these metabolites provided essential data for further pharmacological and clinical studies of rhubarb and related preparation.

5. Introduction

The root of *Scutellaria baicalensis*, called Huangqin in Chinese, is one of the most commonly used traditional Chinese medicines for the treatment of hepatitis, tumors, diarrhea, and inflammatory diseases [15]. It originated from Shennong Materia Medica, the earliest pharmacopoeia of China in Eastern Han (24-220 A.D.), and has been officially listed in the Chinese Pharmacopoeia for a long time. The major chemical constituents of Huangqin are flavonoids. Modern pharmacological studies have demonstrated that flavones have wide biological activities, such as anti-oxidants, anti-cancer, anti-inflammatory, *etc* [16,17,18]. Few data are available on the metabolism and metabolites of *S. baicalensis* extract *in vivo*. Therefore it is important to explicate the biotransformation of flavonoids *in vivo* so as to clarify the mechanism of pharmacological action and to promote its availability as well.

A simple and rapid high-performance liquid chromatographic-electrospray ionization (ESI) tandem mass spectrometric method has been developed for elucidation of the structures of the metabolites in rat plama, urine samples. LC-MS/MS is a more powerful analytical tool for the identification of durg metabolites in biological matrices by comparing changes in molecular masses (ΔM), retention-times, and spectral patterns of product ions with those of the parent drug [19,20].

6. Experimental

6.1 Chemicals and reagents

The roots of *Scutellaria baicalensis* Georgi were collected from Xi'an, ShanXi province, China, and authenticated by Professor Shen Jingui of Shanghai Institute of Materia Medica, Chinese Academy of Sciences. HPLC grade acetonitrile was purchased from Dikma Company (Dikma, USA). Water was deionized and double distilled. Other reagents used are of analytical grade.

6.2 Instrumentation

HPLC-MS experiments were performed with a Finnigan LCQ Advantage ion trap mass spectrometer (Thermo Finnigan, San Jose, CA) was connected to a Agilent 1100 HPLC instrument via an ESI source. The software Xcalibur version 1.2 (Finnigan) was applied for system operation and data collection. A high-speed desktop centrifuge (TGL-16C, Shanghai Anting Scientific Instrument Factory, Shanghai, China) was used to centrifuge urine, plasma sample. The urine, plasma sample were extracted on a C18 solid-phase extraction (SPE) cartridge (1ml/100mg, Supelco).

6.3 Chromatographic and mass spectrometric conditions

An Agilent series 1100 HPLC instrument (Agilent, Waldbronn, Germany) equipped with a quaternary pump, a UV detector, and a column compatment was used for analyses. The samples were separated on a Apollo C_{18} column (5μm, 4.6 × 250mm, Grace), including an EasyGuad Kit C_{18} (4 × 2mm) guard column. The column was maintained at 25°C. Detection wavelengths were set at 280nm. The flow rate was 0.8m/min. A gradient elution of 0.5% aqueous formic acid (A) and acetonitrile (B) was used as follows: 20% B in the first 10min, 20%~25% B at 10~11 min, then B held at 25% for 14min, linearly gradient to 35% B at 26 min and hold for 15min, 35%~55% B at 41~45 min, linearly gradient to 100%B at 50min and hold for 5min. The mass spectra were recorded in negative modes, drying gas flow rate 10L/min, drying gas temperature 35°C, nebulizer 35 psig., capillary voltage 4000V, fragmentor 100V, mass range 50-1500 m/z.

6.4 Administration

Male Sprague-Dawley (SD) rats (220 ± 10g body weigh, laboratory Animal Center of Shanghai University of Tradition Chinese Medicine) were divided into a blank group and drug group. Prior to oral administration, each rat was fasted for 24h in a metabolic cage with free access to water, and were then administered 1.2g/Kg the extract of S. baicalensis by i.g. Urine were collected separately at 2h, 4h, 6h, 8h, 10h and 24h. Samples were stored at -20°C until analysis. Blood samples were collected at 0.25, 0.5, 1, 3, 5, 7, and 24h after dosing from the caudal vein of the rats, then shaken and centrifuged at 4000rpm for 10min. The supernatant was decanted, and immediately frozen at -20°C until analysis.

6.5 Sample preparation

Solid phase extraction (SPE) with C18 cartridge (1ml/100mg, Supelclean™, Dikma) was used to purify the above supernatants of urine, plasma samples, for LC-MS/MS analysis. Before use, SPE columns were conditioned by 4ml methanol, 2ml deionized water. Then the selected supernatant sample was loaded, and the column was washed with 3ml deionized water to elute the impurity and 1ml methanol to elute the analytes in turn. The eluent was evaporated to dryness at 37°C in vacuum, and the residue dissolved in 100μl of 100% methanol. After centrifugation at 8000rpm. for 10min, 10μl of the supernatant was introduced into the HPLC system for HPLC-MS.

7. Results and discussion

7.1 Identification of metabolites

To elucidate the active constituents responsible for the pharmacological action, it is necessary to perceive the metabolic changes *in vivo* and chemical constituent profile in biological system. Therefore, the full-scan mass spectrum total-ion current chromatogram obtained from rat urine and plasma (Figs. 8(c), 9(b)) after *i.g.* of extract of *S. baicalensis* was compared with that from blank urine to find probable metabolites. The results show that the total peaks and corresponding peak areas in metabolic chromatograms were different when collected at different periods, and the most abundant metabolites were found at 4-6h in urine samples. These compounds were then analyzed by LC-MS/MS. Using negative ion electrospray tandem mass spectrometry, a total of 12 and 6 metabolites were detected in drug-containing urine and plasma samples in comparison with the extract of *S. baicalensis* and blank sample.

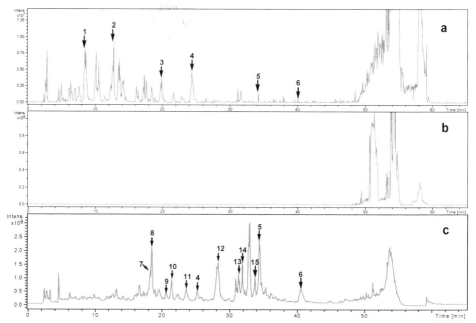

Fig. 8. HPLC-MS total ion current of the *S. baicalensis* decoction and its metabolites in negative mode. (a) The decoction of *S. baicalensis*; (b) Blank rat urine; (c) Urine sample after oral administration.

Peak 4 and 5 , 6 were confirmed as original components, baicalin (4) , wogonoside (5) and baicalein (6). The [M-H]- ion of baicalein at m/z 269 produced an ion at m/z 251, which should result from the loss of H_2O. The ion at m/z 241 was due to the loss of CO, and the m/z 223 ion was due to the successive loss of H_2O and CO.

Peak 6 showed [M-H]- m/z 445.3, with retention a Baicalin is an O-glucuronide. Upon CID, the glycosidic bond was easily cleaved to generate an ion at m/z 269, which resulted from the neutral loss of a glucuronic acid (Δm = 176u). In the MS^3 experiment, ion at m/z 269 produced the same ions as baicalein described above.

Wogonin is a methoxylated flavone. It exhibited a significant radical anion [M-H-CH3]-• as the base peak. In MS^3 spectra, we observed the significant ion at m/z 239 [M-H-CH3-• - COH•]-, and the low signal intensity ions at m/z 163 (^{0,2}A-), 212 [M-H-CH3•-2CO]-•, 223 [M-H-CH3•-CO2H•]-, 240 [M-H-CH3•-CO]-•, which is identical with the previous report.

Peak 7 showed a [M-H]- m/z 607.4, with retention time at 18.3min on HPLC. Its MS^2 produced an ion at m/z 431 [M-H-176]-, indicating the existence of a glucuronic acid.

Additionally, the successive yielded the ion at m/z 269 [M-H-176-162]⁻. Based on these data and by the knowledge on the flavones in S. *baicalensis*, compounds 1 were identified as Baicalein glucoside glucuronide conjugate.

Peak 8 gave a [M-H]⁻ ion at m/z 621.4, with retention time at 18.5min on HPLC. CID of this compound produced an ion of [M-H-176]⁻ at m/z 445, which resulted from the neutral loss of a glucuronic acid residue. In the MS³ of m/z 445, fragments of m/z 430 and 269 indicated the presence of a H_2O and a glucuronic acid, respectively. Therefore, this compound was thus proposed as Baicalin glucuronide conjugate.

With a retention time at 19.6min on HPLC, peak 9 generated a [M-H]⁻ at m/z 635.3 in MS spectrum and a [M-H]⁻ at m/z 459 ([M-H]⁻ -176, loss of a glucuronic acid) in MS². In the MS³ experiment, ion at m/z 283 produced the same ions as wogonoside described above. Therefore, compound 9 was thus proposed as Wogonoside glucuronide conjugate.

Peak 10 displayed a [M-H]⁻ ion at m/z 577.4, with retention time at 20.6min on HPLC. The MS² and MS³ spectra gave ions at m/z 401 and 269, suggesting sequential losses of glucuronic acid (176 Da) and arabinose (132 Da) residues. This compound was thus identified as Baicalein xyloside glucuronide conjugate.

Peak 11 showed a [M−H]⁻ ion at m/z 417.3, with retention time at 21.4min on HPLC. In the MS² speetrum of m/z 417.3, the fragment ion of 241 and 399 was generated by natural loss of a glucuronic acid and a H_2O, then the successive yielded the ion at m/z 199 [M-H-GlcA-C_2H_2O]⁻ in MS³. Therefore, it was tentatively identified as pinosylvin 2-hydroxymethyl glucuronide conjugate.

Peaks 12 and 15 are sulfation metabolites. Peak 12 with a retention at 23.6 min on HPLC, showed a [M−H]⁻ m/z 539.4. In the MS² speetrum, the fragment ion of 363 and 459, indicating loss of a glucuronic acid and SO_3, respectively. Based on these data and by the knowledge on the flavones in S. *baicalensis*, this compound were identified as wongonoside sulfate conjugate. Peak 16 with a retention time at 33.7min on HPLC, yield MS fragments at m/z 363.2 and [M-H]⁻ m/z 282.9 ([M-H]⁻ - 80 Da, loss of a SO_3) in MS². Based on these data and by the knowledge on the flavones in S. *baicalensis*, this compound could be confirmed as wogonin sulfate conjugate.

Peak 13 gave a [M-H]⁻ ion at m/z 447.3, with retention time at 31.3min on HPLC. CID of this compound produced an ion of [M-H-176]⁻ at m/z 270.9, which resulted from the neutral loss of a glucuronic acid residue. Based on these data and by the knowledge on the flavones in S. *baicalensis*, this compound was thus proposed as baicalein glucuronide conjugate.

Peak 14, appearing at 31.8min on HPLC , had a [M-H]- at m/z 446 and yield a major ion at m/z 268.9 ([M-H]- - 176 Da, loss of a glucuronic acid unit) in MS² and a MS³ fragment [M-H]⁻ at m/z 251.0 ([M-H]⁻ -176 Da–18 Da, loss of a glucuronic acid unit and one molecule of H_2O). Therefore it was presumed as apigenin glucuronide conjugate, which acts as one of the major apigenin metabolites in urine.

7.2 Plasma metabolites

The direct comparison of the TIC chromatograms of the blank rat plasma and the rat plasma samples collected at 0.5, 1, 2, 3, 4h after the oral administration of the extract of S. *baicalensis*. It showed that the information in the chromatogram at 1h post administration was more sufficient (Fig.9(b)). Including two original components, two metabolites, were tentatively elucidated as baicalin glucuronide conjugate (16), baicalin (4), norwogonoside glucuronide conjugate (17), wogonoside sulfate conjugate (18), wogonoside (5).

Peak 17 with retention time at 33.7min on HPLC, showed a [M-H]- ion of m/z 621.1. The MS[2] and MS[3] spectra gave ions at m/z 445 and 269, suggesting sequential losses of two glucuronic acid (2 ×176 Da) residues. In the MS[3] experiment, ion at m/z 225 produced [M-2Glc A-CO-H]-. Base on these data, the structrue of 17 could be identified as norwogonoside glucuronide conjugate.

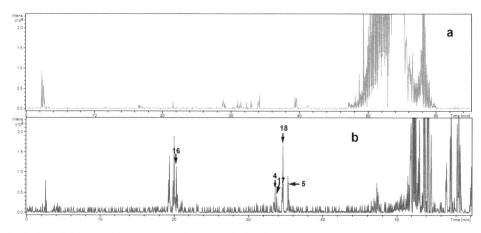

Fig. 9. HPLC-MS total ion current of the *S. baicalensis* decoction and its metabolites in negative mode. (a) Blank rat plasma; (b) Plasma sample after oral administration.

7.3 Identification of Baicalin metabolites in rat blood

Some reported that baicalin are the main active components of *S. baicalensis* [21]. In order to further study of baicalin metabolism *in vivo*. The metabolites of baicalin were studied further in rat plasma.

We identified three metabolites and the parent drug in rat plasma after administration of baicalin by healthy rats. Their protonated molecular ions ([M-H]-) were at m/z 621, 643, and 564, respectively. MS[n] spectra of motabolites, obtained by CID of their molecular ions, were used for more precise structural identification of metabolites. Among them, the retention time, the MS[2] and MS[3] spectra of the molecular ion at m/z 445 (M0) were the same as those of baicalin. Therefore, M0 is the unchanged parent drug.

M1 was observed at the retention time of 19.9 min and gave an deprotonated molecule [M-H]- at m/z 621. The ion at m/z 621 was increased by 176Da compared to that of unchanged baicalin and glucuronidation was a very common metabolic pathway of drug in vivo, indicating that M1 might be a conjugate of baicalin with glucuronic acid, which was confirmed by the characteristic fragment ions presented in the following MS[n] spectrum. The [M-H]- ion at m/z 621 of M1 generated the base peak at m/z 445 in the MS/MS spectrum, attributed to the loss of 176 Da, suggesting the loss of a glucuronic acid. Then the product ion at m/z 445 was subjected to MS[3] analysis and produced an intense ion at m/z 268 by loss of a glucuronic acid group (176Da) again. Therefore, M1 was elucidated as baicalin glucuronide conjugate.

M2, eluted at 20.1 min, exhibited [M-H]- signal at m/z 643 which was 198 Da greater than that of parent compound, which indicated that M2 was a Na glucuronide metabolite of baicalin. The MS[2] spectrum of m/z 643 produced a significant radical ion at m/z 467 (Fig.10) via the loss of glucuronic acid (176Da). Then the ion at m/z 467 was successively subjected to MS^3 analysis and produced ion at m/z 269 by the loss of Na and glucuronic acid (198 Da). At the same time, the bask peak at m/z 241 was observed in the MS^4 spectrum by the loss of CO (28Da) from the ion at m/z 269. Therefore, M2 was tentatively proposed to be the baicalin Na glucuronide conjugate.

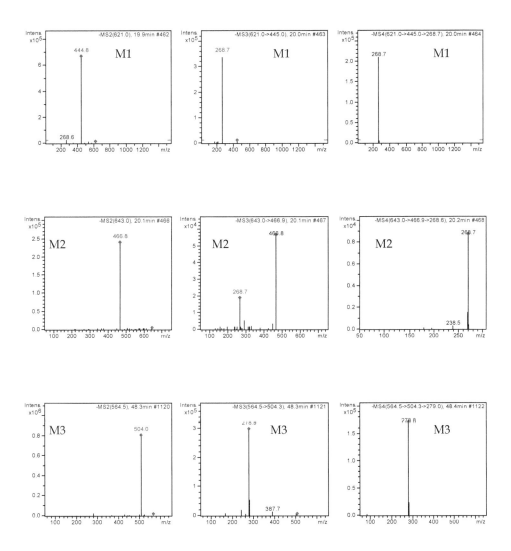

Fig. 10. Negative ion ESI-MS^n spectra of baicalin metabolites in rat plasma

M3 was detected as a deprotonated molecule [M-H]$^-$ at m/z 564, with the retention time of 48.3 min. The molecular ion at m/z 564 was increased by 119 Da compared to that of the parent compound and there may be cysteine (119Da) reactions occurring at the baicalin skeleton. The molecular ion at m/z 564 by loss of the neutral fragment $C_2O_2H_3N$(60Da) produced the product ion at m/z 504 (Fig.10C) in the MS^2 spectrum. The obtained ion was subjected to MS^3 fragmentation, in which the base peak at m/z 389 was observed by the losing a glucuronic acid(176 Da). Based on the above results, M3 could be characterized as the baicalin cysteine conjugate.

8. Conclusion

In this paper, we discribe a strategy using liquid chromatogrphic-electrospray ionization (ESI) tandem ion trap mass spectrometric for fast analysis of the metabolic profile of *S. baicalensis* and baicalin. Using negative ion mode and applying the MS fragmentation rules of flavonoids reported before, 3 organic components, 9 metabolites in urine, 2 organic and 3 metabolites in plasma, were identified or tentatively identified in the extracts of *S. baicalensis*. 3 metabolites were identified in bacailin. However, several new analogues were identified in the present study, which proved that HPLC-MS is a powerful and rapid method to discover new constituents in Chinese medicinal herbs and its metabolites, help to lay the foundation of further study *in vivo*.

9. Acknowledgements

We thank the National Science & Technology Major Project "Key New Drug Creation and Manufacturing Program" (no. 2009ZX09301-001; 2009ZX09501-030; 2009ZX09308-005) and the National Natural Science Foundation of China (no. 20805054; 81030065) for financial support of this work.

10. References

[1] J. Wang, H. Zhao, W. Kong, C. Jin, Y. Zhao, Y. Qu, X. Xiao (2010). Microcalorimetric assay on the antimicrobial property of five hydroxyanthraquinone derivatives in rhubarb (*Rheum palmatum* L.) to *Bifidobacterium adolesentis*. *Phytomedicine*, 17: 684-689.

[2] K. Suresh Babu, P.V. Srinivas, B. Praveen, K. Hara Kishore, U. Suryanarayana Murty, J. Madhusudana Rao (2003). Antimicrobial constituents from the rhizomes of Rheum emodi. *Phytochemistry*, 62: 203-207.

[3] Mi Kyoung Moon, Dae Gill Kang, Jun Kyong Lee, Jin Sook Kim, Ho Sub Lee (2006). Vasodilatory and anti-inflammatory effects of the aqueous extract of rhubarb via a NO-cGMP pathway. *Life Sciences*, 78: 1550-1557.

[4] Sook-Kyoung He, Hyun-Jeong Yun, Eui-Kyu Noh, Sun-Dong Park (2010). Emodin and rhein inhibit LIGHT-induced monocytes migration by blocking of ROS production. *Vasc Pharmacol*, 53: 28-37.

[5] Hai-Rong Xiong, Jun Luo, Wei Hou, Hong Xiao, Zhan-Qiu Yang (2011). The effect of emodin, an anthraquinone derivative extracted from the roots of Rheum

tanguticum, against herpes simplex virus in vitro and in vivo. *J Ethnopharmacol*, 133: 718-23.

[6] Zhi-Heng He, Ming-Fang He, Shuang-Cheng Ma, Paul Pui-Hay But (2009). Anti-angiogenic effects of rhubarb and its anthraquinone derivatives. *J Ethnopharmacol*, 121: 313-317.

[7] Akira Iizuka, Osamu T. Iijima, Kazuo Kondo, Hiroshige Itakura, Fumihiko Yoshie, Hiroko Miyamoto, Masayoshi Kubo, Masami Higuchi, Hiroshi Takeda, Teruhiko Matsumiya (2004). Evaluation of Rhubarb using antioxidative activity as an index of pharmacological usefulness. *J Ethnopharmacol*, 91: 89–94.

[8] Li Liu, Shifang Yuan, Yin Long, Zhenjun Guo, Yang Sun, Yuhua Li, Yinbo Niu, Chen Li, Qibing Mei (2009). Immunomodulation of Rheum tanguticum polysaccharide (RTP) on the immunosuppressive effects of dexamethasone (DEX) on the treatment of colitis in rats induced by 2, 4, 6-trinitrobenzene sulfonic acid. *Int Immunopharmacol*, 9: 1568-1577.

[9] Jiabo Wang, Yanling Zhao, Xiaohe Xiao, Huifang Li, Haiping Zhao, Ping Zhang, Cheng Jin (2009). Assessment of the renal protection and hepatotoxicity of rhubarb extract in rats. *J Ethnopharmacol*, 124: 18-25.

[10] Jianfeng Xue, Wenjun Ding, Yan Liu (2010). Anti-diabetic effects of emodin involved in the activation of PPARγ on high-fat diet-fed and low dose of streptozotocin-induced diabetic mice. *Fitoterapia*, 81: 173–177.

[11] Chun-Hui Ma, Zhi-Xiong Li, Long-Xing Wang, Yi-Hong Tang, Hong-Bin Xiao, Cheng-Gang Huang (2009). Identification of Major Alkaloids in Rat Urine by HPLC/DAD/ESI-MS/MS Method Following Oral Administration of Cortex Phellodendri Decoction. *Helv Chim Acta*, 92: 379-397.

[12] Guan Ye, Hai-Yan Zhu, Zhi-Xiong Li, Chun-Hui Ma, Ming-Song Fan, Zhao-Lin Sun, Cheng-Gang Huang (2007). LC-MS characterization of efficacy substances in serum of experimental animals treated with Sophora flavescens extracts. *Biomed Chromatogr*, 21: 655-660.

[13] Rui Song, Lei Xu, Fengguo Xu, Zhe Li, Haijuan Dong, Yuan Tian, Zunjian Zhang (2010). *In vivo* metabolism study of rhubarb decoction in rat using high-performance liquid chromatography with UV photodiode-array and mass-spectrometric detection: A strategy for systematic analysis of metabolites from traditional Chinese medicines in biological samples. *Journal of Chromatography A*, 1217: 7144–7152.

[14] Susana González-Manzano, Ana González-Paramás, Celestino Santos-Buelga and Montserrat Dueñas (2009). Preparation and Characterization of Catechin Sulfates, Glucuronides, and Methylethers with Metabolic Interest. *J Agric Food Chem*, 57: 1231-1238.

[15] Pharmacopoeia of the People's Republic of China. Beijing: China Medical Technology Press. *National Commission of Chinese Pharmacopoeia*, 2010: 282.

[16] D.F. Birt, S. Hendrich, W.Q. Wang (2001). *Pharmacol Therapeut*, 90: 157.

[17] C.A. Williams, J.B. Harborne, H. Geiger, J. Robin, S. Hoult (1999). *Phytochemistry*, 51: 417

[18] A. Mantas, E. Detetey, F.H. Ferretti, M.R. Estrada, I.G. Csizmadia (2000). *J Mol Struct (Theochem)*, 504: 171.

[19] Y. Li, D. F. Zhong, S. W. Chen, I. Maeba (2005). *Acta Pharmacol Sin*, 26: 1519.

[20] A. Li, M. P. May, J. C. Bigelow (2006). *J Chromatogr B: Anal Technol Biomed Life Sci*, 836: 129.

[21] J. Han, M. Ye, M. Xu, J.H. Sun, B.R. Wang, D. Guo (2007). *J Chromatogr B*, 848: 355.

11

Therapeutic Effects of Lignans and Blend Isolated from *Schisandra chinesis* on Hepatic Carcinoma

Dae Youn Hwang
Pusan National University,
Republic of Korea

1. Introduction

Schisandra chinesis (*S. chinesis*) is widely used as one of the 50 fundamental herbs in traditional Oriental medicine; the species is a member of the *Schisandra* genus of shrub, which grows commonly in the native forests of Northern China, Korea, Japan and Russia. The *Schisandra* are deciduous climbers that thrive in any type of soil, so long as it is moist, shaded, and well-drained (Panossian and Wikman, 2008). The female *S. chinesis* plant can produce the fruit via fertilization with pollen from a male plant (Shilova, 1963). It is harvested in most countries, including Korea, by the cutting of half-matured berries between August and September. The berries of *S. chinesis* are called omija (translated as "five-flavor fruit") in Korea, because this fruit has all five of the basic flavors-salty, sweet, sour, pungent, and bitter (Gutnikova, 1951; Panossian and Wikman, 2008). Generally, its dried fruits have been used for a variety of purposes, including as a therapeutic drug, teas and wines. In many countries, it has been used as a therapeutic drug, and is purported to have liver-protective and immune-modulatory abilities. A variety of key constituents including schizandrin, deoxyschizandrin, gomisin, and pregomisin have been isolated from the seeds of the fruit. Additionally, *S. chinesis* berries have been used in the manufacture of several foods. A wine was using the berries of *S. chinesis* has been produced in China, whereas in Korea, the berries are made into a tea. Meanwhile, in Japan, these berries are referred to as "gomishin", and have been used for medicinal purposes, to treat colds and sea sickness. In Russia, dozens of tons of berries are used annually in the commercial production of juices, wine, extracts and sweets (Gutnikova, 1951; Agejenko and Komisssarenko, 1960).

A variety of previous pharmacological studies have suggested that *S. chinesis* may exert beneficial biological effects on liver tissue, the central nervous system, the respiratory system, the cardiovascular system and the endocrine system (Table 1) (Panossian and Wikman, 2008). The major and characteristic components of *Schisandraceae* berries have been previously isolated, and are referred to as lignans. The lignans are categorized into the five following classes: dibenzocyclooctadiene lignans (type A), spirobenzofuranoid dibenzocyclooctadiene lignans (type B), 4-aryltetralin lignans (type C), 2,3-dimethyl-1,4-diarylbutane lignans (type D), and 2,5-diaryltetrahydrofuran lignans (type E)(Table 2)(Lu and Chen, 2009). Thus far, a total of 43 lignans have been isolated from *S. chinesis* in various

studies; a list is provided in Table 2. Among these lignans, most of the lignans isolated from
S. *chinesis* exhibit a dibenzocyclooctadiene lignan (type A) structure, with the exception of
three lignans: pregomisin, meso-dihydroguaiaretic acid and nordihydroguaiaretic acid. The
three lignans described in this chapter are of the type A structural group. Additionally, the
dibenzocyclooctadiene lignans are further divided into two types based on their
stereostructures-S- and R-biphenyl configuration. Structural elucidation studies have shown
that the cyclooctene rings of dibenzocyclooctadiene lignans evidence a twist-boat-chair
(TBC) or twist-boat (TB) conformation (Lu and Chen, 2009). Approximately half of the
lignans from S. *chinesis* evidence an S-biphenyl configuration and the other half exhibit an R-
biphenyl configuration. According to the conformation with cyclooctene rings, only four
lignans exhibited a TB conformation, but the rest of the lignans had the TBC conformation.
Among the three lignins described in this chapter, only gomisin N exhibits an S-biphenyl
configuration, whereas tigloylgomisin H and schisandrin A has an R-biphenyl
configuration.

Body system	Regulatory system: stress-system	Pharmacological effect: adaptogenic effect
Cardiovascular system	Central and vegetative nervous system	Stimulating effect
Gastrointestinal system	Endocrine system	Stress-mimetic and stress-protective effect
Respiratory system	Immune system	Stress-protective effect

Table 1. Summary of the pharmacological activities of S. *chinensis* (Panossian and Wikman,
2008).

Compounds	Structure type	Configuration/ conformation	References
Gomisin N	A	S/TBC	Ikeya et al., 1978a
Schizandrin C(wuweizisu C, schisandrin C)	A	S/TBC	Chen and Shu, 1976
(-)-Gomisin K1	A	S/TBC	Ikeya et al., 1980
Gomisin J	A	S/TBC	Ikeya et al., 1978b
(-)-Gomisin L2	A	S/TBC	Ikeya et al., 1982
(-)-Gomisin L1	A	S/TBC	Ikeya et al., 1982
Gomisin S	A	S/TBC	Ikeya et al., 1988
Epigomisin O	A	S/TBC	Ikeya et al., 1991; Ikeya et al., 1979
Tigloylgomisin P	A	S/TBC	Ikeya et al., 1990; Ikeya et al., 1980
Angeloylgomisin P	A	S/TBC	Ikeya et al., 1990; Ikeya et al., 1980
Gomisin D	A	S/TBC	Ikeya et al., 1976
Gomisin E	A	S/TBC	Ikeya et al., 1979
Gomisin O	A	S/TBC	Ikeya et al., 1979
6-o-benzoylgomisin O	A	S/TB	Chen et al., 1994
Angeloylgomisin O	A	S/TB	Ikeya et al., 1982

Angeloyl isogomisin O	A	S/TB	Ikeya et al., 1982
Benzoyl isogomisian O	A	S/TB	Ikeya et al., 1982
Schisandrene	A	S/TBC	Choi et al., 2006
Angeloylgomisin Q	A	S/TBC	Ikeya et al., 1979
Gomisin F	A	S/TBC	Taguchi and Ikeya, 1977
Gomisin G	A	S/TBC	Taguchi and Ikeya, 1977
Schisantherin A(gomisin C, wuweizi ester A)	A	S/TBC	Ikeya et al., 1990; Taguchi and Ikeya, 1977
Schisantherin B(gomisin B, wuweizi ester B)	A	S/TBC	Ikeya et al., 1990; Taguchi and Ikeya, 1977
Schisantherin D	A	S/TBC	Liu et al., 1978; Ikeya et al., 1982
Gomisin R	A	S/TB	Ikeya et al., 1982
Deoxyschizandrin (wuweizisu A, schisandrin A, deoxyschisandrin)	A	R/TBC	Chen and Shu, 1976; Yue et al., 1994
(+)-Gomisin K2	A	R/TBC	Ikeya et al., 1980
Schisanhenol [(+)-gomisin K3]	A	R/TBC	Ikeya et al., 1980; Ikeya et al., 1990
γ-Schizandrin(γ-schisandrin)	A	R/TBC	Liu et al., 1978
Schizandrin B(wuweizisu B, schisandrin B, (±)- γ-schizandrin)	A	R/TBC	Chen and Shu, 1976
(±)-Gomisin M1	A	R/TBC	Ikeya et al., 1982
(+)-Gomisin M2	A	R/TBC	Ikeya et al., 1982
Schizandrin(schisandrol A, schisandrin, wuweizi alcohol A)	A	R/TBC	Chen and Shu, 1976
Gomisin A(schisandrol B, wuweizi alcohol B)	A	R/TBC	Taguchi and Ikeya, 1977
Gomisin H	A	R/TBC	Ikeya et al., 1979
Angeloylgomisin H	A	R/TBC	Ikeya et al., 1979
Tigloylgomisin H	A	R/TBC	Ikeya et al., 1979
Benzoylgomisin H	A	R/TBC	Ikeya et al., 1979
Gomisin T	A	R/TBC	Ikeya et al., 1988
Isoschizandrin	A	R/TBC	Ikeya et al., 1991; Ikeya et al., 1988
Pregomisin	D	/	Ikeya et al., 1978
Meso-dihydroguaiaretic acid	D	/	Ikeya et al., 1979
Nordihydroguaiaretic acid	D	/	Sakurai et al., 1992

Table 2. Lignans isolated from the fruits of *S. chinensis*. A: Dibenzocyclooctadiene lignan; D: 2,3-dimethyl-1,4-diarylbutane lignan; S or R: the configuration of the biphenyl unit; TBC or TB: the conformation of the cyclooctane ring (Lu and Chen, 2009).

Meanwhile, hepatocellular carcinoma is a primary malignancy of the hepatocytes, and generally leads to death within 6-20 months. The disease is the fifth most common cancer in men and the eighth most common cancer in women worldwide (Bosch et al., 2004). Cirrhosis of any etiology is known to be the major risk factor for hepatocellular carcinoma (Adami et al., 2008). Thus far, approximately 80% of patients with newly diagnosed hepatocellular carcinoma have preexisting cirrhosis in the liver organ, caused mainly by excessive alcohol use, hepatitis C infection and hepatitis B infection (El-Serang and Mason, 2000). Additionally, many therapeutic strategies have been attempted to medically treat hepatocellular carcinoma, including surgical resection and liver transplantation, although the available treatment options depend on the specific characteristics of the tumor (Thomas and Zhu, 2005; Bruix and Sherman, 2005).

There has been some very interesting research conducted to determine whether the lignans isolated from *S. chinensis* may improve and prevent a variety of human diseases, including cardiac disease, respiratory disease, immune disease, endocrine disease and neuronal disease. However, only a few investigations have been conducted to determine the therapeutic effects of lignans isolated from *S. chinensis* on hepatic carcinoma. Therefore, this chapter describes the important results of an experiment using three lignans (gomisin N, tigloylgomisin H (TGH) and schisandrin A) and one blend (KY88 Liver-Livo) which may prove valuable in the development of a therapeutic drug for the treatment of hepatic carcinoma.

2. Therapeutic effects of lignans and blend isolated from *S. chinensis* on hepatic carcinoma

This main section described experimental data regarding the biological effects of three lignans and a blend on hepatic carcinoma, and the potential for the use of those lignins as therapeutic drugs.

2.1 Effects of gomisin N

Gomisin N (Fig. 1) is already well known as a member of the schisandrin B family, and the most abundant lignin in the fruit lignins of *S. chinensis*. Among the various functions of gomisin N, its ability to increase antioxidant capacity and protect against mitochondria decay was initially identified by a biochemical mechanism study (Ko and Lam, 2002). Additionally, gomisin N could induce an increase in heat shock protein, which performed an important function when cells and tissues were affected by a variety of stressful stimuli from the external environment. Recently, a stereoisomer of gomisin N, (-) schisandrin B, was identified and its function in cell protection was investigated. These results demonstrated that schisandrin B and (-) schisandrin B were the most potent in enhancing antioxidant protection. Therefore, these two lignans may be employed for the protection against and reversal of tissue damage induced by environmental hazards, physical exercise, and aging (Chiu et al., 2006). However, we found a new function of gomisin N, particularly its effects against hepatic carcinoma.

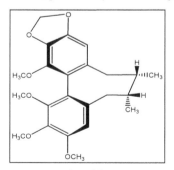

Fig. 1. Chemical structure of gomisin N isolated from *S. chinensis*.

2.1.1 Preparation of gomisin N

The dried fruits of *S. chinensis* (2.5 kg) were ground to a fine powder and were successively extracted at room temperature with *n*-hexane, EtOAc, and MeOH. The hexane extract (308 g) was evaporated under vacuum and chromatographed on a silica gel (40 μm, J.T. Baker, NJ, USA) column (70 x 8.0 cm) with a step gradient of 0%, 5%, 10%, 20%, and 30% EtOAc in hexane (each 1 L). Of these extracts, Fraction 11IA, one of 5 subfraction originated from fraction 11 was further purified by column chromatography on silical gel eluting with CHCl₃-acetone (19:1) to give a gomisin N (774 mg)(Yim et al., 2009).

2.1.2 Effects of gomisin N on cell proliferation

The therapeutic effects of gomisin N on hepatic carcinomas was initially suggested by Yim et al. (2009). First, they extracted lignans including gomisin N (Seo et al., 2004), schisandrin (Ikeya et al., 1979a), schisandrin C (Seo et al., 2004) and gomisin A (Ikeya et al., 1979b; Park et al., 2007) from *S. chinensis* via *n*-hexane, EtOAc and MeOH extraction techniques. Their structures were analyzed via LC-MS and NMR analysis for identification. Proliferation activity was screened for all groups that had received one of the four lignans of varying concentrations via an MTT assay to select the lignan with the highest apoptotic effect on hepatic carcinoma. For schisandrin C, the MTT assay demonstrated that this lignan induced cell proliferation rather than cell death in hepatic carcinoma cells in a concentration range of 40 μM to 160 μM, whereas the gomisin A-treated group maintained a stable cell population (Fig. 2). However, the MTT screening also demonstrated that two lignans, gomisin N and schisandrin, significantly induced cell death in relation to other lignans. In the gomisin N-treated group, cell proliferation in the 40 μM-treated groups was slightly increased compared to the vehicle. However, cell proliferation decreased rapidly in a gomisin N concentration range from 80 μM to 320 μM (Fig. 2). Schisandrin also induced cell death at the higher concentrations, but the cell death ratio was lower than that observed with gomisin N (Fig. 2). These results indicated that gomisin N treatment was highly effective in inducing the death of hepatic carcinoma cells at higher concentrations, but not at low concentrations. Yim et al. selected gomisin N as the candidate lignan for further analysis, owing to its anti-proliferation and pro-apoptosis functions.

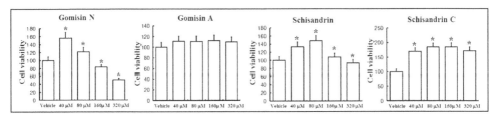

Fig. 2. Anti-proliferative effect of gomisin N, schisandrin, schisandrin C and gomisin A isolated from *S. chinensis* (Yim et al., 2009).

Additionally, phase-contrast microscope analysis was conducted to determine whether the cell death effects observed in the MTT assay were concurrent with the observed cell morphological changes. In the 40 μM-treated group, the number and morphology of hepatic carcinoma evidenced greater crowding than was observed in the vehicle-treated group. The hepatic carcinoma cell line in the 80 μM-treated groups evidenced a pattern similar to that observed with the vehicle-treated group. In the 160 μM-treated group, few dead cells were observed in the microscopic images of the hepatic carcinoma cell line. The numbers of these cells were increased markedly in the 320 μM-treated groups (Fig. 3). These results demonstrated that the results observed on cell morphology analysis under gomisin N-treated conditions were consistent with the results of an MTT assay under the same conditions (Yim et al., 2009).

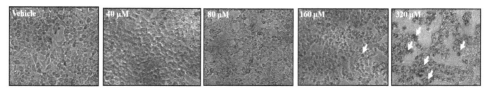

Fig. 3. Microscope images of hepatic carcinoma cell lines after 24 hrs of treatment with gomisin N at various concentrations (Yim et al., 2009).

2.1.3 Effects of gomisin N on apoptosis

Apoptosis, or programmed cell death, performs a critical role in a variety of physiological processes during fetal development and in adult life. Defects in the apoptotic process lead to the progress of many diseases involving progressive cell accumulation and cancer in most cases. Yim et al. (2009) further investigated the correlation between gomisin N and apoptosis. To achieve this, a hepatic carcinoma cell line treated with various concentrations of gomisin N were stained with FITC Annexin V, and fluorescence activity was determined via flow cytometry. Gomisin N significantly induced the increase in the number of cells undergoing apoptosis, from 15% to 98%, in 24 hrs. However, this reaction was induced even at low gomisin N concentrations, and this level of induction remained at a constant level up to and throughout higher concentrations (Fig. 4). Therefore, these results indicated that gomisin N could induce the apoptosis of hepatic carcinoma cell lines in a dose-independent manner. Specifically, gomisin N may induce the loss of plasma membrane asymmetry, one of the early events in the apoptosis process, for most cells treated at a concentration of 40 μM.

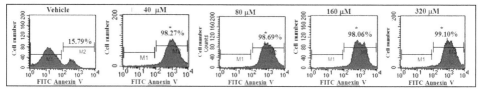

Fig. 4. Identifying apoptotic cells affected with gomisin N treatment. Hepatic carcinoma cells were incubated with gomisin N at various concentrations for 24 hrs, and stained with FITC Annexin V to detect the apoptotic cells (Yim et al., 2009).

Additionally, the apoptosis process involves many families of proteins. Among these proteins, the Bcl-2 proteins are one of the key molecules in inducing the anti-apoptotic process (Apakama et al., 1996). The results of previous studies have shown that this protein was overexpressed in many solid tumors, and that it contributes to chemotherapy resistance and radiation-induced apoptosis (Apakama et al., 1996; Joensuu et al., 1994). Unlike many other known human oncogenes, Bcl-2 exerts its influence by enhancing cell survival rather than by stimulating cell division (Joensuu et al., 1994). Yim et al. (2009) attempted to determine whether the expression level of Bcl-2 protein would be affected by gomisin N treatment in a hepatic carcinoma cell line. Additionally, Yim et al. (2009) assessed the effects of gomisin N treatment on proteins associated with the apoptosis signaling pathway. To achieve this, the expression levels of Bcl-2 and Bax proteins were determined in the vehicle-treated and gomisin N-treated groups via Western blot analysis. The expression level of Bcl-2 protein did not change in the low concentration range as compared to the vehicle. However, the high concentration range-namely the 160 μM and 320 μM-treated groups-evidenced higher levels of Bcl-2 protein expression than was observed in the low concentration range. In the case of Bax, the expression level of this protein was markedly increased only in the 320 μM treated group compared to the vehicle and the other concentration groups. Furthermore, in order to determine whether the tumor suppressor gene would be affected by gomisin N in the hepatic carcinoma cell line, the expression level of p53 protein was detected in the vehicle and gomisin N-treated groups. The expression level of p53 protein remained unchanged in the four treatment groups and the vehicle (Fig. 5). These results indicate that gomisin N may simultaneously induce an increase in the levels of the proteins associated with the anti-apoptotic and pro-apoptotic processes, but does not alter the level of expression of the tumor suppressor protein, p53.

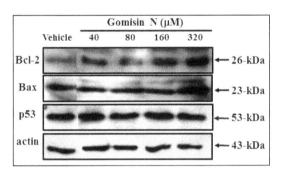

Fig. 5. Effects of gomisin N on Bcl-2, Bax and p53 protein expression to investigate the mechanism underlying apoptosis (Yim et al., 2009).

2.2 Effects of KY88 liver-livo (KY88)

KY88 was one of herbal blends containing *Schizandrae fructus* (Chow et al., 2001). Thus far, three major functions of this drug have been demonstrated; the modulation of the immune system, the induction of apoptosis, and the induction of cytokines by lymphocytes and liver cancer cells (Chow et al., 2004). However, a thorough determination of the therapeutic effects of KY88 against hepatic carcinoma will require further research into its action mechanism.

2.2.1 Preparation of KY88

KY88 is a blend containing the herbal extract of *Schizandrae fructus, Bupleuri radix, Artemisiae capillaris, Desmodii herba, Poria sclerotium, Lithospermi radix, Paeoniae radix, Phellodendri cortex, Scutellariae radix* and *Trichosanthis radix*. Ten grams of each of all ingredients of above herbs were primarily washed and concentrated and purified with the process of extraction. Then, the essence of the herbal extracts -KY88- was assembled. Also, this capsule had been verified by SGS Hong Kong Ltd (Socie´te´ Ge´ne´rale de Surveillance) to be free of heavy metals and microorganisms. Before the study for inhibition ability, KY88 (50 g) was extracted with three times using MeOH. The solid residue obtained from the crude extract was then dissolved in dimethyl sulphoxide to a concentration of 92 mg/ml and stored at 4°C until use (Loo et al. 2007).

2.2.2 Effects of KY88 on cell proliferation and HBeAg/HBsAg secretion

Loo et al. (2007) was the first to investigate whether KY88 has an ability to inhibit hepatocellular carcinoma cell proliferation and the secretion ability of HBsAg (hepatitis B virus surface antigen) and HBeAg (hepatitis B virus core antigen). For this assessment, KY88 was applied to the HB-8064 hepatocellular carcinoma cell line, and the cell proliferation rate and HBsAg/HBeAg secretion were measured on days 1, 3, 5 and 7. The MTT assay showed that the treatment of 0.1, 0.5 and 1 mg/ml KY88 for 7 days induced the significant suppression of hepatic carcinoma. Additionally, the cell proliferation rate of all KY88-treated cells was significantly lower than that of the control-treated group (Fig. 6). In particular, a remarkable suppression of cell proliferation was detected at three concentrations from day 5. Therefore, these data demonstrated that KY88 may potentially exert an effect in inhibiting the cellular proliferation of hepatocellular carcinoma.

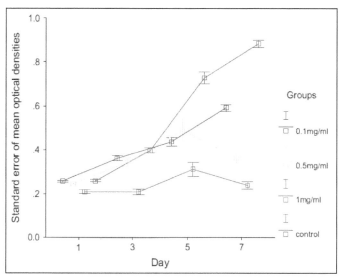

Fig. 6. Dose-dependent inhibition of cell proliferation at three concentrations of KY88 (Loo et al., 2007).

Furthermore, the secretions of HBsAg and HBeAg from the hepatocellular carcinoma cell line were dramatically inhibited by KY88 treatment (Fig. 7). The observation of HBsAg and HBeAg reflected the cell's infection with hepatitis B virus and their replication activity (Loo et al., 2007). This data indicated that KY88 may potentially have the ability to inhibit the proliferation of hepatocellular carcinoma cells, as well as the reduced secretions of HBsAg and HBeAg to restrict tumor growth.

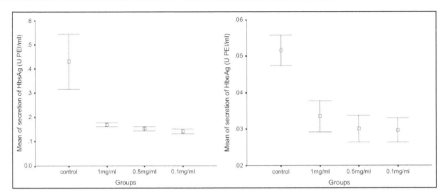

Fig. 7. Secretion level of HBsAg and HBeAg from hepatocellular carcinoma cell line after KY88 treatment (Loo et al., 2007).

2.2.3 Effects of KY88 on apoptosis and cytokine secretion

Chow et al. (2004) previously evaluated the effects and action mechanism of KY88 on liver cancer cells using methanol extracts of KY88 to develop a novel therapeutic drug for the treatment of hepatoma. After methanol extracts of KY88 were applied to a hepatocellular carcinoma cell line, the cell proliferation, DNA laddering and cytokine secretion were detected in these cells. KY88 induced a significant inhibition of cell proliferation and an increase in the DNA ladder pattern, which is a marker that indicates apoptosis in hepatocellular carcinoma cells (Fig. 8).

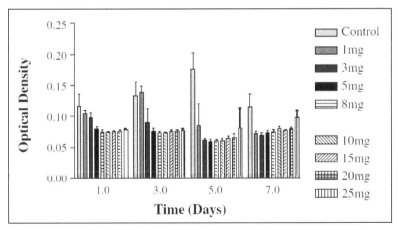

Fig. 8. Inhibition effect of KY88 methanol extracts on hepatocellular carcinoma cell (Chow et al., 2004).

Additionally, cytokine ELISA assay results demonstrated that IL-4 and TNF-α concentrations were increased significantly by KY88 treatment when compared against the control group at 24 hrs. However, IL-2, IL-6 and INF-γ concentrations were maintained at constant levels (Fig. 9). Therefore, this data indicates that the methanol extracts of KY88 may induce apoptosis via the regulation of IL-4 and TNF-α secretion.

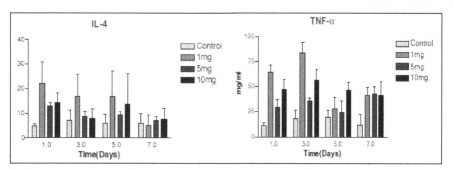

Fig. 9. Significant change of IL-4 and TNF-α level in hepatocellular carcinoma cell after KY88 treatment (Chow et al., 2004).

2.3 Effects of schizandrin A

Schizandrin A is referred to by several other names, including deoxyschizandrin, wuweizisu A, and deoxyschisandrin (Lu and Chen, 2009), and is one of the most effective lignins isolated from *S. chinensis* (Fig. 10). Previous studies have also demonstrated that schizandrin A may have the hepatoprotective, antioxidative, neurobiological performance-improving and anti-tumor activities (Deng et al., 2008; Huang et al., 2008). For the first time, the function of schizandrin A was found to protect against liver injuries, activate liver regeneration and supress liver carcinogenesis (Zheng et al., 1997). Additionally, this lignan was partially used as a Ca^{2+} modulator which induced the synchronization of Ca^{2+} oscillation via the influx inhibition of extracellular Ca^{2+} and the initiation of action potential (Fu et al., 2008). However, only a small amount of research has been conducted regarding the possible inhibitory effects of schizandrin A on hepatocellular carcinoma. This chapter also describes recent key results regarding the possible anti-liver cancer effects of schizandrin A.

Fig. 10. Chemical structure of schizandrin A isolated from *S. chinensis*.

2.3.1 Preparation of schizandrin A

Generally, schizandrin A was prepared with a methods suggested by Chen et al. (1976) and Yue et al. (1994). Firstly, *S. chinensis* Baill (10 kg) was extracted with 50 L of hexane for 1.5 hr and the obtained extract was dried under a reduced pressure. The 978.8 g of hexane extract were dissolved in 9.8 L of hexane and sequentially extracted two times with 9.8 L of 60% (v/v) MeOH. The mixture obtained from above extraction was dried under a reduced pressure and finally 112.2 g of a fraction having a high lignan content were obtained. These fraction having a high lignan content was subjected to the fractionation high-speed liquid chromatography [column: Kiesel Gel 60 (230 to 400 mesh) supplied by Merk, diameter=10 cm, length=100 cm, moving phase: n-hexane/ethyl acetate (7/3), flow rate: 200 ml/min, apparatus: Waters Prep LC/System 500A]. Fractions eluted at 63 to 70 minutes in the fractionation high-speed liquid chromatography were combined and dried under a reduced pressure. The obtained residue (schizandrin A) was recrystallized from methanol to obtain 1.05 g of a colorless prism crystal.

2.3.2 Effects of schizandrin A and LCC (five schizandrins and crud extract from *Fructus shizandrae*) on human hepatocellular carcinoma

Huang et al. (2008) evaluated the reversal effects of five schizandrins (schizandrin A, schizandrin B, schizandrin C, schizandrol A and schizandrol B) and LCC on multidrug resistance (MDR) in several cancer cells, including hepatocellular carcinoma and epidermal carcinoma *in vitro* and *in vivo*. After treatment with various concentrations of five schizandrins and LCC into cancer cell lines, drug sensitivity, apoptosis, doxorubicin (Dox) accumulation and protein kinas C (PKC) expression were measured in cancer cell lines. Various levels of MDR reversal activity were noted at a 25 µM concentration of the five tested compounds. The most potent compound found was schizandrin A. The reversal activity of MDR was also induced by 25 µg/ml of LCC in KBV200, MCF-7/Dox cells, and human hepatic cellular carcinoma Bel7402 cells. The flow cytometry analysis results demonstrated that both schizandrin A and LCC treatment induced an increase in apoptosis in human hepatocellular carcinoma cells. As shown in Fig. 11, the sub-G1 peak, which is one of the characteristics of apoptosis, was increased significantly from 1.8% in the Bel7402 cells treated with Dox only to 10-14% in the schizandrin A + Dox-treated cells or the LCC + Dox-treated cells. Additionally, chromatin condensation, another marker of apoptosis, was enhanced in cells treated with schizandrin A + Dox or with LCC + Dox. Furthermore, downregulations of PKC and P-glycoprotein expression were noted in cells treated with schizandrin A + Dox or LCC + Dox (Fig. 11). These data showed that schizandrin A and LCC may induce a reversal of MDR in cancer cells via the inhibition of P-glycoprotein and PKC expression.

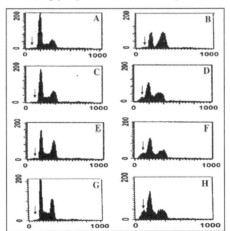

Fig. 11. Enhancing effects of schizandrin A and LCC on apoptosis in human hepatocellular carcinoma cells. **A** Control, **B** Dox 1,250 ng/ml, **C** Verapamil (VPL) 20 µM, **D** Dox 1,250 ng/ml + VPL 20 µM, **E** Schizandrin A 25 µM, **F** Dox 1,250 ng/ml + Schizandrin A 25 µM, **G** LCC 25 µg/ml, **H** Dox 1,250 ng/ml + LCC 25 µg/ml (Huang et al., 2008).

2.3.3 Effects of LCC on the tumor growth of mice

In order to confirm the MDR-reversing effects of LCC and schizandrin A detected *in vitro*, tumor growth was measured in nude mice bearing KBv200 xenografts. Following 10 days of vincristine injection, tumor growth was inhibited significantly-by approximately 12%-when tumor size was compared to that of the control group (Huang et al., 2008). Furthermore, co-treatment with LCC and vincristine at 100, 200 and 300 mg/kg BW increased the anti-tumor activity induced by vincristine in a dose-dependent manner (Fig. 12). In particular, LCC 300 mg/kg BW co-treatment for 15 days resulted in dramatic differences-most notably, a 41.9% inhibition of tumor size (Huang et al., 2008). These results indicate that LCC has potential for use in the development of a therapeutic drug for hepatoma *in vivo*.

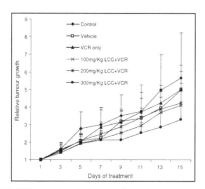

Fig. 12. Inhibition effects of LCC on vincristine-induced anti-tumor activity in nude mice bearing the KBv200 xenograft (Huang et al., 2008).

2.4 Effects of TGH

The structure of TGH (Fig. 13) was firstly assessed by Ikeya et al. (1978a). In Korea, this lignin was initially identified via gas chromatography/mass spectrometry (GC/MS) from *S. chinensis* harvested in Muju, Korea (Sohn and Bock, 1989). However, many things remain unknown regarding the functions of this lignan. Recently, several important study results suggesting a possible function of TGH in cancer therapy have caused an increase in interest in the compound.

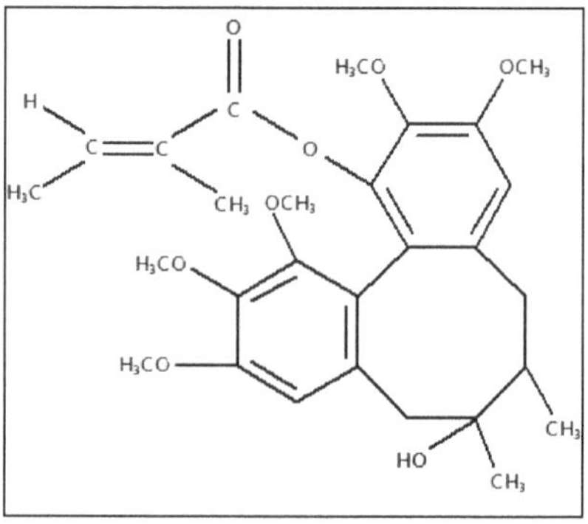

Fig. 13. Chemical structure of TGH isolated from *S. chinensis*.

2.4.1 Preparation of TGH

In order to prepare TGH, the fruit of *S. chinensis* (250 g) was firstly extracted three times using 500 mL of MeOH with sonication for 1 hr. The dried MeOH extract was collected from filtered solution with dryness under reduced pressure. Then, MeOH extract (50 g) was suspended in water and sequentially fractionated with *n*-hexane and CH_2Cl_2. The purified *n*-hexane fraction (10 g) was subjected to chromatography on an RP-18 column (4.5 x 20 cm, 5:5 - 9:1 MeOH:water, v/v) to yield fractions 1-8. Furthermore, fraction 4 (650 mg) was dissolved in MeOH and subjected to isocratic semi-preparative HPLC using an YMC J-sphere ODS column (20 x 250 mm, 4 µm; YMC). TGH was separated with MeCN-0.1% TFA in H2O (50:50 in 50 min, 10 mL/min, 254 nm) to yield 62.0 mg of compound 4 (93.65%). The identity of TGH was confirmed by 1H- and 13C-NMR spectroscopy (Lee et al., 2009).

2.4.2 Effects of TGH on cell survival

Lee et al. (2009) initially investigated the anti-cancer functions and action mechanisms of nine lignans isolated from the fruit of *S. chinensis*. Firstly, nine lignans including schisandrol A, schisandrol A, TGH, angeloylgomisin H (AGH), schisandrin A, schisandrin B, gomisin J, gomisin N and schisandrin C were isolated from *S. chinensis* and the effects of each lignin on the cell survival rate were determined. Among the nine lignans, TGH induced a reduction in cell survival at concentrations ranging from 31.3 µM to 250.0 µM, whereas the AGH samples maintained a steady level in terms of cell survival (Fig. 14). During this period, the quinone reductase activity was dramatically increased in hepatocarcinoma cells and evidenced a high chemoprevention index. Additionally, the mechanism study results demonstrated that the expression of genes mediated by the antioxidant response element (ARE), an important regulatory region in the promoter of the detoxification enzyme gene which is regulated by the nuclear accumulation of Nrf2, was enhanced significantly by TGH. Therefore, all study results appear to indicate that TGH may be considered as a potential liver cancer-preventive compound that specifically induces increases in antioxidant enzyme expression via the formation of the Nrf2-ARE binding complex.

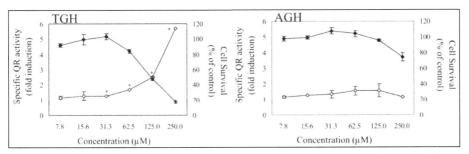

Fig. 14. Effects of TGH treatment on the quinone reductase activity and cell survival (Lee et al., 2009).

3. Conclusion

The development of novel therapeutic drugs for hepatic carcinoma is a very important objective in the field of pharmacological research. Among the variety of approaches thus far pursued to develop novel drugs, identification and screening of natural compounds from medical herbs has proven a very effective one-not least, because this method saves a great deal of time and cost. Recently, many institutes and companies in advanced countries have focused on an approach to novel drugs for hepatic carcinoma via the use of various lignins isolated from *S. chinensis*. This chapter introduces three lignans and one blend which may prove valuable in efforts to combat hepatic carcinoma. Gomisin A at high concentration was found to significantly induce anti-proliferative and pro-apoptotic effects in hepatic carcinoma. Schizandrin A markedly increased vincristine-induced hepatic carcinoma apoptosis and anti-tumor activity. Additionally, TGH induced the death of hepatic carcinoma cells and inhibited quinone reductase activity. Furthermore, KY88 was a blend composed of 10 herbal extracts and effects a dose-dependent inhibition of hepatocellular carcinoma cellular proliferation (Table 3).

Collectively, the results of these studies demonstrated that these lignins and the blend from *S. chinensis* were regarded as an anti-cancer drug candidate capable of inducing apoptosis and inhibiting the cell proliferation of hepatocellular carcinoma via a variety of mechanisms.

Compounds	Function on hepatocellular carcinoma	References
Gomisin N	· Induction of hepatic carcinoma apoptosis · Increase of Bcl-2 protein expression	Yim et al., 2009
KY88	·Dose-dependent inhibition of hepatocellular carcinoma proliferation and secretion of HBsAg and HBeAg ·Induction of hepatic carcinoma apoptosis and IL-4/TNF-α secretion	Loo et al., 2007 Chow et al., 2004
Schizandrin A	·Induction of hepatic carcinoma apoptosis and PKC down regulation ·Increase of anti-tumor activity induced by vincristine	Huang et al., 2008
TGH	·Induction of hepatic carcinoma death and inhibition of quinone reductase activity	Lee et al., 2009

Table 3. Summary therapeutic function of three lignins and one blend from *S. chinensis* on hepatocellular carcinoma.

4. Acknowledgments

I would like to express my gratitude to students, including JE Kim, SH Nam, SI Choi, IS Hwang, HR Lee and YJ Lee in our laboratory, for helping to compile this paper and with the graphics and charts herein.

5. References

Print Books

Adami, HO.; Hunter, D. & Trichopoulos, D. (2008): *Cancer of the Liver and Biliary Tract. In: Textbook of Cancer Epidemiology* (Second edition), Oxford University Press, ISBN 978-0-19-531117-4, Oxford England, pp. 308-332

Agejenko, AS. & Komissarenko, BT. (1960). *Schizandra and its Therapeutic Administration.* Sakhalinsk Book Press, Yuzhno-Sakhalinsk, p. 38

Gutnikova, ZI. (1951). Schizandra chinensis in the Far East. In: Lazarev,N.V. (Ed.), Materials for the Study of Ginseng and Schizandra Roots. Far East Branch of USSR Academy of Science, Vladivostok, pp. 23–43

Shilova, LM. (1963). *On the problem of sexual dimorphism and pollination in Schizandra chinensis.* In: Brekhman, I.I., Belikov, I.F., Kuznetsova, G.E. (Eds.), Materials for the Study of Ginseng and Schizandra. Far East Branch of the USSR Academy of Science, Primorsk Book Publisher, Vladivostok, pp. 267–270

Papers in Journals

Apakama, I.; Robinson, MC.; Walter, NM.; Charlton, RG.; Royds, JA.; Fuller, CE.; Neal, DE. & Hamdy, FC. (1996) Bcl-2 overexpression combined with p53 accumulation correlates with hormone refractory prostate cancer. *British Journal of cancer,* Vol. 74, No. 8, (October 1996), pp. 1258-1262, ISSN 0007-0920

Bosch, FX.; Ribes, J.; Díaz, M. & Cléries, R. (2004) Primary liver cancer: worldwide incidence and trends. *Gastroenterology,* Vol. 127, No. 5, (November 2004), pp. S5-S16, ISSN 0016-5085

Bruix, J. & Sherman, M. (2005) Management of hepatocellular carcinoma. *Hepatology,* Vol. 42, No. 5, (November 2005), pp. 1208-1236, ISSN 1527-3350

Chen, CC.; Shen, CC.; Shih, YZ. & Pan, TM. (1994) 6-O-Benzoylgomisin O, a New Lignan from the Fruits of Schizandra chinensis. *Journal of Natural Products,* Vol. 57, No. 8, (August 1994), pp. 1164-1165, ISSN 0163-3864

Chen, YY.; Shu, ZB. & Li, LN. (1976) Studies of Fructus schizandrae. IV. Isolation and determination of the active compounds (in lowering high SGPT levels) of Schizandra chinensis Baill. *Scientia Sinica,* Vol. 19, No. 2, (April 1976), pp. 276-290, ISSN 0250-7870

Chiu, PY.; Leung, HY.; Poon, MK.; Mak, DH. & Ko, KM. (2006) Effects of schisandrin B enantiomers on cellular glutathione and menadione toxicity in AML12 hepatocytes. *Pharmacology,* Vol. 77, No. 2, (April 2006), pp. 63-70, ISSN 0031-7012

Choi, YW.; Takamatsu, S.; Khan, SI.; Srinivas, PV.; Ferreira, D.; Zhao, J.P. & Khan I.A. (2006) Schisandrene, a Dibenzocyclooctadiene Lignan from *Schisandra chinensis*: Structure–Antioxidant Activity Relationships of Dibenzocyclooctadiene Lignans. *Journal of Natural Products,* Vol. 69, No. 3, (December 2005), pp. 356-359, ISSN 0163-3864

Chow, CW.; Loo, TY.; Sham, ST. & Cheung, NB. (2004) *Radix bupleuri* containing compound (KY88 liver-livo) induces apoptosis and production of interleukin-4 and tumor necrosis factor-alpha in liver cancer cells in vitro. *The American Journal of Chinese Medicine,* Vol. 32, No. 2, (February 2004), pp. 185-93, ISSN 0192-415X

Chow, LW.; Loo, WY. & Sham, JS. (2001) Effects of a herbal compound containing bupleurum on human lymphocytes. *Hong Kong Medical Journal,* Vol. 7, No. 4, (December 2001), pp. 408–413, ISSN 1024-2708

Deng, X.; Chen, X.; Yin, R.; Shen, Z.; Qiao, L. & Bi, K. (2008) Determination of deoxyschizandrin in rat plasma by LC-MS. *Journal of Pharmaceutical Biomedical Analysis,* Vol. 46, No. 1, (January 2008), pp. 121-126, ISSN 0731-7085

El-Serang, HB. & Mason, AC. (2000) Risk factors for the rising rates of primary liver cancer in the United States. *Archives of Internal Medicine,* Vol. 160, No. 21, (November 2000), pp. 3227-3230, ISSN 0003-9926

Fu, M.; Sun, ZH.; Zong, M.; He, XP.; Zuo, HC. & Xie, ZP. (2008) Deoxyschisandrin modulates synchronized Ca2+ oscillations and spontaneous synaptic transmission of cultured hippocampal neurons. *Acta Pharmacologica Sinica,* Vol. 29, No. 8, (August 2008), pp. 891-898, ISSN 1671-4083

Huang, M.; Jin, J.; Sun, H. & Liu, GT. (2008) Reversal of P-glycoprotein-mediated multidrug resistance of cancer cells by five schizandrins isolated from the Chinese herb Fructus Schizandrae. *Cancer Chemotherapy and Pharmacology,* Vol. 62, No. 6, (November 2008), pp. 1015-1026, ISSN 0344-5704

Ikeya, Y.; Kanatani, H.; Hakozaki, M.; Taguchi, H. & Mitsuhashi, H. (1988) The constituents of Schizandra chinensis Baill. XV. Isolation and structure determination of two new lignans, gomisin S and gomisin T. *Chemical & Pharmaceutical Bulletin,* Vol. 36, No. 10, (October 1988), pp. 3974-3979, ISSN 0009-2363

Ikeya, Y.; Miki, E.; Okada, M.; Mitsuhashi, H. & Chai, JG. (1990) Benzoylgomisin Q and benzoylgomisin P, two new lignans from Schisandra sphenanthera Rehd. et Wils. *Chemical & Pharmaceutical Bulletin,* Vol. 38, No. 5, (May 1990), pp. 1408-1411, ISSN 0009-2363

Ikeya, Y.; Ookawa, N.; Taguchi, H. & Yosioka, I. (1982b) The constituents of Schizandra chinensis Baill. XI. The structures of three new lignans, angeloylgomisin O, and angeloyl- and benzoylisogomisin O. *Chemical & Pharmaceutical Bulletin,* Vol. 30, No. 9, (September 1982b), pp. 3202-3206, ISSN 0009-2363

Ikeya, Y.; Sugama, K.; Okada, M. & Mitsuhashi, H. (1991) Two lignans from Schisandra sphenanthera. *Phytochemistry,* Vol. 30, No. 3, (March 1991), pp. 975-980, ISSN 0031-9942

Ikeya, Y.; Taguchi, H. & Litaka, Y. (1976) The constituents of Schizandra chinensis Baill. The structure of a new lignin, gomisin D. *Tetrahedron Letters,* Vol. 17, No. 17, (April 1976), pp. 1359-1362, ISSN 0040-4039

Ikeya, Y.; Taguchi, H. & Yosioka, I. (1979d) The constituents of Schizandra chinensis Baill. The cleavage of the methylenedioxy moiety with lead tetraacetate in benzene, and the structure of angeloylgomisin Q. *Chemical & Pharmaceutical Bulletin,* Vol. 27, No. 10, (October 1979d) pp. 2536-2538, ISSN 0009-2363

IKeya, Y.; Taguchi, H. & Yosioka, I. (1980a) The constituents of Schizandra chinensis Baill. VII. The structures of three new lignans, (-)-gomisin K1 and (+)-gomisins K2 and K3. *Chemical & pharmaceutical bulletin,* Vol. 28, No. 8, (August 1980a), pp. 2422-2427, ISSN 0009-2363

IKeya, Y.; Taguchi, H. & Yosioka, I. (1982a) The constituents of Schizandra chinensis BAILL. X. The structures of γ-schizandrin and four new lignans, (-)-gomisins L1 and L2, (±)-gomisin M1 and (+)-gomisin M2. *Chemical & pharmaceutical bulletin,* Vol. 30, No. 1, (January 1982a), pp. 132-139, ISSN 0009-2363

Ikeya, Y.; Taguchi, H. & Yosioka, I. (1982c) The Constituents of Schizandra chinensis BAILL. XII. Isolation and Structure of a New Lignan, Gomisin R, the Absolute Structure of Wuweizisu C and Isolation of Schisantherin D. *Chemical & Pharmaceutical Bulletin,* Vol. 30, No. 9, (September 1982c) pp. 3207-3211, ISSN 0009-2363

Ikeya, Y.; Taguchi, H.; Yosioka, I. & Kobayashi, H. (1978a) The constituents of *Schizandra chinensis* BAILL. The structures of two new lignans, pre-gomisin and gomisin J. *Chemical & Pharmaceutical Bulletin,* Vol. 26, No. 2, (February 1978a), pp. 682-684, ISSN 0009-2363

Ikeya, Y.; Taguchi, H.; Yosioka, I. & Kobayashi, H. (1978b) The Constituents of Schizandra chinensis BAILL. The Structures of Two New Lignans, Gomisin N and Tigloylgomisin P. *Chemical & pharmaceutical bulletin,* Vol. 26, No. 10, (October 1978b), pp. 3257-3260, ISSN 0009-2363

Ikeya, Y.; Taguchi, H.; Yosioka, I. & Kobayashi, H. (1979a) The constituents of *Schizandra chinensis* Baill. I. Isolation and structure determination of five new lignans, gomisin A, B, C, F and G, and the absolute structure of schizandrin. *Chemical & pharmaceutical bulletin,* Vol. 27, No.6, (November 1979a), pp. 1383-1394, ISSN 0009-2363

Ikeya, Y.; Taguchi, H.; Yosioka, I. & Kobayashi, H. (1979b) The constituents of Schizandra chinensis Baill. III. The structures of four new lignans, gomisin H and its derivatives, angeloyl-, tigloyl- and benzoyl-gomisin H. *Chemical & pharmaceutical bulletin,* Vol. 27, No. 7, (July 1979b), pp. 1576-1582, ISSN 0009-2363

Ikeya, Y.; Taguchi, H.; Yosioka, I. & Kobayashi, H. (1979c) The constituents of Schizandra chinensis Baill. IV. The structures of two new lignans, pre-gomisin and gomisin J. *Chemical & Pharmaceutical Bulletin,* Vol. 27, No. 7, (July 1979c) pp. 1583-1588, ISSN 0009-2363

Ikeya, Y.; Taguchi, H.; Yosioka, I. & Kobayashi, H. (1979e) The constituents of Schizandra chinensis Baill. V. The structures of four new lignans, gomisin N, gomisin O, epigomisin O and gomisin E, and transformation of gomisin N to deangeloylgomisin B. *Chemical & Pharmaceutical Bulletin,* Vol. 27, No. 11, (December 1979e), pp. 2695-2709, ISSN 0009-2363

Ikeya, Y.; Taguchi, H.; Yosioka, I.; Yosioka, I. & Kobayashi, H. (1980b) The constituents of Schizandra chinensis Baill. VIII. The structures of two new lignans,tigloylgomisin P and angeloylgomisin P. *Chemical & Pharmaceutical Bulletin,* Vol. 28, No. 11, (November 1980b), pp. 3357-3361, ISSN 0009-2363

Joensuu, H.; Pylkkänen, L. & Toikkanen, S. (1994) Bcl-2 protein expression and long-term survival in breast cancer. *The American Journal of pathology,* Vol. 145, No. 5, (May 1994), pp. 1191-1198, ISSN 0002-9440

Ko, KM. & Lam, BY. (2002) Schisandrin B protects against tert-butylhydroperoxide induced cerebral toxicity by enhancing glutathione antioxidant status in mouse brain. *Molecular & Cellular Biochemistry,* Vol. 238, No. 1-2, (September 2002), pp. 181-186, ISSN 0300-8177

Lee, SB.; Kim, CY.; Lee, HJ.; Yun, JH. & Nho, CW. (2009) Induction of the phase II detoxification enzyme NQO1 in hepatocarcinoma cells by lignans from the fruit of Schisandra chinensis through nuclear accumulation of Nrf2. *Planta Medica,* Vol. 75, No. 12, (October 2009), pp. 1314-1318

Liu, CS.; Fang, SD.; Huang, MF.; Kao, YL. & Hsu JS. (1978) Studies on the active principles of Schisandra sphenanthera Rehd. et Wils. The structures of schisantherin A, B, C, D, E, and the related compounds. *Scientia Sinica,* Vol. 21, No. 4, (July-August 1978), pp. 483-502, ISSN 0250-7870

Loo, WT.; Cheung, MN. & Chow, LW. (2007) Fructus schisandrae (Wuweizi)-containing compound inhibits secretion of HBsAg and HBeAg in hepatocellular carcinoma cell line. *Biomedicine & Pharmacotherapy*, Vol. 61, No. 9, (October 2007), pp. 606-610, ISSN 0753-3322

Lu, Y. & Chen, DF. (2009) Analysis of Schisandra chinensis and Schisandra sphenanthera. *Journal of Chromatography A*, Vo. 1216, No. 11, (March 2009), pp. 1980-1990, ISSN 0021-9673

Panossian, A. & Wikman, G. (2008) Pharmacology of Schisandra chinensis Bail.: an overview of Russian research and uses in medicine. *Journal of Ethnopharmacology*, Vol. 118, No. 2, (July 2008), pp. 183-212, ISSN 0378-8741

Park, JY.; Lee, SJ.; Yun, MR.; Seo, KW.; Bae, SS.; Park, JW.; Lee, YJ.; Shin, WJ.; Choi, YW. & Kim, CD. (2007) Gomisin A from *Schisandra chinensis* induces endothelium-dependent and direct relaxation in rat thoracic aorta. *Planta Medica*, Vol. 73, No. 15, (December 2007), pp. 1537-1542, ISSN 0032-0943

Sakurai, H.; Nikaido, T.; Ohmoto, T.; Ikeya, Y. & Mitsuhashi, H. (1992) Inhibitors of adenosine 3',5'-cyclic monophosphate phosphodiesterase from Schisandra chinensis and the structure activity relationship of lignans. *Chemical & Pharmaceutical Bulletin*, Vol. 40, No. 5, (May 1992), pp. 1191-1195, ISSN 0009-2363

Seo, SM.; Lee, HJ.; Park, YK.; Lee, MK.; Park, JI.; Paik, KH. & Park, JI. (2004). Lignans from the fruits of *Schizandra chinensis* and their inhibitory effects on dopamine content in PC12 cells. *Natural Product Sciences*, Vol.10, No.3, (June 2004), pp. 104-108, ISSN 1226-3907

Sohn, HJ. & Bock, JY. (1989) Identification of lignan compounds in fruits of *Schizandra chinensis* BAILLON by gas chromatography/mass spectrometry. *Journal of the Korean Agricultural Chemical Society*, Vol. 32, No. 4, (December 1989), pp. 344-349, ISSN 0368-2897

Taguchi, H. & Ikeya, Y. (1977) The Constituents of Schizandra chinensis BAILL. The Structures of Two New Lignans, Gomisin F and G, and the Absolute Structures of Gomisin A, B, and C. *Chemical & Pharmaceutical Bulletin*, Vol. 25, No. 2, (February 1977), pp. 364-366, ISSN 0009-2363

Thomas, MB. & Zhu, AX. (2005) Hepatocellular carcinoma: the need for progress. *Journal of Clinical Oncology*, Vol. 23, No. 13, (May 2005), pp. 2892-2829, ISSN 0732-183X

Yim, SY.; Lee, YJ.; Lee, YK.; Jung, SE.; Kim, JH.; Kim, HJ.; Son, BG.; Park, YH.; Lee, YG.; Choi, YW. & Hwang, DY. (2009) Gomisin N isolated from Schisandra chinensis significantly induces anti-proliferative and pro-apoptotic effects in hepatic carcinoma. *Molecular medicine reports*, Vol. 2, No. 5, (October 2009), pp. 725-732, ISSN 1791-2997

Yue, JM.; Jun, X. & Chen, YZ. (1994) Triterpenoids of Schisandra sphenanthera. *Phytochemistry*, Vol. 35, No. 4, (April 1994), pp. 1068-1069, ISSN 0031-9422

Zheng, RL.; Kang, JH.; Chen, FY.; Wang, PF.; Ren, JG. & Liu, QL. (1997) Difference in antioxidation for schisandrins and schisantherin between bio- and chemo-systems. *Phytotherapy Research*, Vol. 11, No. 8, (December 1997), pp. 600-602, ISSN 1099-1573

12

Traditional Chinese Medicine Active Ingredient-Metal Based Anticancer Agents

Zhen-Feng Chen, Hong Liang and Yan-Cheng Liu
Guangxi Normal University,
China

1. Introduction

Traditional Chinese medicine (TCM) possesses a rich and ancient history, tracing its roots back several thousand years. The practice of TCM, highly influenced by the development of Chinese culture, involves physical therapy using acupuncture, moxibustion (application of heat to the acupuncture point by burning a piece of the Chinese plant Artemisia moxa on the skin or the acupuncture needle), and chemical therapy. TCM natural products are isolated as decoctions of animal, mineral and herbal materials (Chan, 1995; Shibata, 1985;). The objective of the system of TCM is on the patient rather than disease, which fundamentally intention to promote health and enhance the quality of life, with therapeutic strategies for treatment of specific disease or symptoms in holistic fashion. TCM represents an old Chinese philosophical thinking, where the human is considered the centre of the universe and acts as an antenna between celestial and earthly elements of the world. The world is a single unit and its movement affords yin and yang, the two main antithetic aspects. Moreover, Chinese believe that yin and yang are not absolute but relative. Consistent with the modern view of homeostasis, yin and yang are interchanged to meet the view that yang decline and yin rises? Or yang is raised to produce a decline of yin? The four bodily humors (qi, blood, moitsture and essence) and internal organ systems (zang fu) play an important role in balancing the yin and yang in human body. Proper formation, maintenance and circulation of these energies are essential for health. When the two energies fall out of harmony, and the balance is broken, disease develops (Patwardhan et al., 2005). The physician takes into account this concept while treating patients. Drugs or herbs are used to correct this imbalance of yin-yang in the human body (Cheng, 2000; Gibert, 1998).

Different from TCM, western science and medicine are focused on the mechanism, which belongs to reductionism. Rather than addressing the overall well being of a patient, it is only the disease that is analyzed at the cellular, molecular, and pharmacological level. The history, philosophy, theory and practice of TCM can been seen in recent reviews (Liu, 1988), herein, we do not give unnecessary details.

Although medicinal herbs have played an important role in Western medicine from ancient to modern times, medicinal plants gradually lost their importance as synthetic pharmaceuticals advanced in Western countries during the 20th century. Currently, there is a revival of interest in bioactive natural products as chemical lead compounds for the generation of semi-synthetic derivatives, namely regression nature.

Traditional Chinese medicine (TCM) has held, and still holds, an important position in primary health care over vast rural areas of China and is appreciated in urban and well-developed areas because of its 5000-year-old tradition. Recently, the Chinese government has undertaken enormous efforts to modernize TCM by investing capital in scientific research, technology programs, and in the economic development of TCM therapies. In the Western world, interest in TCM is increasing due to the belief that it may lead to novel TCM-Western hybrid medicines and treatments.

Since the discovery of cisplatin (**1**, Fig. 1) in 1969, great progress has been made expanding the diversity of platinum anticancer drugs and the conditions they treat (Alt et al., 2007; Clark et al., 1999; Giandomenico, 1999; Jung & Lippard, 2007; Orvig & Abrams, 1999; Rosenberg et al., 1969; Wataru et al., 2008; Wong & Jamieson & Lippard, 1999; Zutphen & Reedijk, 2005). Cisplatin is currently used to treat bladder, non-small cell lung, head and neck, ovarian, cervical, and other cancers, being curative in nearly all cases of testicular cancers. Several similar platinum complexes with fewer toxic side effects, carboplatin (**2**, Fig.1) and oxaliplatin (**3**, Fig.1) were approved as a first-line treatment for colorectal cancer. Nedaplatin (**4**, Fig. 1) was approved for use in Japan, and lobaplatin (**5**, Fig.1) was approved for use in China (Lovejoy & Lippard, 2009). During the past three decades, medicinal chemists have investigated many approaches to enhance antitumor activity, reduce side effects, and overcome drug resistances. To data, thousands of platinum compounds have been synthesized, characterized, and their antitumor activity investigated; however, only 30 platinum compounds have entered clinical trials. Moreover, none have exceeded the anticancer activity of cisplatin. Obviously, current synthetic strategies for development of metal-based anticancer are inefficient (Kelland, 2007). Although non-platinum antitumor metal complexes exhibit different action mechanisms and structural characteristics compared to platinum drugs, the antitumor activity of these non-platinum compounds needs to be determined and their action mechanisms await further investigation. Recent research has shown that metal complexes based on TCMs afforded a novel approach to a potential (pro-) drugs (Chen et al., 2009; Ho et al., 2001; Liu et al., 2009).

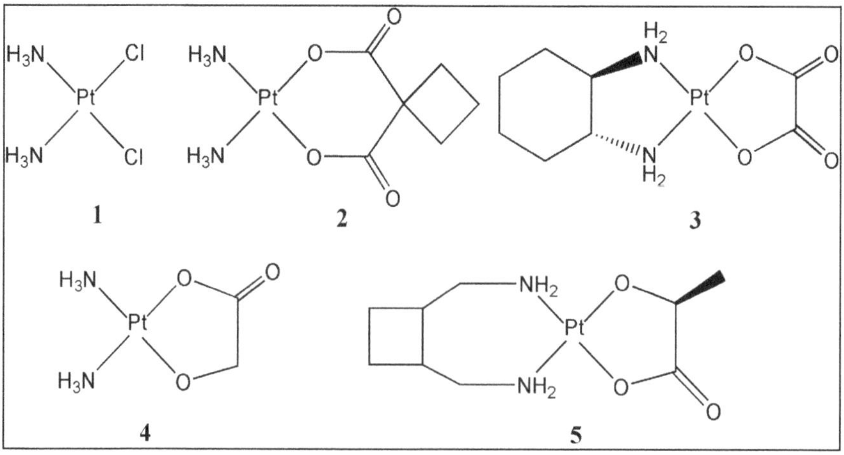

Fig. 1. Strucutres of platinum compounds currently in clinical use. 1: cisplatin, 2: carboplatin, 3: oxaliplatin, 4: nedaplatin, 5: lobaplatin.

2. The anticancer metal-based agents based on TCM active ingredients

Considering the low success rate of current metal-based anticancer synthetic strategies, some bioinorganic chemists have shifted focus to TCM derivatives. There are many successful examples of TCM-derived anticancer agents through organic modification of the active TCM constituents, which is considered a shortcut to discover new anticancer drugs, however, the TCM-metal based anticancer agents are still lack of enough attention, which represent another approach of modification. It is well known that metals and metal complexes can make significant contributions to drug development, but are not receiving the attention they merit. Metal complexes are relative easy to prepare, and the additional geometric possibilities resulting from the use of six-coordinate metal centres (compared to four-coordinate carbon) make this an attractive approach for the rapid development of new species, either as drugs or as probes of the geometric requirements of active sites (Hambley, 2007). Along with the TCM coordination chemistry theory springs up, it is convinced of that metal ion existence plays important role in TCM. Moreover, due to many active compounds containing hydroxyl, carboxylic acid, and amine groups, they are excellent donor atoms that may easily form coordination bonds. Developing TCM coordination complexes may lead to novel therapies that synergistically combine the functions of TCM and metals, generating a novel strategy that bridges traditional Chinese medicine to rational cancer therapy. This concept has attracted increased interest in TCM-metal based antitumor agents. Herein, we review the progress in TCM-metal based anticancer agents according to the TCM active gradient category.

2.1 Alkaloid-metal based anticancer agents

Alkaloids, which are generally defined as nitrogen-containing natural molecules independently of the basic character of the nitrogen, are abundant secondary metabolites in plants and represent one of the most widespread class of compounds endowed with multiple, varied pharmacological properties, including anticancer, antibacterial, anti-fungi, and even anti-virus activities. Up to now, the alkaloid-metal based anticancer agents mainly include oxoaporphine, matrine, β-carboline alkaloid-metal based anticancer agents.

2.1.1 Liriodenine-metal based anticancer agents

Among alkaloids, the aporphinoids constitute a broad subgroup of benzylisoquinoline compounds, with more than 500 alkaloids isolated up to now. They are widely distributed in a large number of plant families including *Annonaceae, Magnoliaceae, Monimiaceae, Menispermaceae, Hernandiaceae, Renunculaceae.* Our group has widely carried out a series of investigations on oxoaporphine-metal based anticancer agents. Liriodenine (**6**, Fig. 2), as an oxoaporphine alkaloid, was isolated for the first time form Liriodendron *tulipifera L.* and was subsequently found mainly in the family of *Annonaceae, Rutaceae, Magnoliaceae, Monimiaceae, Menispermaceae,* ect. (Bentley, 2001; Lan et al., 2003; Lin et al., 1994; Hsien et al., 2005; Nissanka et al., 2001; Woo et al., 1997; Wu et al., 1990). Liriodenine has a wide range of pharmacological activities, such as anti-bacterial, anti-fungi, antitumour and even anti-virus activities. Due to its planar aromatic structure, liriodenine can intercalate into the neighbouring base pairs of DNA double helix, to which its significant antitumor activity can be primarily attributed. Moreover, it also catalytically inhibits topoisomerase to block DNA synthesis and increase p53 and iNOS expression to induce cell cycle G1 arrest (Chang et al, 2004). Liriodenine has been isolated by our group from a classical Chinese herb richly yield in Guangxi Province of China, *Zanthoxylum nitidum* Var. *Fastuosum*, known for its significant anticancer properties. Based on the planar character of liriodenine and its N-7/O-8 donor sites, it can ligate metal ions (M^{n+}) to form metal-based bifunctional compounds with potential synergistic effects on antitumor activity.

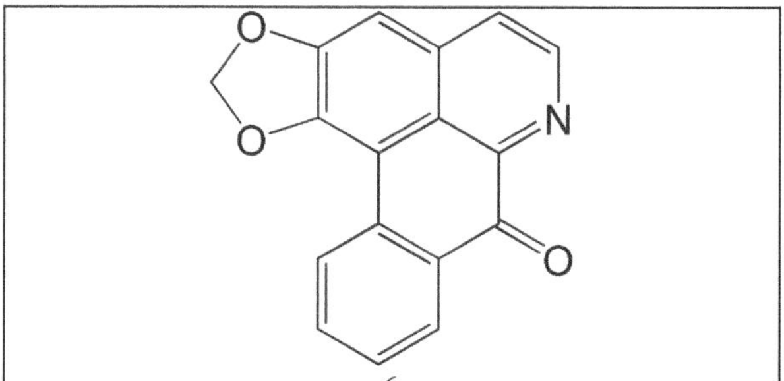

Fig. 2. Structure of liriodenine.

Reaction of liriodenine (L) with Pt(II), Ru(II), Mn(II), Fe(II), and Zn(II) as well as a series of lanthanides afforded a series of metal complexes. The crystal structures of *cis*-[Pt(L)(DMSO)Cl$_2$] (**7**), *cis*-[Ru(L)(DMSO)Cl$_2$]·1.5H$_2$O (**8**) (Chen et al., 2009); [MnCl$_2$(L)$_2$] (**9**), [FeCl$_2$(L)$_2$] (**10**), [Zn$_2$(L)$_2$(μ_2-Cl)$_2$Cl$_2$] (**11**) (Fig.3) (Liu et al., 2009); [Ce(L)$_2$(NO$_3$)$_3$] (**12**), [Pr(L)$_2$(NO$_3$)$_3$] (**13**), [Sm(L)$_2$(NO$_3$)$_3$] (**14**), [Eu(L)$_2$(NO$_3$)$_3$] (**15**) (Fig. 4) (Chen et al., 2011), were determined by single crystal X-ray diffraction methods. These complexes were fully characterized by elemental analysis, IR, ^{1}H and ^{13}C NMR spectroscopy, and ESI-MS spectrometry.

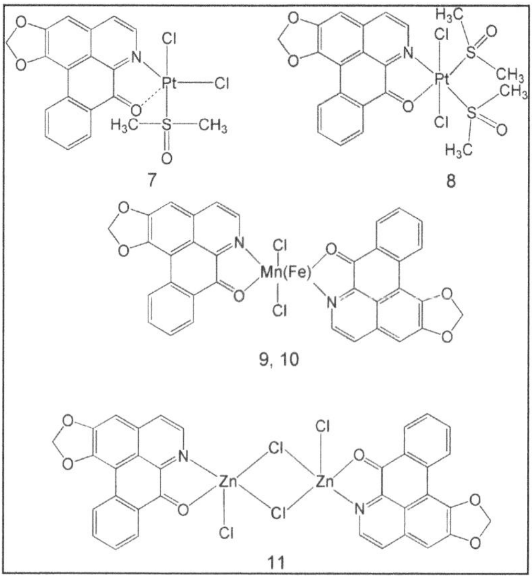

Fig. 3. Crystal structures of *cis*-[PtCl$_2$(L)(DMSO)] (**7**), *cis*-[RuCl$_2$(L)(DMSO)$_2$] (**8**), MnCl$_2$(L)$_2$ (**9**), [FeCl$_2$(L)$_2$] (**10**), and [Zn$_2$(L)$_2$(μ_2-Cl)$_2$Cl$_2$] (**11**).

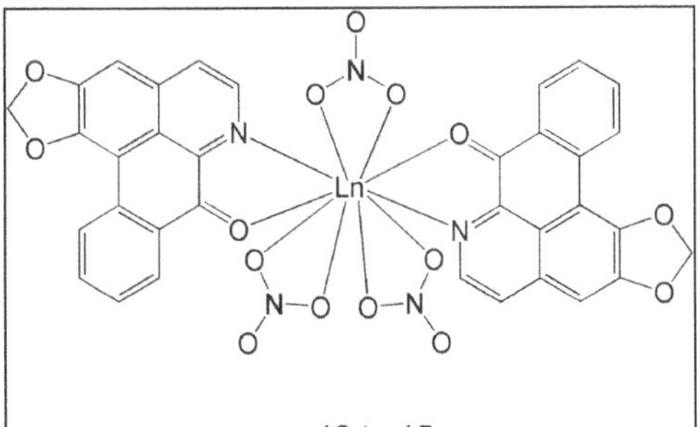

Fig. 4. Structures of four lanthanide complexes (**12** to **15**) with liriodenine.

The *in vitro* cytotoxicity of L and a series of its metal complexes against a panel of tumour cell lines have been evaluated by MTT method. The results show that these liriodenine metal-based compounds exhibit enhanced cytotoxicity *vs.* free L in most cases, and the IC_{50} values are in range of μM, suggesting that these compounds display synergic effect in the combination of metal ions and liriodenine. Although there is some evidence to suggest that other biological targets, including RNA or proteins, may be important in the cisplatin action mechanism, it is generally accepted that DNA is the primary target. Similarly, interactions between small molecules and DNA rank among the primary action mechanisms of anticancer activity. DNA replication in tumour cells will be blocked by the small molecule intercalation of the neighboring base pairs of DNA. On the other hand, topoisomerases are ubiquitous molecules that relieve the torsional stress in the DNA helix generated as a result of replication, transcription, and other nuclear processes; they are also specific targets for a number of anticancer agents (Baraldi et al., 2004), including the camptothecins, indolocarbazoles, and indenoisoquinolines. These compounds bind to a transient topoisomerase I (TOPO I)-DNA covalent complex and inhibit the resealing of a single-starnd nick that the enzyme creates to relieve superhelical tension in duplex DNA (Holfalnd et al, 2000; Staker et al., 2005). Therefore, in our researches, we investigated the interactions of these compounds with DNA and TOPO I. The interactions between ct-DNA and L or its Pt(II) and Ru(II) complexes through UV-Vis, fluorescence, EB competition binding, CD spectra, viscosity and agarose gel electrophoretic experiments reveal that these compounds mostly adopted a classical intercalation mode with DNA, but the metal complexes may bind covalently to DNA simultaneously because they easily hydrolyze to give coordinate active sites. Based on quantitative analysis of spectral titration experiments, it can conclude that the Pt(II) and Ru(II) complexes have higher binding ability than L itself does, suggesting that the metal complexes of planar L reinforce the binding ability. Although these results do not display a good coherence with what has been revealed in quantitative spectral analysis, however, it still confirms that DNA is an important target in cellular systems for these metal-based compounds derived from TCM. To introduce a TCM as a ligand to form bifunctional metal-based anticancer compounds (Herein, bifunction means TCM moiety intercalation and complex covalent binding to DNA, and differs from the meaning appearing in previous literature (Song et al., 2002; Wu et al., 2005) is a new effective strategy to achieve promising potential metal-based anticancer drug.

The *in vitro* cytotoxicity of three divalent transition metal (Mn(II), Fe(II), Zn(II)) complexes against 10 human tumor cell lines shows that most of these metal complexes exhibit higher cytotoxicity than L or cisplatin does, suggesting a probable synergistic effect upon liriodenine (L) coordinated to metal ions. The interactions between ct-DNA and L or its four divalent later transition metal complexes studied by UV-Vis, fluorescence, EB competition binding and CD spectra, as well as viscosity measurements and gel mobility shift assay experiments, reveal that these compounds mostly adopted an intercalation mode with DNA. Complexes **9**, **10** have higher binding affinity than L itself, suggesting that the metal complexes of planar L reinforce the binding ability. But it is lower than that of typical metallointercalator, which could be attributed to dichloride complex species (neutral) without chloride ligand exchange for water in short incubation period. In contrast, for biological assay on tumor cell lines, the long period incubation could allow (inside the cell) the conversion to diaqua species (dicationic) with a better interaction with NDA, and exhibit satisfied cytotoxicity. The electrostatic interactions between complex **11** and the polyanionic backbone of DNA helix should be considered simultaneously. Complex **11** tends to hydrolyze to form coordination unsaturated species, $[Zn(L)]^{2+}$, which can covalently bound to DNA. In addition, complexes **9–11** exhibit significant topoisomerase I inhibition ability at lower concentrations in contrast to L, implying topoisomerase I may be another molecular target. Although the exact molecular mechanism (including the real complex species in these metal complexes interacting with ct-DNA and tumour cell lines) needs further more detailed investigation, anyway, the three synthesized divalent later transition metal complexes of liriodenine exhibit significant enhanced cytotoxicity, offering a new effective strategy to achieve promising potential dual targeting cytotoxic agents by combining bioactive non-cytotoxic metal ions with cytotoxic active components from TCM.

The *in vitro* cytotoxicity of the lanthanide complexes **12–15** of liriodenine against four selected cell lines (7702, SK-OV-3, 7404, NCI-H460) were tested using MTT colorimetric method. The results indicate that the metal complexes exhibit enhanced cytotocicity against the four selected cell lines than that of liriodenine, which display the synergistic effects. All the complexes exhibit higher cytotoxicity to the tested tumor cells than ligand and cisplatin does. Remarkably, among these complexes, complexes **13** and **14** exhibit the highest cytotoxicity to tumour cells SK-OV-3, with IC_{50} values of 0.22±0.09 and 0.23±0.05 μM. The interactions between the liriodenine, its complexes and DNA were investigated by using various spectroscopic methods such as UV-Vis, fluorescence, CD, as well as viscosity and agarose gel electrophoresis experiments. The results indicate that liriodenine and its metal complexes interacted with DNA in an intercalation binding mode due to the liriodenine having good planarity and the π cyclic conjugated system. DNA has negative charge, there exist electrostatic interactions between liriodenine, its complexes. The interaction of complexes and DNA are stronger than that of liriodenine, it is agreed well with the results of antitumor activity tests. Overall, these liriodenine-metal complexes interact with DNA mainly by intercalation and electrostatic interaction, which blocks DNA synthesis and replication and induces cytotoxicity.

2.1.2 Oxoglaucine-metal based anticancer agents

Oxoglaucine (OG, **16**, Fig. 5) is an oxoaporphine alkaloid that has been isolated from overground parts of plants belonging to different families such as *Annonaceae* (Chang et al., 1998; Chen et al., 1996), *Lauraceae* (Chen et al., 1998), *Magnoliaceae* (Chen et al., 1976), *Fumariaceae* (Blanco et al., 1993; Tojo et al., 1991), *Menispermaceae* (Ohiri et al., 1982) and *Papveraceae* (Sari, 1999), which is also found widely exist in many traditional Chinese medicine, such as *aquilegia ecalcarata Maxim* (*Ranunculaceae*) mainly distributed in Sichuan and Yunnan Provinces of China and used for the treatment of necrotic boils, pustulosis and other infections (Wu et al., 1998). The primary screening results reveal that oxoglaucine possesses strong anticancer activity, such as against HCT-8 (ED$_{50}$ = 1.00 µg/ml) and K$_B$ (ED$_{50}$ = 2.00 µg/ml) (Chang et al., 2002; Chen et al., 2002; Wu et al., 1989). In addition, oxoglaucine exhibits other important pharmacological activities including antiplatelet aggregation (Chang et al., 1998; Jantan et al., 2006), immunomodulatory activity (Ivanovska et al., 1997 and 2000), treatment of adjuvant arthritis (Ivanovska & Hristova, 2000), anti-inflammatory (Remichkova et al., 2009), antifungal activity (Clark et al., 1987).

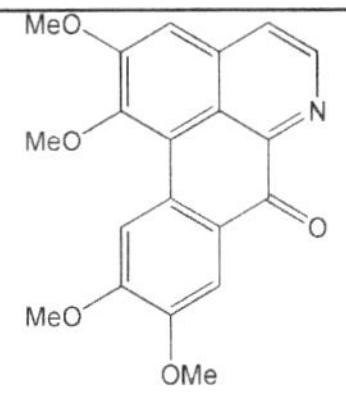

16

Fig. 5. Structure of oxoglaucine (**16**).

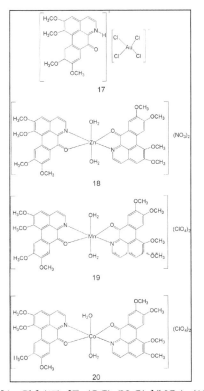

Fig. 6. Structures of [OGH][AuCl$_4$] (**17**), [Zn(OG)$_2$(H$_2$O)$_2$](NO$_3$)$_2$ (**18**), [Mn(OG)$_2$(H$_2$O)$_2$](ClO$_4$)$_2$ (**19**), [Mn(OG)$_2$(H$_2$O)$_2$](ClO$_4$)$_2$ (**20**).

Oxoglaucine alkaloid (OG) was synthesized via a two-step reaction route. Using OG as ligand to react with corresponding transition metal salts gave rise to four metal-based compounds: [OGH][AuCl$_4$]·DMSO   (17),   [Zn(OG)$_2$(H$_2$O)$_2$](NO$_3$)$_2$ (18), [Mn(OG)$_2$(H$_2$O)$_2$](ClO$_4$)$_2$ (19), [Co(OG)$_2$(H$_2$O)$_2$](ClO$_4$)$_2$ (20, Fig. 6), whose structures were determined by X-ray single crystal diffraction analysis. The *in vitro* cytotoxicity of 17–20 against various tumour cell lines was assayed by MTT method. The results show that most of these metal-based compounds of oxoglaucine exhibit enhanced cytotoxicity *vs.* oxoglaucine and corresponding metal salts, with IC$_{50}$ values ranging from 1.4 to 32.7 μM for sensitive cancer cells, implying a positive synergistic effect. Moreover, these complexes seem to be selectively active against certain cell lines. The interactions of oxoglaucine and its metal complexes with DNA and topoisomerase I were investigated by spectroscopic, viscosity and agarose gel electrophoresis measurements, which indicate that these OG metal–based compounds interact with DNA mainly *via* intercalation mode. Of special note, these metal-based compounds effectively inhibit Topoisomerase I even at low concentration, implying topoisomerase I may be another molecular target. However, the exact molecular mechanism requires further detailed investigation. Cell-cycle analysis revealed that these OG-metal complexes cause S-phase cell arrest.

2.1.3 Matrine-metal based anticancer agents

Matrine, a quinolizidine alkaloid matrine (MT), a main component found in roots of the Chinese herb *Sophora* including *Sophora flavescens* and *Sophora tonkinensis*, was selected as an active ligand. Matrine has been extensively used in China for the treatment of viral hepatitis and cardiac diseases (Liu et al., 2007). Matrine also exhibits inhibition activity toward many tumour cells (such as HeLa cell and gastric cancer MKN45 cell) (Galasso et al., 2006; Luo et al., 2007; Ruan et al., 2006; Zhang et al., 2001 & 2007).

Three TCM-metal compounds of Ga(III), Au(III), with Sn(IV) and matrine (MT), [H-MT][GaCl$_4$] (21), [H-MT][AuCl$_4$] (22) and [SnCl$_5$(H-MT)] (23, Fig. 7), have been synthesized and characterized. The crystal structure analyses reveal that 21 and 22 are ionic compounds, while 23 is a coordination compound formed by monodentate MT *via* its carbonyl O (Fig.7). But the ESI-MS results show that they may exist with ionic species: [H-MT]$^+$, [GaCl$_4$]$^-$, [AuCl$_4$]$^-$ and [SnCl$_5$]$^-$ in water solution. The *in vitro* cytotoxicities of 21, 22 and 23 against eight selected human tumour cell lines are different. In some case, they exhibit significant enhanced antitumour activity, such as 21 to SW480, 22 to HeLa, HepG2 and MCF-7, which exceed matrine and cisplatin, and display synergistic contribution of their components. However, in the case of 23, such synergistic effect could not be observed due to the electronic structure alteration of lactam group of matrinium, thus 23 exhibits lower antitumour activity than that of compounds 21 and 22. Although the spectroscopic and agarose gel electrophoresis assay show that these compounds bind to DNA inducing only small structural changes in the duplex, it could lead to a different cellular response. The cell cycle analyses show that compounds 21, 23 and MT exhibit cell cycle arrest at the G2/M phase. Their interactions with ct-DNA indicate that these metal-matrine compounds may be act mainly via intercalation mode of H-MT. In addition, 21 and 22 exhibit potent TOPO I inhibition ability, implying topoisomerase I may be another molecular target. However, the exact molecular mechanism requires further detailed investigation (Chen et al., 2011).

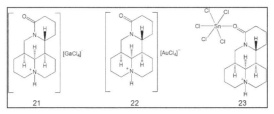

Fig. 7. Structures of [H-MT][GaCl₄] (**21**), [H-MT][AuCl₄] (**22**) and [SnCl₅(H-MT)] (**23**).

2.1.4 β-Carboline alkaloid-metal based anticancer agents

β-Carboline alkaloids, naturally occurring nitrogen-containing ligands, for example, harmaline (4,9-dihydro-7-methyl-3H-pyrido[3,4-b]indole), harmalol (4,9-dihydro-1-methyl-3H-pyrido[3,4-b] indole-7-ol), harmine (7-methoxy-1-methyl-9H-pyrido[3,4-b]indole), and harmane (1-methyl-9H-pyrido[3,4-b]indole), are extremely effective as antituberculosis, analgesic, and antimicrobial agents. Al-Allaf and co-worker reported the synthesis and cytotoxic evaluation of a series of novel biologically active platinum(II) (**24**, **26**, **28**, **30**) and palladium(II) (**25**, **27**, **29**, **31**, **32**, Fig. 8) complex of some β-carboline alkaloids (harmaline, harmine, and harmane). These complexes exhibited promising antitumour activity. The IC₅₀ of the complexes varied from 0.2 to 2.0 µg/mL in the antiproliferative assays against three tumour cell lines, and the calculated therapeutic index varied again from 10 to 20 µg/mL (Al-Allaf et al., 1990; Al-Allaf & Rashan, 1998).

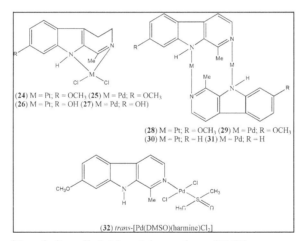

(**24**) M = Pt; R = OCH₃ (**25**) M = Pd; R = OCH₃
(**26**) M = Pt; R = OH (**27**) M = Pd; R = OH)

(**28**) M = Pt; R = OCH₃ (**29**) M = Pd; R = OCH₃
(**30**) M = Pt; R = H (**31**) M = Pd; R = H

(**32**) *trans*-[Pd(DMSO)(harmine)Cl₂]

Fig. 8. Structures of β-carboline alkaloid-metal complexes (**24-32**).

2.2 Flavonoid-metal based anticancer agents

Flavonoids are found in many plants and belong to a group of natural substances occurring in TCM with variable phenolic structures. Their therapeutic effects were known long before they were isolated (Nijveldt et al., 2001). Flavonoids display many important biological effects including antitumour, antioxidative, anti-inflammatory (inhibition of cyclooxygenase and lipoxygenase), antiviral, antibacterial, and antifungal actions. They also were shown to be effective inhibitors of platelet aggregation (Narayana et al., 2001; Nijhoff et al., 1995).

2.2.1 Chrysin, morin-metal based anticancer agents

Chrysin (5, 7-di-OH-flavone) is one flavonoid occurring in TCM, a natural ligand for benzodiazepine receptors with anticonvulsant properties. Complexes with Co(II), Ni(II), Cu(II), Pb(II), Fe(III) and Y(III) etc., have been synthesized and characterized. [Ansari, 2008; Engelmann et al., 2005; Pusz et al., 1997, 2000] Recently, Tang et al. reported chrysin-La(III) complex, La(chrysin)$_2$(OAc)·7H$_2$O (**33**, Fig. 9), which exhibited high inhibition rate (*in vitro*) to A549 and P388 with 74.5% and 42.4 at 10μM, respectively; and higher too much than that of chrysin (4.9% and 16.7%). The intrinsic binding constants of La(III) complex and chrysin are 1.29×10^6 and 5.44 ×10^{5}M^{-1}, respectively, which are considered both them bind to DNA by intercalation (Zeng et al., 2003).

Morin (2', 3, 4', 5, 7-pentahydroxyflavone) occurs in TCM and has antitumour activity (Alldrick et al., 1986). Wang et al. synthesized and characterized two complexes, Zn(morin)$_2$·3H$_2$O (**34**, Fig. 9) and Cu(morin)$_2$·2H$_2$O (**35**, Fig. 9) The two complexes exhibit higher *in vitro* antitumour activity to Hep-2, BBHK-2, BHK21 and HL-60 than morin alone, but the antitumour activity of the cobalt(II) complex (**36**, Fig. 9) is lower than morin (Zhang et al., 1996). Song and co-worker investigated the Zn(II) and Co(II) complexes of morin bound to ct-DNA by spectroscopic and voltammetric methods. The results indicate that they have different spectral characteristics and electrochemical behaviour, which suggests that the mode and affinity of Zn(II) and Co(II) complexes of morin bound to ct-DNA, may be responsible to their different antitumor activity (Song et al., 2003).

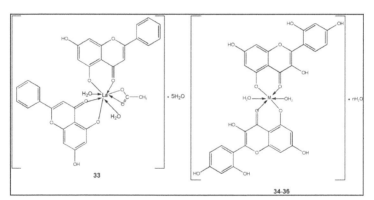

Fig. 9. Structure of La(chrysin)$_2$(OAc)·7H$_2$O (**33**) and the possible structure of the complexes. M = Zn(II) (**34**), Cu(II) (**35**), Co(II) (**36**), n = 0, or 1.

2.2.2 Hesperetin, naringenin, and apigenin-metal based anticancer agents

Hesperetin (5, 7, 3-trihydroxy-4-methoxy-flavanone), naringenin (4, 5, 7-trihydroxyflavanone) and apigenin (4, 5, 7-trihydroxyflavone), are biologically active flavonoids, commonly found in TCM (Tripoli et al., 2007). They have been reported to exhibit antitumour effects against breast cancer and hepatoma HepG2 cell lines (Korkina & Afanasev, 1997; Pereira et al., 2007). In addition, some metal complexes of hesperetin and naringenin have been found to exhibit antioxidant and anticancer activity (Chiang et al., 2006; So et al., 1996). The Naringenin Schiff base La(III) complex is more potent against the A-549 cell line than cisplatin under reasonable experimental concentrations (Li et al., 2008; Wang et al., 2006). Copper(II) complex of naringenin Schiff base possesses potent antioxidant activity, better than standard antioxidants like vitamin C and mannitol (Li et al., 2007). Our group reported three new copper(II) complexes of hesperetin, naringenin, and apigenin of general composition [CuL₂(H₂O)₂]·nH₂O (**37–39**, Fig. 10). The *in vitro* antitumor activity of the copper(II) complexes *vs* free ligand against human cancer cell lines HepG-2, SGC-7901, and HeLa have been assayed. Hesperetin-Cu(II) and apigenin-Cu(II) complexes were found to exhibit growth inhibition of SGC-7901 and HepG2 cell lines with respect to the free ligands; the inhibitory rate of hesperetin-Cu(II) complex is 43.2% and 43.8%, while apigenin-Cu(II) complex is 46% and 36%, respectively. Both hesperetin-Cu(II) complex and hesperetin were found to bind DNA in intercalation modes, and the binding affinity of the complex was stronger than that of free hesperetin (Tan et al., 2009).

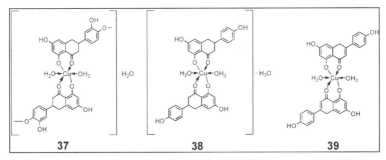

Fig. 10. The possible structure of the hesperetin-Cu(II) (**37**), naringenin-Cu(II) (**38**) and apigenin-Cu(II) (**39**) complexes.

2.2.3 Quercetin-metal based anticancer agents

Quercetin (3, 5, 7, 3', 4'-pentahydroxyflavone), a widely occurring compound in TCM, protects DNA from damage induced by reactive oxygen species (ROS) (Russo et al., 2000). Quercetin can chelate metal ions to form metal complexes that have better antioxidation and antitumour activity than quercetin alone (Zhou et al., 2001). Williams and co-worker reported the synthesis, characterization, antitumoural and osteogenic activities of quercetin vanadyl(IV) complexes. It was found that the free ligand quercetin might be a good candidate to be further evaluated in the treatment of bone tissue tumours because its effect has been more deleterious for tumoural osteoblasts that for the normal cells. However, the complexation of quercetin with vanadium center does not improve its potential anticarcinogenic properties. On the other hand, quercetin vanadyl(IV) complex seems to be a promising compound because it activates type I collagen production and shows a slight inhibitory effect on ALP specific activity, two markers of osteoblastic differentiation. It was believed that the activation of ERK pathways seems to be involved at least as one possible mechanism in the biological effects of quercetin vanadyl(IV) complex (Ferrer et al., 2006). Wang et al. investigated in detail the DNA binding, cytotoxicity, apoptotic inducing activity, and potential molecular mechanism of quercetin zinc(II) (46, Fig. 11) and copper(II) (47, Fig. 11) complexes. The quercetin znic(II) complex exhibits significant cytotoxicity against three tumour cell lines (HepG2, SMMC7721, and A549), which might be related to its intercalation into DNA (Tan et al., 2009). The quercetin zinc(II) complex displays strong DNA hydrolytic cleavage activity, which successfully promotes the cleavage of plasmid DNA, producing single and double DNA strand breaks, supported by evidence from free radical quenching, thiobarbituric acid-reactive substances (TBARS) assay, and T4 ligase ligation (Tan et al.,

2007). Tan et al. systematically investigated the mode of DNA binding, oxidative DNA cleavage activity, and apoptosis-inducing activity of the quercetin copper(II) complex. The results showed that the antitumour mechanism of the quercetin copper(II) complex involves not only its oxidative DNA damage with generation of ROS but also its specific interaction with DNA (Tan et al., 2009).

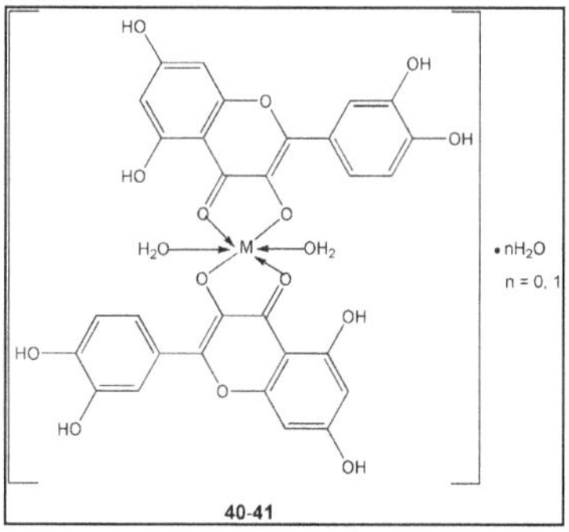

Fig. 11. The possible structures of quercetin metal complexes (M = Zn(II) (**40**), Cu(II)(**41**)).

In conclusion, flavonoids possess many potential pharmacological activity, represent a large type of TCM ligands, but because the flavonoids contain rich phenolic and carbonyl groups, chelate to metal ion, very easily to form polymeric structures, resulting in poor solubility, that limit the actual applications. Therefore, investigation of flavonoid metal-based antitumour agents, the excellent synthetic and characterized techniques is required, the good choice of flavonoids is very important.

2.3 Other TCM active ingredient-metal based anticancer agents
2.3.1 Coumarin-metal based anticancer agents
It is well documented that coumarin and a variety of coumarin derivatives have antitumour and antiproliferative activity. They have been shown to inhibit proliferation of particular human malignant cell lines *in vitro*, as well as affecting tumour activity against several in vitro tumour types (Kostova & Momekov, 2006). Kostova et al. synthesized a series of new zirconium(V) complexes with bis-coumarin ligands containing pyrazole or pyridine rings. The cytotoxic screening by MTT assay to HL-60 and the chronic myeloid leukemia LAMA-84 indicates that the zirconium(V) complexes of coumarins proved to be less potent than the corresponding free ligands (Kostova & Momekov, 2006). Egan and coworker investigated in vitro antitumour and cytoselective effects of coumarin-3-carboxylic acid and three of its hydroxylated derivatives, along with their silver-based complexes using human epithelial carcinoma cell lines (A-498 and Hep-G2). The *in vitro* antitumour assay results indicated that all of the ligands and their silver complexes induced a concentration-dependent cytotoxic effect. Hydroxylation of C-3-COOH and its subsequent complexation with silver led to the production of a series of compounds with dramatically enhanced cytotoxicity, with 6-OH-C-3-COO-Ag having the greatest activity, and all of the metal-based complexes were selectively cytotoxic to both carcinoma-derived cell lines, relative to normal renal and hepatic cells. The IC$_{50}$ values obtained with Hep-G2 cells were between 2 and 5.5 times more cytotoxic than cisplatin. All of the coumarin-silver complexes inhibited the DNA synthesis, which did not appear to be mediated *via* intercalation. These findings suggest that both

hydroxylation, particularly in the 6th position, and complexation with silver give rise to a cytotoxic-selective agent that significantly targets cancer cells, relative to normal cells (Thati et al., 2007). In addition, Kostova and co-worker investigated the cytotoxic activity of new lanthanum (III) and cerium (III) complexes of bis-coumarins. Their findings suggest that the coumarin-lanthanide complexes exhibited cytotoxic activity in micromolar contrations. Their *in vitro* effects are clearly expressed (Kostova et al., 2005, 2006). Recently, Creaven et al. reported the antibacterial and anticancer activities, coordination modes of copper(II) complexes of Schiff based-derived coumarin ligands (Creaven et al., 2010). Therefore, these coumarin-metal compounds have potential to develop as anticancer drugs, which provides hope for the pursuit of non-platinum anticancer drugs.

2.3.2 Cantharidin-metal based anticancer agents

Cantharidin is the active principle of Epicanta gorhami or Mylabris("blister beetles), which has long been applied as a TCM treatment for liver, lung, intestinal and digestive tract tumours (Wang, 1989). Cantharidin has severe side effects such as dysphagia, hematemesis, and dysuria (Wang, 1989). Cantharidin and its derivatives have been reported to have strong affinity and specificity for a protein phosphatase 2A (Li & Casida, 1992). Demethylcantharidin (norcantharidin, DMC) is a synthetic analogue of cantharidin and has potent antitumour activity but without the latter's adverse effects (Wang, 1989). Ho and coworker have carried out systematic, innovative research on the combination of demethylcantharidin with a platinum moiety to give a series of TCM-based platinum compounds $[Pt(C_8H_8O_5)(NH_2R)_2]$ (**42-46**, Fig. 12). These platinum complexes exhibit selective cytotoxicity toward SK-Hep-1 (human liver cell line), and circumvention of cross-resistance. They may possess a novel dual mechanism of antitumour action: inhibition of PP2A and platination of DNA (Ho et al., 2001 & 2003; To et al., 2004). Ho et al. determined the release of hydrolyzed demethylcantharidin from norcantharidin-Pt(II) compounds with anticancer activity by gas chromatography, in which the TCM component was slowly released from the norcantharidin-Pt(II) compounds over 24h, leading to PP2A inhibition. These complexes may prove to be new anticancer agents with novel mechanisms of cytotoxic action (To et al., 2002). The *in vitro* anti-proliferative activity of compounds **42-46** was investigated in human hepatocellular carcinoma (HCC) cell lines using MTT assay, which showed that compounds **42-46** were approximately 2-20 and 20-200 times more potent than cisplatin and carboplatin, respectively, in SK-Hep1 and HepG2 cells. The *in vivo* antitumour efficacies of **42-46** were evaluated in a s.c. inoculated SK-Hep1 xenograft model in nude mice. Compounds **42-46** exhibited definite *in vivo* activity without undue toxicity, contrasting the lack of activity of cisplatin and carboplatin. For *in vivo* cisplatin resistance model of human HCC, compounds **42-46** performed the same level of tumour growth suppression as in the control tumours, indicating the circumvention of cisplatin (To et al., 2005). Further studies indicated that compounds **42-46** were considerably less reactive to sulfur-containing nucleophiles than cisplatin, implying that they had reduced toxicity when compared with cisplatin, but the antitumour activity still remained (To et al., 2006). In order to determine the influence of the isomers on their anticancer activity, a series of platinum complexes integrating demethylcantharidin (CMC) with isomers of 1, 2-diaminocyhexane (DACH) have been synthesized. These compounds exhibit superior *in vitro* anticancer activity against colorectal and human hepatocellular cancer cell lines comparing with oxaliplatin, cisplatin, and carboplatin. The flow cytometric analysis results showed that the *trans*-DACH-Pt-DMC analogues presented similar behaviour to oxaplatin on affecting the cell cycle of the HCT116 colorectal cancer cells, but different from that of cisplatin or carboplatin. The DACH component obviously dictates the *trans*-DACH-Pt-DMC complexes to act similar to oxaliplatin, whereas the DMC ligand enhanced the compounds' overall anticancer activity. It was speculated these compounds accelerated the cell cycle from G1 to S-phase with subsequent onset of G2/M arrest and accompanying apoptosis (Yu et al., 2006). Ho's group also studied the pharmacokinetics and tissue distribution of these DMC-Pt anticancer agents in rats. Their findings suggested that the novel DMC-Pt compounds might afford higher clinical efficacy and reduced systemic side effects in contrast to cisplatin (Wang et al., 2007).

Moreover, the synergistic interaction between platinum-based antitumour agents and demethylcantharidin were investigated *in vitro* and *in vivo*, which demonstrated that synergistic effects occurred by combining demethylcantharidin with platinum-based antitumour agents. The demethylcantharidin might play a role in enhancing the efficacy of cisplatin in the treatment of various solid human tumours such as HCC, and overcoming cisplatin resistance. The demethylcantharidin has considerable promise as an adjuvant to chemotherapy (To et al., 2005).

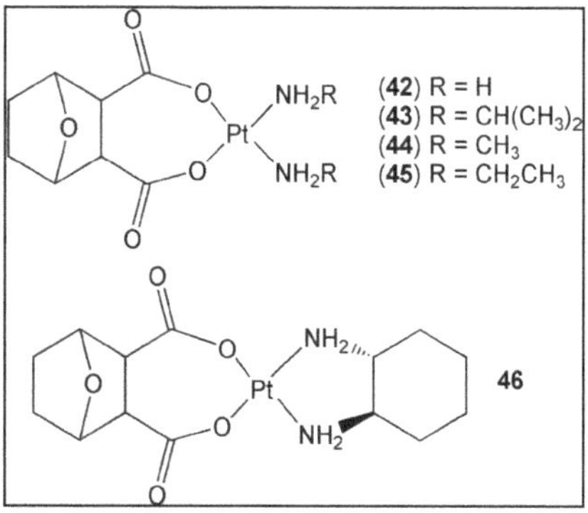

Fig. 12. Structures of [Pt(C$_8$H$_8$O$_5$)(NH$_2$R)$_2$] (**42-46**) .

The systematic work carried out by Ho's group on cis-DMC-Pt anticancer agents provides a successful paradigm for future research of TCM metal-based anticancer agents by utilization of multi-targets and multi-mechanisms of TCM-metal based compounds. Their achievement make us to believe that innovative metal-based anticancer drugs enable to develop by integration of the multiple advantages of metals and metal complexes with TCM's multi-target and multi-mechanism features.

2.3.3 Plumbagin-metal based anticancer agents

Plumbagin (PLN) is a potent toxic natural product extracted from TCM *Plumbago Zeylanica* L. (*Plumbaginaceae*), which has been used in China as well as other Asian countries for the treatment of rheumatoid arthritis, dysmenorrhea, injury by bumping, and even cancer. The anticancer property of PLN against HeLa, P388 lymphocytic, leukemia, colon cancer and hepatoma has been reported (Aziz et al., 2008; Kuo et al., 2006; Lin et al., 2003; Olagunju et al., 1999; Srinivas et al., 2004). Our group carried out the studies on plumbagin metal-based antitumour agents. The anticancer TCM, plumbagin (PLN), was isolated from *Plumbago Zeylanica*. Reaction of plumbagin with Cu(II) salt, afforded [Cu(PLN)$_2$]·2H$_2$O (47, Fig.13).

With 2,2'-bipyridine (bipy) as a co-ligand, PLN reacts with Cu(II) to give rise to [Cu(PLN)(bipy)(H$_2$O)]$_2$(NO$_3$)$_2$·4H$_2$O (48, Fig. 13). The two complexes were characterized by elemental analysis, IR, and ESI-MS. Their crystal structures were determined by single crystal X-ray diffraction methods (Fig. 13) And the *in vitro* cytotoxicity of PLN and the two copper complexes against seven human tumour cell lines was assayed. The metal-based compounds exhibit enhanced cytotoxicity vs. that of PLN, suggesting that these compounds display synergy in the combination of metal ions with PLN. The binding properties of PLN and the two copper complexes to DNA were investigated with UV-vis, fluorescence, CD spectroscopy, and gel mobility shift assay, which indicated that the two copper complexes of plumbagin were non-covalently binding and mainly intercalated in the neighboring base pairs of DNA. PLN and its copper complexes exhibit inhibition activity to topoisomerase I (TOPO I), but the metal complexes were more effective than PLN (Chen et al., 2009).

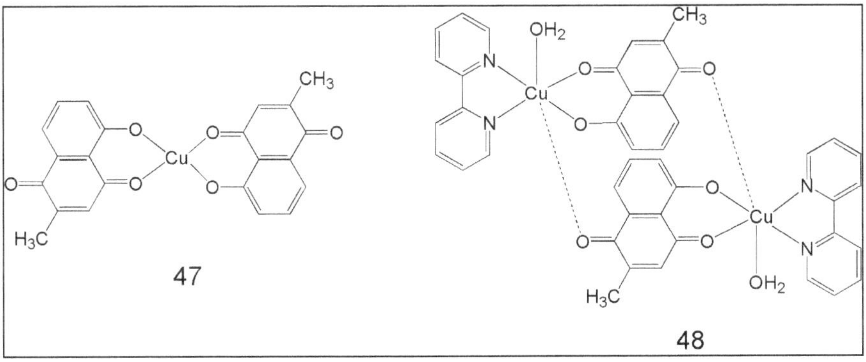

Fig. 13. Crystal structures of [Cu(PLN)$_2$] (**47**) and [Cu(PLN)(bpy)(H$_2$O)](NO$_3$)$_2$ (**48**).

This work has recently been reviewed by Professor Roy Planalp. He thought that this work is very exciting with regards to the enhanced antitumour properties of a natural substance by complexation with a common biometal (Saxton, 2010).

In order to investigate the cytotoxicity of plumbaginate lanthanide complexes, five new lanthanide(III) complexes of deprotonated plumbagin: [Y(PLN)$_3$(H$_2$O)$_2$] (**49**), [La(PLN)$_3$(H$_2$O)$_2$] (**50**), [Sm(PLN)$_3$(H$_2$O)$_2$]·H$_2$O (**51**), [Gd(PLN)$_3$(H$_2$O)$_2$] (**52**), and [Dy(PLN)$_3$(H$_2$O)$_2$] (**53**, Fig. 14) were synthesized by the reaction of plumbagin with the corresponding lanthanide salts, in amounts equal to ligand/metal molar ration of 3:1. The PLN-lanthanide(III) complexes were characterized by different physicochemical methods: elemental analyses, UV-visible, IR and 1H NMR and ESI-MS as well as TGA. The plumbagin and its lanthanide(III) complexes **49–53**, were tested for their in vitro cytotoxicity against BEL7404 (liver cancer) cell lines by MTT assay. The five PLN-lanthanide (III) complexes **49–53** effectively inhibited BEL7404 cell lines growth with IC$_{50}$ values of 11.0±3.5, 5.1±1.3, 6.1±1.1, 6.4±1.3, and 9.8±1.5μM, respectively, and exhibited a significantly enhanced cytotoxicity compared to plumbagin and the corresponding lanthanide salts, suggesting a synergistic effect upon plumbagin coordination to the Ln(III) ion. The lanthanide complexes under investigation also exerted dose- and time-dependent cytotoxic activity. [La(PLN)$_3$(H$_2$O)$_2$] (**50**) and plumbagin interact with calf thymus DNA (ct-DNA) mainly via intercalation mode, but for [La(PLN)$_3$(H$_2$O)$_2$] (**50**), the electrostatic interaction should not be excluded; the binding affinity of [La(PLN)₃(H₂O)₂] (**50**) to DNA is stronger than that of free plumbagin, which may correlate with the enhanced cytotoxicity of the PLN-lanthanide(III) complexes (Chen et al. 2011).

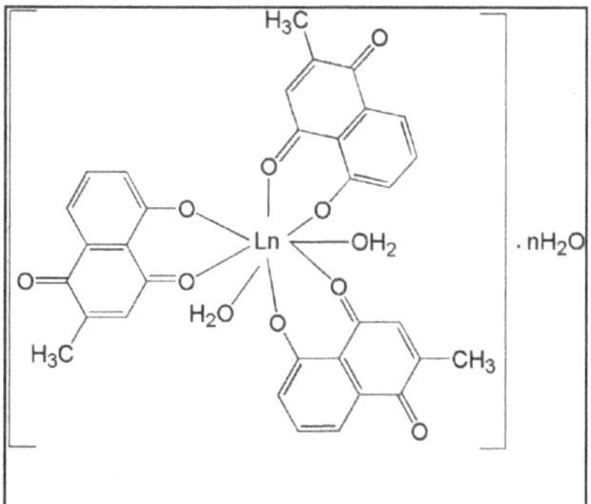

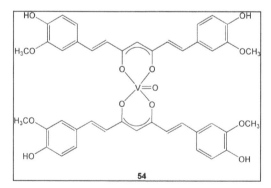

49 to 53

Fig. 14. The possible structure of complexes **49–53** (n=0, Ln = Y(III) (**49**), La(III) (**50**), Gd(III) (**52**), Dy(III) (**53**); n = 1, Ln = Sm(III) (**51**)).

2.3.4 Curcumin-metal based anticancer agents

Curcumin, an extract of turmeric, Curcuma longa L., has been used for centuries in variety of TCM pharmaceutical applications (Sharma, 1976), including treatment of arthritis (Deodhar et al., 1980), as an anti-inflammatory agent (Rao et al., 1982; Srimal & Dhawan, 1973) and as an orally available treatment for diabetes (Arun & Nalini, 2002). Thompson and co-worker synthesized a novel vanadyl curcumin complex (VO(cur)₂) (**54**, Fig. 15) and studied its anticancer potential in inhibiting mouse lymphoma cell growth. The complex was more effective than uncoordinated curcumin (Thompson et al., 2004).

54

Fig. 15. Structure of vanadyl curcumin complex (VO(cur)₂ **54**).

2.3.5 Camphorato-metal based anticancer agents

Camphor has long been used as TCM to relieve pain, stop tickle, anti-inflammation, cure ulcers and sores, dental caries, and kill worms and acariasis as early as the Ming Dynasty. Camphoric acid can be obtained by the oxidation of camphor and is used in pharmaceuticals as exciting centre and respiration analeptic agent. Gou and coworker synthesized eight new camphorato platinum complexes (**55**, Fig. 16) and evaluated their in vitro cytotoxicity against HL-60, 2AO, BEL-7402 and A549 cells. The results show that most complexes exhibited good cytotoxic activity against the selected cell lines. One complex displayed not only higher *in vivo* antitumour activity, but also less toxicity than oxaliplatin when it was administered intravenously at a dose of 6 mg/Kg three times. Gou and coworkers research provides a new selection to find chiral leaving groups from TCM (Wang et al., 2005).

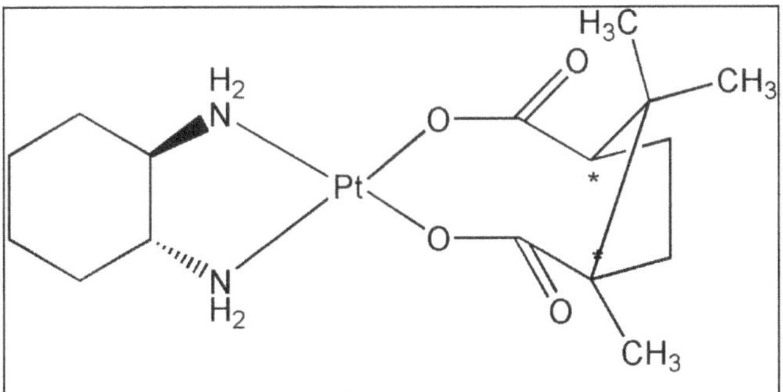

Fig. 16. *trans*-1R, 2R-Daiminocyclohexane camphorate-Pt complex (**55**).

3. Conclusion

TCM is a natural "combination chemical resources armoury", which has undergone several thousands years worth of clinical practice and screening. TCM possess multi-component, multi-target and co-regulatory features which meet the view points of multi-target drugs through the network approach (Csermely et al., 2005) and robustness-based approach to systems-oriented drug design (Kitano, 2007). TCM metal-based antitumor agents have at least two remarkable advantages: either TCM playing key role or metal complex making multiple contributions in development of drugs. In this review, the alkaloids, flavonoids, cantharidin, coumarins, plumbagin, curcumin and camphoric acid metal-based compounds with antitumor activity were summarized. Generally, TCM-metal based compounds formed *via* metal ions coordinating to TCM with O, N donors, exhibiting enhanced activity and synergistic effect with multi-targets and multi-mechanisms. With the Chinese government promotion of the modernization of TCM (Normile, 2003) and carrying out the *herbalome* (Stone, 2008), as well as the advancements of genome, proteome, metabolome, there is the possibility to design new TCM metal-based anticancer drugs and develop modern TCM, which will benefit to overcoming multidrug resistance (MDR). The promising trends have been supported by great potential of TCM metal-based antitumor agents mentioned above. We believe that innovative metal-based anticancer drugs enable to develop by integration of the multiple advantages of metals and metal complexes with TCM's multi-target and multi-mechanism features. But the action species and multi-target and multi-mechanism in cell and *in vivo* of the TCM metal-based antitumor agents still need to be widely and deeply investigated by adopting modern genome, proteome, metabolome technologies.

4. Acknowledgment

This work was supported National Basic Research Program of China (Nos. 2009CB526503, 2010CB534911), the National Natural Science Foundation of China (20861002), and Natural Science Foundation of Guangxi Province of China (Nos. 0991012Z, 0991003, and 2010GXNSFF013001).

5. References

Al-Allaf, T. A. K.; Ayoub, M. T.; Rashan, L. J. (1990). Synthesis and characterization of novel biologically active platinum(II) and palladium(II) complexes of some β-carboline alkaloids. *J. Inorg. Biochem.*, Vol.38, No.1, (January 1990), pp. 47-56, ISSN 0162-0134.

Al-Allaf, T. A. K.; Rashan, L. J. (1998). Synthesis and cytotoxic evaluation of the first trans-palladium(II) complex with naturally occurring alkaloid harmine. *Eur. J. Med. Chem.*, Vol.33, No.10, (October 1998), pp. 817-820, ISSN 0223-5234.

Alldrick, A. J.; Flynn J.; Rowland, I. R. (1986). Effects of plant-derived flavonoids and polyphenolic acids on the activity of mutagens from cooked food. *Mutat. Res.*, Vol.163, No.3, (December 1986), pp. 225-232, ISSN 0027-5107.

Alt, A.; Lammens, K.; Chiocchini,C.; Alfred Lammens, A.; Pieck, J. C.; Kuch, D.; Karl-Peter Hopfner, K.-P.; Carell, T. (2007). Bypass of DNA lesions generated during anticancer treatment with cisplatin by DNA polymerase eta. *Science*, Vol. 318, No.5852, (November, 2007), pp. 967-970, ISSN 0036-8075.

Ansari, A. A.(2008). ^{1}H NMR and spectroscopic studies of biologically active yttrium (III)-flavonoid complexes. *Main Group Chem.*, Vol.7, No.2, (February 2008), pp. 133-145, ISSN 1024-1221.

Arun, N.; Nalini, N. (2002). Efficacy of turmeric on blood sugar and polyol pathway in diabetic albino rats. *Plant Foods Hum. Nutr.*, Vol.57, No.1, (January 2002), pp. 41-52, ISSN 0921-9668.

Aziz, M. H.; Dreckschmidt, N. E.; Verma, A. K. (2008). Plumbagin, a medicinal plant-derived naphthoquinone, is a novel inhibitor of the growth and invasion of hormone-refractory prostate cancer. *Cancer Res.*, Vol.68, No.21, (November 2008), pp. 9024-9032, ISSN 0008-5472.

Baraldi, P. G.; Bovero, A.; Fruttarolo, F.; Preti, D.; Tabrizi, M. A.; Pavani, M. G.; Romagnoli, R. (2004). *Med. Res. Rev.*, Vol.24, No.4, (April 2004), pp. 475-496, ISSN 0198-6325.

Bentley, K. W. (2001). β-Phenylethylamines and the isoquinoline alkaloids. *Nat. Prod. Rep.*, Vol.18, No.2, (February 2001), pp. 148-170, ISSN 0265-0568.

Blanco, O. M.; Castedo, L.; Villaverde, M. C. (1993). *Phytochemistry*, Vol.32, No.4, (March 1993), pp. 1055–1057, ISSN 0031-9422.

Chan, K. (1995). Progresseses in traditional Chinese medicine. *Trends Pharmacol. Sci.*, Vol.16, No.6, (June 1995), pp. 182-187, ISSN 0165-6147.

Chang, F.-R.; Hsieh, T.-J.; Huang, T.-L.; Chen, C.-Y.; Kuo, R.-Y.; Chang, Y.-C.; Chiu, H.-F.; Wu, Y.-C. (2002). Cytotoxic constituents of the stem bark of neolitsea *acuminatissima*. *J. Nat. Prod.*, Vol.65, No.3, (March 2002), pp. 255–258, ISSN 0163-3864.

Chang, H. C.; Chang, F. R.; Wu, Y. C.; Lai, Y. H. (2004). Anti-cancer effect of liriodenine on human lung cancer cells. *Kaohsiung J. Med. Sci.*, Vol.20, No.8, (August 2004), pp. 365-371, ISSN 1607-551X.

Chen, C.-L.; Chang, H.-M.; Cowling, E. B.; Huang Hsu, C.-Y.; Gates, R. P. (1976). *Phytochemistry*, Vol.15, No.7, (July 1976), pp. 1161–1167, ISSN 0031-9422.

Chen, K.-S.; Chang, F.-R.; Chia, Y.-C.; Wu, T.-S.; Wu, Y.-C. (1998). Chemical constituents of Neolitsea parvigemma and Neolitsea konishii. J. Chin. Chem. Soc., Vol.45, No.1, (January 1998), pp. 103–110, ISSN 0009-4536.

Chen, S.-B.; Gao, G.-Y.; Yu, S.-C.; Xiao, P.-G. (2002). Cytotoxic Constituents from *Aquilegia ecalcarata*. *Planta Med.*, Vol.68, No.6, (June 2002), pp. 554–556, ISSN 0032-0943.

Chen, Z.-F.; Liu, Y.-C.; Liu, L.-M.; Wang, H.-S.; Qin, S.-H.; Wang, B.-L.; Bian, H.-D.; Yang, B.; Fun, H.-K.; Liu, H.-G.; Liang, H.; Orvig, C. (2009). Potential new inorganic antitumour agents from combining the anticancer traditional Chinese medicine (TCM) liriodenine with metal ions, and DNA binding studies. *Dalton Trans.*,Vol.38, No.2, (January 2009), pp. 262-272, ISSN 1477-9226.

Chen, Z.-F.; Mao, L.; Liu, L.-M.; Liu, Y.-C.; Peng, Y.; Hong, X.; Wang, H.-H.; Liu, H.-G.; Liang, H. (2011). Potential new inorganic antitumour agents from combining the anticancer traditional Chinese medicine (TCM) matrine with Ga(III), Au(III), Sn(IV) ions, and DNA binding studies. *J. Inorg. Biochem.*, Vol.105, No.2, (February 2011), pp.171-180, ISSN 0162-0134.

Chen, Z.-F.; Shi, Y.-F.; Liu, Y.-C.; Hong, X.; Geng, B.; Peng, Y.; Liang H. (2011). Unpublish results.

Chen, Z.-F.; Tan, M.-X.; Liu, L.-M.; Liu, Y.-C.; Wang, H.-S.; Yang, B.; Peng, Y.; Liu, H.-G.; Liang H. and Orvig, C. (2009). Cytotoxicity of the traditional Chinese medicine (TCM) plumbagin in its copper chemistry. *Dalton Trans.*, Vol.38, No.48, (December 2009), pp. 10824-10833, ISSN 1477-9226.

Chen, Z.-F.; Tan, M.-X.; Liu, Y.-C.; Peng, Y.; Wang, H.-H.; Liu, H.-G.; Liang, H. (2011). Synthesis, characterization and preliminary cytotoxicity evaluation of five lanthanide-plumbagin complexes. *J. Inorg. Biochem.*, Vol.105, No.2, (February 2011), pp. 308–316, ISSN0162-0134.

Chen, Z.-F.; Tao, L.; Liu, Y.-C.; Liang, H. (2011), unpulish results.

Cheng, J. T. (2000). Review: drug therapy in Chinese traditional medicine. *J. Clin. Pharmacol.*, Vol.40, No.5, (May, 2000), pp. 445-450, ISSN 0091-2700.

Chiang, L.-C.; Ng, L. T.; Lin, I.-C.; Kuo, P.-L.; Lin, C.-C. (2006). Anti-proliferative effect of apigenin and its apoptotic induction in human Hep G2 cells. *Cancer Lett.*, Vol.237, No.2, (June 2006), pp. 207–214, ISSN 0304-3835.

Clark, A. M.; Watson, E. S.; Ashfaq, M. K.; Hufford, C. D. (1987). *In vivo* efficacy of antifungal oxoaporphine alkaloids in experimental disseminated candidiasis. *Pharmaceutical Res.*, Vol.4, No.6, (December 1987), pp. 495–498, ISSN 0724-8741.

Clarke, M. J.; Zhu, F.; Frasca, D. R. (1999). Non-platinum chemotherapeutic metallopharmceuticals. *Chem. Rev.*, Vol.99, No.9, (August 1999), pp. 2511-2533, ISSN 0009-2665.

Creaven, B. S.; Czegledi, E.; Devereux, M.; Enyedy, E. A.; Kia, A. F.-A.; Karcz, D.; Kellett, A.; McClean, S.; Nagy, N. V.; Noble, A.; Rockenbauer, A.; Szabo-Planka, T.; Walsh, M. (2010). Biological activity and coordination modes of copper(II) complexes of Schiff based-derived coumarin ligands. *Dalton Trans.*, Vol.39, No.45, (December 2010), pp. 10854–10865, ISSN 1477-9226.

Csermely, P.; Ágoston, V.; Pongor, S. (2005). The efficiency of multi-target drugs: the network approach might help drug design. *Trends Pharmacol. Sci.*, Vol.26, No.4, (April2005), pp. 178-182, ISSN 0165-6147.

Deodhar, S. D.; Sethi, R.; Srimal, R.C. (1980). Preliminary study on antirheumatic activity of curcumin (diferuloyl methane). *Indian J. Med. Res.*, Vol.71, No.4, (April 1980), pp. 632-634, ISSN 0971-5916.

Engelmann, M. D.; Hutcheson, R.; Cheng, I. F. (2005). Stability of ferric complexes with 3-hydroxyflavone (flavonol), 5,7-dihydroxyflavone (chrysin), and 3',4'-dihydroxyflavone. *J. Agric. Food Chem.*, Vol.53, No.8, (March 2005), pp. 2953-2960, ISSN 0021-8561.

Ferrer, E. G.; Salinas, M. V.; Correa, M. J.; Naso, L.; Barrio, D. A.; Etcheverry, S. B.; Lezama, L.; Rojo, T.; Williams, P. A. M. (2006). Synthesis, characterization, antitumoral and osteogenic activities of quercetin vanadyl(IV) complexes. *J. Biol. Inorg. Chem.*, Vol.11, No.6, (October 2006), pp. 791-801, ISSN 0949-8257.

Galasso, V.; Asaro, F.; Berti, F.; Pergolese, B.; Kovac, B.; Pichierri, F. (2006). On the molecular and electronic structure of matrine-type alkaloids. *Chem. Phys.*, Vol.330, No.3, (November 2006), pp. 457-468, ISSN 0301-0104.

Gibert, T. F. (1998). Thought on traditional Chinese medicine and its pharmacopeia. *Ann. Pharm. Fr.*, Vol.56, No.6, (November 1998), pp. 282-285, ISSN 0003-4509.

Hambley, T. W. (2007). Metal-based therapeutics. *Science*, Vol.318, No.5855, (November 2007), pp. 1392-1393, ISSN 0036-8075.

Hofland, K.; Petersen, B. O.; Falck, J.; Helin, K.; Jensen, P. B.; Sehested, M. (2000). Differential cytotoxic pathways of topoisomerase I and II anticancer agents after overexpression of the E2F-1/DP-1 transcription factor complex. *Clin. Cancer Res.*, Vol.6, No.4, (April 2000), pp. 1488-1498, ISSN 1078-0432.

Ho, Y.-P.; Au-Yeung, S. C. F.; To, K. K. W. (2003). Platinum-based anticancer agents: innovative design strategies and biological perspectives. *Med. Res. Rev.*, Vol.23, No.5, (September 2003), pp. 633-655, ISSN 0198-6325.

Ho, Y.-P.; To, K. K. W.; Au-Yeung, S. C. F.; Wang, X.; Lin, G.; Han, X. Potential new antitumor agents from an innovative combination of demethylcantharidin, a modified traditional Chinese medicine, with a platinum moiety. *J. Med. Chem.*, Vol.44, No.13, (June, 2001), pp. 2065-2068, ISSN 0022-2623.

Hsieh, T. J.; Liu, T. Z.; Chern, C. L.; Tsao, D. A.; Lu, F. J.; Syu, Y. H.; Hsien, P. Y.; Hu, H. S.; Chang, T. T.; Chen, C. H. (2005). Liriodenine inhibits the proliferation of human hepatoma cell lines by blocking cell cycle progressesesion and nitric oxide-mediated activation of p53 expression. *Food and Chem. Toxicol.*, Vol.43, No.7, (July 2005), pp. 1117-1126, ISSN 0278-6915.

Ivanovska, N.; Hristova, M.; Philipov, S. (2000). Immunosuppression and recovery of drug-impaired host resistance against Candida albicans infection by oxoglaucine. *Pharmacol. Res.*, Vol.41, No.1, (January 2000), pp. 101–107, ISSN 1043-6618.

Ivanovska, N.; Hristova, M. (2000). Treatment with oxoglaucine can enhance host resistance to Candida albicans infection of mice with adjuvant arthritis. *Diagnostic Microbiology and Infectious Disease*, Vol.38, No.1, (September 2000), pp. 17–20, ISSN 0732-8893.

Ivanovska, N.; Philipov, S.; Georgieva, P. (1997). *Pharmacol. Res.*, Vol.35, No.4, (April 1997), pp. 267–272, ISSN 1043-6618.

Jamieson, E. R.; Lippard, S. J. (1999). Structure, recognition, and processing of cisplatin-DNA adducts. *Chem. Rev.*, Vo.99, No.9, (August, 1999), pp. 2467-2498, ISSN 0009-2665.

Jantan, I.; Raweh, S. M.; Yasin, Y. H. M.; Murad, S. (2006). Antiplatelet activity of aporphine and phenanthrenoid alkaloids from Aromadendron elegans Blume. *Phytother. Res.*, Vol.20, No.6, (June 2006), pp. 493–496, ISSN 0951-418X.

Jung, Y.; Lippard, S. J. (2007). Direct cellular responses to platinum-induced DNA damage. *Chem. Rev.*, Vol.107, No. 5, (May, 2007), pp. 1387-1407, ISSN 0009-2665.

Kelland, L. (2007). The resurgence of platinum-based cancer chemotherapy. *Nature Rev.*, Vol.7, No.8, (August 2007), pp. 573-584, ISSN 1474-175X.

Kitano, H. (2007). A robustness-based approach to systems-oriented drug design. *Nature Rev. Drug Discovery*, Vol.6, No. 3, (March 2007), pp. 202-210, ISSN 1474-1776.

Korkina, L. G. & Afanasev, I. B. (1997). Antioxidant and chelating properties of flavonoids. *Adv. Pharmacol.*, Vol.38, No.2, (February 1997), pp. 151–163, ISSN 1054-3589.

Kostova, I.; Manolov, I.; Momekov, G.; Tzanova, T.; Konstantinov, S.; Karaivanova, M. (2005). Cytotoxic activity of new cerium (III) complexes of bis-coumarins. *Eur. J. Med. Chem.*, Vol.40, No.12, (December 2005), pp. 1246-1254, ISSN 0223-5234.

Kostova, I.; Momekov, G. (2006). New zirconium (IV) complexes of coumarin with cytotoxic activity. *Eur. J. Med. Chem.*, Vol.41, No.6, (June 2006), pp. 717-726, ISSN 0223-5234.

Kostova, I.; Momekov, G.; Zaharieva, M.; Karaivanova, M. (2005). Cytotoxic activity of new lanthanum (III) complexes of bis-coumarins. *Eur. J. Med. Chem.*, Vol.40, No.6, (June 2005). pp. 542-551, ISSN 0223-5234.

Kostova, I.; Momekov, G.; Tzanova, T.; Karaivanova, M. (2006). Sythesis, characterization, and cytotoxic activity of new lanthanum (III) complexes of bis-coumarins. *Bioinorg. Chem. Appl.*, Doi 10.1155/BCA?2006/25651, ISSN 1687-479X.

Kuo, P.-L.; Hsu, Y.-L.; Cho, C.-Y. (2006). Plumbagin induces G2-M arrest and autophagy by inhibiting the AKT/mammalian target of rapamycin pathway in breast cancer cells. *Mol. Cancer Ther.*, Vol.5, No.12, (December 2006), pp. 3209-3221, ISSN 1535-7163.

Lan, Y. H.; Chang, F. R.; Yu, J. H.; Yang, Y. L.; Chang, Lee, Y. L.; S. J.; Wu, Y. C. (2003). Cytotoxic styrylpyrones from Goniothalamus amuyon. *J. Nat. Prod.*, Vol.66, No.4, (April 2003), pp.487-490, ISSN 0163-3864.

Li, T.-R.; Yang, Z.-Y.; Wang, B.-D. (2007). Synthesis, characterization and antioxidant activity of naringenin Schiff base and its Cu(II), Ni(II), Zn(II) complexes. *Chem. Pharm. Bull.*, Vol.55, No.1, (January 2007), pp. 26-28, ISSN 0009-2363.

Li, T.-R.; Yang, Z.-Y.; Wang, B.-D. Qin, D.-D. (2008). Synthesis, characterization, antioxidant activity and DNA-binding studies of two rare earth(III) complexes with naringenin-2-hydroxy benzoyl hydrazone ligand. *Eur. J. Mod. Chem.*, Vol.43, No 8, (August 2008), pp. 1688–1695, ISSN 0223-5234.

Li, Y. M.; Casida, J. E. (1992). Cantharidin-binding protein: identification as protein phosphatase 2A. *Proc. Natl. Acad. Sci. USA*, Vol.89, No.24, (December 1992), pp. 11867-11870, ISSN 1091-6490.

Lin, C. H.; Chang, G. J.; Su, M. J.; Wu, Y. C.; Teng, C. M.; Ko, F. N. (1994). Pharmacological characteristics of liriodenine, isolated from Fissistigma glaucescens, a novel muscarinic receptor antagonist in guinea-pigs. *Br. J. Pharmacol.*, Vol.113, No.1, (September 1994), pp. 275-281, ISSN 0007-1188.

Lin, L. C.; Yang L. L. and Chou C. J. (2003). Cytotoxic naphthoquinones and plumbagic acid glucosides from Plumbago zeylanica. *Phytochemistry*, Vol.62, No.4, (February 2003), pp. 619-622, ISSN 0031-9422.

Liu, Y.-C.; Chen, Z.-F.; Liu, L.-M.; Peng, Y.; Hong, X.; Yang, B.; Liu, H.-G.; Liang, H. and Orvig, C. (2009). Divalent later transition metal complexes of the traditional chinese medicine (TCM) liriodenine: coordination chemistry, cytotoxicity and DNA binding studies. *Dalton Trans.*, Vol.38, No.48, (December 2009), pp. 10813-10823, ISSN 1477-9226.

Liu, J. Y.; Hu, J. H.; Zhu, Q. G.; Li, F. Q.; Wang, J.; Sun, H. J. (2007). Effect of matrine on the expression of substance P receptor and inflammatory cytokines production in human skin keratinocytes and fibroblasts. *International Immunopharmacol.*, Vol.7, No.6, (June 2007), pp. 816-823, ISSN 1567-5769.

Liu, Y. C. (1988). *The essential book of traditional Chinese medicine: theory, clinical practice*, Columbia University Press.

Lovejoy, K. S. and Lippard, S. J. (2009). Non-traditional platinum compounds for improved accumulation, oral bioavailability, and tumor targeting. *Dalton Trans.*, Vol.38, No.48, (December 2009), pp. 10651-10659, ISSN 1477-9226.

Luo, C.; Zhu, Y. L.; Jiang, T. J.; Lu, X. Y.; Huang, J. (2007). Matrine induced gastric cancer MKN45 cells apoptosis via increasing pro-apoptotic molecules of Bcl-2 family. *Toxicology*, Vol.229, No.3, (January 2007), pp. 245-252, ISSN 0300-483X.

Narayana, K. R.; Reddy, M. S.; Chaluvadi, M. R.; Krishna, D. R. (2001). Bioflavonoids classification, pharmacological, biochemical effects and therapeutic potential. *Indian J. Pharmacol.*, Vo.33, No.1, (February 2001), pp. 2-16, ISSN 0253-7613.

Nijveldt, R. J.; van Nood, E.; Hoorn, D. E. C.; Norren, K.; Leeuwen, P. A. M. (2001). Flavonoids: a review of probable mechanisms of action and potential applications. *Am. J. Clin. Nutr.*, Vol.74, No.4, (October 2001), pp. 418-425, ISSN 0002-9165.

Nijhoff, W. A.; Bosboom, M. A.; Smidt, M. H.; Peters, W. H. M. (1995). Enhancement of rat hepatic and gastrointestinal glutathione and glutathione S-transferases by alpha-angelicalactone and flavone. *Carcinogenesis*, Vol.16, No.3, (March 1995), pp. 607-612, ISSN 0143-3334.

Nissanka, A. P. K.; Karunaratne, V.; Bandara, B. M. R.; Kumar, V.; Nakanishi, T.; Nishi, M.; Inada, A.; Tillekeratne, L. M. V.; Wijesundara, D. S. A.; Gunatilaka, A. A. L. (2001). Antimicrobial alkaloids from Zanthoxylum tetraspermum. and caudatum.. *Phytochemistry*, Vol.56, No.8, (April 2001), pp. 857-861, ISSN 0031-9422.

Normile, D. (2003). The new face of traditional Chinese medicine. *Science*, Vol.299, No.5604, (October 2003), pp. 188-190, ISSN 0036-8075.

Ohiri, F. C.; Verpoorte, R.; Baerheim Svendsen, A. (1982). Alkaloids from Chasmanthera dependens. *Planta Med.* Vol.46, No.12, (December 1982), pp. 228–230, ISSN 0032-0943.

Olagunju, J. A.; Jobi, A. A.; Oyedapo, O. O. (1999). An investigation into the biochemical basis of the observed hyperglycaemia in rats treated with ethanol root extract of plumbago zeylanica. *Phytother. Res.*, Vol.13, No.4, (June 1999), pp. 346-348, ISSN 0951-418X.

Orvig, C.; Abrams, M. J. (1999). Medicinal inorganic chemistry: introduction. *Chem. Rev.*, Vol.99, No.9, (August 1999), pp. 2201-2203, ISSN 0009-2665.

Patwardhan, B.; Warude, D.; Pushpangadan, P. and Bhatt, N. (2005). Ayurveda and traditional Chinese medicine: a comparative overview. *Evid. Based Complement. Altern. Med.*, Vol.2, No.4, (December 2005), pp. 465-473, ISSN 1741-427X.

Pereira, R. M. S.; Andrades, N. E. D.; Paulino, N. Sawaya, A.C. H.; Eberlin, M. N.; Marcucci, M. C.; Favero, G. M.; Novak., E. M.; Bydlowski, S. P. (2007). Synthesis and characterization of a metal complex containing naringin and Cu, and its antioxidant, antimicrobial, antiinflammatory and tumor cell cytotoxicity. *Molecules*, Vol.12, No.7, (July 2007), pp. 1352–1366, ISSN 1420-3049.

Pusz, J.; Nitka, B. (1997). Synthesis and physicochemical properties of the complexes of Co(II), Ni(II), and Cu(II) with chrysin. Microchem. J., Vol.56, No.3, (July 1997), pp. 373-381, ISSN 0026-256x.

Pusz, J.; Nitka, B.; Zieliska, A.; Wawer, I. (2000). Synthesis and physicochemical properties of the Al(III), Ga(III) and In(III) complexes with chrysin. Microchem. J., Vol.65, No.3, (October 2000), pp. 245-253, ISSN 0026-265X.

Rao, T. S.; Basu, N.; Siddiqui, H. H. (1982). Anti-inflammatory activity of curcumin analogues. *Indian J. Med. Res.*, Vol.75, No.2, (April 1982), pp. 574-578, ISSN 0971-5916.

Remichkova, M.; Dimitrova, P.; Philipov, S.; Ivanovska, N. (2009). Toll-like receptor-mediated anti-inflammatory action of glaucine and oxoglaucine Fitoterapia, Vol.80, No.7, (July 2009), pp. 411–414, ISSN 0367-326X.

Rosenberg, B.; VanCamp, L. V.; Trosko, J. E.; Mansour, V. H. (1969). Platinum compounds: a new class of potent antitumour agents. *Nature*, Vol.222, No.5191, (April 1969), pp. 385-386, ISSN 0028-0836.

Ruan, L.-P.; Chen, S.; Yu, B.-Y.; Zhu, D.-N.; Cordell, G. A.; Qiu, S. X. (2006). Prediction of human absorption of natural compounds by the non-everted rat intestinal sac model. *Eur. J. Med. Chem.*, Vol.41, No.5, (May 2006), pp. 605-610, ISSN 0223-5234.

Russo, A.; Acquaviva, R.; Campisi, A.; Sorrenti, V.; Di Giacomo, C.; Virgata, G.; Barcellona, M. L.; Vanella, A. (2000). Bioflavonoids as antiradicals, antioxidants and DNA cleavage protectors. *Cell Biol. Toxicol.*, Vol.16, No.2, (April 2000), pp. 91-98, ISSN 0742-2091.

Sakai, W.; Swisher, E. M.; Karlan, B. Y.; Agarwal, M. K.; Higgins, J.; Friedman, C.; Villegas, E.; Jacquemont, C.; Farrugia, D. J.; Couch, F. J.; Nicole Urban, N.; Taniguchi, T. (2008). Secondary mutations as a mechanism of cisplatin resistance in BRCA2-mutated cancers. *Nature*, Vol.451, No.7182, (February 2008), pp. 1116-1120, ISSN 1476-4687.

Sarl, A. (1999). Alkaloids from *Glaucium leiocarpum*. *Planta Med.*, Vol.65, No.5, (June 1999), pp. 492, ISSN 0032-0943.

Saxton, C. (2010). Natural remedy shows anticancer activity. *Highlights in Chemical Science*, 01.

Sharma, O. P. (1976). Antioxidant activity of curcumin and related compounds. *Biochem. Pharmacol.*, Vol.25, No.5, (August 1976), pp. 1811-1812, ISSN 0006-2952.

Shibata, S. (1985). In *Advances in Chinese Medicinal Materials Research* (Chang, H. M.; Yeung, H. W.; Tso, W. W. and Koo, A.; eds), pp3-16, World Scientific Publishing.

So, F. V.; Guthrie, N.; Chambers, A. F.; Moussa, M. and Carroll, K. K. (1996). Inhibition of human breast cancer cell proliferation and delay of mammary tumorigenesis by flavonoids and citrus juices. *Nutr. Cancer*, Vol.26, No.2, (August 1996), pp. 167–181, ISSN 0163-5581.

Song, Y.; Kang, J.; Wang, Z.; Lu, X.; Gao, J.; Wang, L. (2002). Study on the interactions between CuL2 and Morin with DNA. *J. Inorg. Biochem.*, Vol.91, No.3, (August 2002), pp. 470-474, ISSN 0162-0134.

Song, Y.; Yang, P.; Yang, M.; Kang, J.; Qin, S.; Lü, B. (2003). Spectroscopic and vlotammetric studies of the cobalt(II) complex of morin bound to calf thymus DNA. *Transition Met. Chem.*, Vol.28, No.6, (June 2003), pp. 712-716, ISSN 0340-4285.

Srimal, R. C.; Dhawan, B.N. (1973). Pharmacology of diferuloyl methane (curcumin) a non-steroidal anti-inflammatory agent. *J. Pharm. Pharmacol.*, Vol.25, No.6, (June 1973), pp. 447-452, ISSN 0022-3573.

Srinivas, P.; Gopinath, G.; Banerji, A.; Dinakar, A.; Srinivas, G. (2004). Plumbagin induces reactive oxygen species, which mediate apoptosis in human cervical cancer cells. *Mol. Carcinogen.*, Vol.40, No.4, (August 2004), pp. 201-211, ISSN 1098-2744.

Staker, B. L.; Feese, M. D.; Cushman, M.; Pommier, Y.; Zembower, D.; Stewart, L.; Burgin, A. B. (2005). Structures of three classes of anticancer agents bound to the human topoisomerase I–DNA covalent complex. *J. Med. Chem.*, Vol.48, No.7, (February, 2005), pp. 2336-2346, ISSN 0022-2623.

Stone, R. (2008). Lifting the veil on traditional Chinese medicine. *Science*, Vol.319, No.5864, (February 2008), pp. 709-710, ISSN 0036-8075.

Tan, M.-X.; Zhu, J.-C.; Pan, Y.M.; Chen, Z.-F.; Liang, H.; Liu, H.-G.; Wang, H.-S. (2009). Synthesis, cytotoxic activity, and DNA binding properties of copper (II) complexes with hesperetin, naringenin and apigenin. *Bioinorg. Chem. Appl.*, doi:10.115/2009/347872, ISSN 1687-479X.

Tan, J.; Wang, B. C.; Zhu, L. C. (2007). Hydrolytic cleavage of DNA by quercetin zinc(II) complex. *Bioorg. Med. Chem. Lett.*, Vol.17, No.5, (March 2007), pp. 1197-1199, ISSN 0960-894X.

Tan, J.; Wang, B. C.; Zhu, L. C. (2009). DNA binding and oxidative DNA damage induced by a quercetin copper(II) complex: potential mechanism of its antitumor properties. *J. Biol. Inorg. Chem.*, Vol.14, No.5, (June 2009), pp. 727-739, ISSN 0949-8257.

Tan, J.; Wang, B. C.; Zhu, L. C. (2009). DNA binding, cytotoxicity, apoptotic inducing activity, and molecular modeling study of quercetin zinc(II) complex. *Bioorg. Med. Chem.*, Vol.17, No.2, (January 2009), pp. 614–620, ISSN 0968-0896.

Thati, B.; Noble, A.; Creaven, B. S.; Walsh, M.; McCann, M.; Kavanagh, K.; Devereux, M.; Egan, D. A. (2007). In vitro anti-tumour and cyto-selective effects of courmarin-3-carboxylic acid and three of its hydroxylated derivatives, along with their silver-based complexes, using human epithelial carcinoma cell lines. *Cancer Lett.*, Vol.248, No.2, (April 2007), pp. 321-331, ISSN.

Thompson, K. H.; Böhmerle, K.; Polishchuk, E.; Martins, C.; Toleikis, P.; Tse, J.; Yuen, V.; McNeill, J. H.; Orvig, C. (2004). Complementary inhibition of synoviocyte, smooth muscle cell or mouse lymphoma cell proliferation by a vanadyl curcumin complex compared to curcumin alone. *J. Inorg. Biochem.*, Vol.98, No.12, (December 2004), pp. 2063-2070, ISSN 0162-0134.

To, K. K. W.; Wang, X.; Yu, C.-W.; Ho, Y.-P.; Au-Yeung, S. C. F. (2004). Protein phosphatase 2A inhibition and circumvention of cisplatin cross-resistance by novel TCM-platinum anticancer agents containing demethylcantharidin. *Bioorg. Med. Chem.*, Vol.12, No.17, (September 2004), pp. 4565-4573, ISSN 0968-0896.

To, K. K. W.; Ho, Y.-P.; Au-Yeung, S. C. F. (2002). Determination of the release of hydrolyzed demethylcantharidin from novel traditional Chinese medicine-platinum compounds with anticancer activity by gas chromatography. *J. Chromatogr. A*, Vol.947, No.2, (February 2002), pp. 319-326, ISSN 0021-9673.

To, K. K. W.; Ho, Y.-P.; Au-Yeung, S. C. F. (2005). *In vitro* and *in vivo* suppression of growth of hepatocelular carcinoma cells by novel traditional Chinese medicine-platinum anti-cancer agents. *Anti-cancer Drugs*, Vol.16, No.8, (September 2005), pp. 825-835, ISSN 0959-4973.

To, K. K. W.; Au-Yeung, S. C. F.; Ho, Y.-P. (2006). Differential nephrotoxicity of cis-platin and a novel series of traditional Chinese medicine-platinum anticancer agents correlates with their chemical reactivity towards sulfur-containing nucleophiles. *Anti-cancer Drugs*, Vol.17, No.6, (July 2006), pp. 673-683, ISSN 0959-4973.

To, K. K. W.; Ho, Y.-P.; Au-Yeung, S. C. F. (2005). Synergistic interaction between platinum-based antitumor agents and demethylcantharidin. *Cancer Lett.*, Vol.223, No.2, (June 2005), pp. 227-237, ISSN 0304-3835.

Tojo, E.; Dominguez, D.; Castedo, L. (1991). *Phytochemisrry*, Vol.30, No.3, (March 1991), pp. 1005–1010, ISSN 0031-9422.

Tripoli, E.; Guardia, M. L.; Giammanco, S.; Majo, D. D. and Giammanco, M. (2007). Citrus flavonoids: Molecular structure, biological activity and nutritional properties: A review. *Food Chem.*, Vol.104, No.2, (September 2007), pp. 466–479, ISSN 0308-8146.

Wang, B.-D.; Yang, Z.-Y.; Wang, Q.; Cai, T.-K.; Crewdson, P. (2006). Synthesis, characterization, cytotoxic activities, and DNA-binding properties of the La(III) complex with naringenin Schiff-base. *Bioorg. Med. Chem.*, Vol.14, No.6, (March 2006), pp. 1880–1888, ISSN 0968-0896.

Wang, G. S. (1989). Medical uses of mylabris in ancient China and recent studies. *J. Ethnopharm.*, Vol.26, No.2, (September 1989), pp. 147-162, ISSN0378-8741.

Wang, L.; Gou, S.; Chen, Y., Liu, Y. (2005). Potential new antitumour agents from an innovative cmbination of camphorato, a ramification of traditional Chinese medicine, with a platinum moiety. *Bioorg. Med. Chem. Lett.*, Vol.15, No.14, (July 2005), pp. 3417-3422, ISSN 0960-894X.

Wang, X.; Au-Yeung, S. C. F.; Ho, Y.-P. (2007). Pharmacokinetics and tissue distribution of novel traditional Chinese medicine-platinum anticancer agents in rats. *J. Inorg. Biochem.*, Vol.101, No.6, (June 2007), pp. 909-917, ISSN 0162-0134.

Wong, E.; Giandomcnico, C. M. (1999). Current status of platinum based antitumor drugs. *Chem. Rev.*, Vol.99, No. 9, (August 1999), pp. 2451-2466, ISSN 0009-2665.

Woo, S. H.; Reynolds, M. C.; Sun, N. J.; Cassady, J. M.; Snapka, R. M. (1997). Inhibition of topoisomerase II by liriodenine. *Biochem. Pharmacol.*, Vol.54, No.4, (August 1997), pp. 467-473, ISSN 0006-2952.

Wu, J.-Z.; Yuan, L.; Wu, J.-F. (2005). Synthesis and DNA binding of □-[2,9-bis(2-imidazo[4,5-f][1,10]phenanthroline)-1,10-phenanthroline]bis[1,10-phenanthroline-copper(II)]. *J. Inorg. Biochem.*, Vol.99, No.11, (November 2005), pp. 2211-2216, ISSN 0162-0134.

Wu, Y. C.; Duh, C. Y.; Wang, S. K.; Chen, K. S.; Yang, T. H. (1990). Two new natural azafluorene alkaloids and a cytotoxic aporphine alkaloid from Polyalthia longifolia. *J. Nat. Prod.*, Vol.53, No.5, (September 1990), pp. 1327-1331, ISSN 0163-3864.

Wu, Y.-C.; Liou, Y.-F.; Lu, S.-T.; Chen, C.-H.; Chang, J.-J.; Lee, K.-H. (1989). *Planta Med.*, Vol.55, No.2, (April 1989), pp. 163–165, ISSN 0032-0943.

Wu, Z. Y.; Zhou, T. Y.; Xiao, P. G. (1998). *Xin Hua Compendium of Materia Medica (I)*, Sahnghai: Shanghai Science & Technology Press, 1998: pp. 113–117.

Yu, C.-W.; Li, K. K. W.; Pang, S.-K. ; Au-Yeung, S. C. F.; Ho, Y.-P. (2006). Anticancer activity of a series of platinum complexes integrating demethylcantharidin with isomers of 1, 2-diaminocyclohexane. *Bioorg. Med. Chem. Lett.*, Vol.16, No.6, (March 2006), pp 1686-1691, ISSN 0960-894X.

Zeng, Y.-B.; Yang, N.; Liu, W.-S.; Tang, N. (2003). Synthesis, characterization and DNA-binding properties of La(III) complex of chrysin. *J. Inorg. Biochem.*, Vol.97, No.3, (November 2003), pp. 258-264, ISSN 0162-0134

Zhang, Q.; Wang, L.; Liu X. (1996). Synthesis, characterization and antitumour properties of metal(II) solid complexes with morin. *Transition Met. Chem.*, Vol.21, No.1, (January 1996), pp. 23-27, ISSN 0340-4285.

Zhang, L. J.; Wang, T. T.; Wen, X. M.; Wei, Y.; Peng, X. C.; Li, H.; Wei, L. (2007). Effect of matrine on HeLa cell adhesion and migration. *Eur. J. Pharmacol.*, Vol.563, No.1-3, (June 2007), pp. 69-76, ISSN 0014-4285.

Zhang, L. P.; Jiang, J. K.; Tam, J. W. O.; Zhang, Y.; Liu, X. S.; Xu, X. R.; Liu, B. Z.; He, Y. J. (2001). Effects of Matrine on proliferation and differentiation in K-562 cells. *Leuk. Res.*, Vol.25, No.9, (Septmber 2001), pp. 793-800, ISSN 0145-2126.

Zhou, J.; Wang, L.; Wang, J.; Tang, N. (2001). Antioxidative and anti-tumour activities of solid quercetin metal(II) complexes. *Transition Met. Chem.*, Vol.26, No.1-2, (January 2001), pp. 57-63, ISSN 0340-4285.

Zutphen, S.; Reedijk, J. (2005). Targeting platinum anti-tumour drugs: Overview of strategies employed to reduce systemic toxicity. *Coord. Chem. Rev.*, Vol.249, No.24, (December 2005), pp. 2845-2853, ISSN 0010-8545.

13

The Producing Area of Chinese Medicine and Famous Region Drug Research – Magnolia Officinalis

Guo Li

Jiangxi University of Traditional Chinese Medicine, Nanchang, Jiangxi, PRC

1. Introduction

1.1 Producing area

Under the guidance of the theory of the Traditional Chinese Medicine, many plants, animals and minerals in China can be medicines to treat the human diseases. Synchronously, the capacious land, sea and rich mineral deposits supply resources for them. Before they become medicines, they need grow and be gathered in some areas. But in these areas the weather, geographic features and biologic distributions are very different such as the different natural zones. Therefore these comprehensive factors endow Chinese medicines with different biological features and effects. After long time use, the medical practitioners gradually found the quantity or quality of some Chinese medicines which were produced in different areas were also different. An appellation came into being, which was called famous region drug.

1.2 Famous region drug

This appellation means those medicines which have good breeds and higher quality grow in some characteristic regions and feasible growing environments. They are cultivated and processed reasonably and output is great.

One thousand and five hundred years ago, in (Annotated Shen Nong's Herbal), Jinghong Tao had discussed the producing areas of Chinese Medicine. But at Yuan dynasty, famous region drug were first written in (Peony Pavilion) Xianzu Tang wrote. Until Tang dynasty, the government divided the country into ten areas according natural form. So Simiao Sun recorded famous region drugs producing in these areas in(a supplement to the essential prescriptions worth a thousand gold). (commentaries on the illustrations)written by Song Su and (Compendium of Materia Medica)written by Shizhen Li both recorded the regions and quality of Chinese Medicine. Now some places in China are famous regions of Chinese Medicines, such as Sichuan province, Guangdong province, Shandong province where respectively produced Rhizoma Chuanxiong, Fructus Amomi, Equus asinus L.

1.3 Magnolia officinalis

Magnolia officinalis are from the barks of Magnolia officinalis Reha. et Wils. and Magnolia officinalis Reha. et Wils.var. biloba. Reha. et Wils which belong to Magnoliaceae [1]. Its producing areas mainly include Sichuan, Hubei and Jiangxi province [2]. The characters of its medicinal materials usually showed single or double drum, grey outer surface with vertical wrinkles, purple brown inter surface with wiped oil mark and section with fine crystallization. Microstructure of its medicinal materials usually showed stone and oil cells or starch grains. The modern research also showed that its main effective component is magnolol and honokiol.

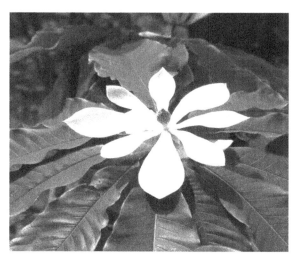

Fig. 1. Medicinal plant of Magnolia officinalis

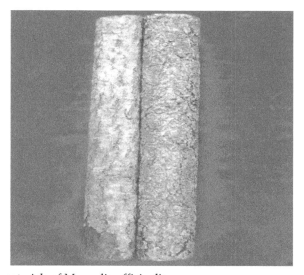

Fig. 2. Medicinal materials of Magnolia officinalis

It is wide used in clinic due to the effect of eliminating dampness and phlegm, promoting qi and removing distention. But the resource of Magnolia officinalis is decreasing and the imbalance between supply and demand is outstanding in recent years. It has been involved in natural protected Chinese medicine. Its variety research seems very urgent for looking for its substitute.

2. Purpose

To explore the exact substitute and the quality evaluation, optimization methods of Magnolia officinalis, the comprehensive varieties researches based on its adulterants and substitutes and quality evaluation methods were reviewed.

3. Methods

The appearance characters, microstructure, physical and chemical(including Thin-Layer Chromatography and high performance liquid chromatography) and randomly amplified polymorphic DNA(RAPD) identification, 1H Nuclear magnetic resonance spectroscopy, powder X-ray diffraction fourier fingerprint, polyamide chromatography of different adulterants and substitutes were applied according to the records. And they were reviewed. The results showed that they totally contained ten families and forty - three varieties. The influence factors on the quality of Magnolia officinalis and the other quality evaluation methods were also reviewed.

4. Result and conclusion

4.1 Families and varieties of plants identified with Magnolia officinalis and identified methods

The difference between Magnolia officinalis and these adulterants and substitutes were significant through the research. Firstly the morphological and(or) histological characters of some varieties were different from Magnolia officinalis, such as sikimmi, aleurites montana, Magnolia rostrata w w smith, Manglietia szechuanica Hu., Neolitsea levinei Merr., phyllanthi fructus, White yulan Magnolia, bigleaf magnolia bark, Wudang yulan magnolia, Magnolia wilsonii, camphortree bark , M.szechuanica Hu, M.insignis(Wal1.)Bl, Manglietia chingii Dandy, Manglietia yuyuanensis Law, sprenger magnolia bark, sargent magnolia bark, Magnolia wilsonii , Magnolia campbellii Hook.f.et Thoms., Mountain yulan Magnolia, M.szechuanica Hu, Manglietia chingii Dandy [3-14]. Secondly some physical and chemical identification showed significant results between Magnolia officinalis, Wudang magnolia bark, Magnolia campbellii Hook.f.et Thoms., albiziae , thinleaf machilus and Ormosia balansae. [15-17].The thin-Layer Chromatography analyzing also showed Magnolia officinalis were very different from the following adulterants and substitutes: (1)Wudang magnolia bark, Xikang magnolia bark and sargent magnolia bark were identified with cyclohexane-chloroform-ethanol (7:3:1) as developer and 5% vanillin sulfuric acid solution as coloration using silica gel G and observed at 254 nm using ultraviolet lamp [18]. (2)White yulan Magnolia, biond magnolia flower, shikimmi, red nanmu, aleurites montana, schima root-bark, Albizziakal Kora(Roxb).Prain., arbutus were identified with benzene-methanol (27:1) as developer and vanillin sulfuric acid solution as coloration using silica gel G and observed at 365 nm using ultraviolet lamp [19]. (3)Magnolia campbellii Hook.f.et Thoms.was identified with benzene-methanol (9:1) as developer and 1% vanillin sulfuric acid solution as coloration using silica gel G [20]. (4) Guangxi Manglietia was identified with benzene-methanol (8:2) as developer and 5% vanillin sulfuric acid solution as coloration

families	varieties numbers	varieties
Magnoliaceae	26	sprenger magnolia bark、 sargent magnolia bark、 Magnolia campbellii Hook.f.et Thoms.、 Xikang magnolia bark 、 Wudang yulan magnolia、white yulanMagnolia、Mountain yulan Magnolia、 Magnolia wilsonii、 Tianmu mountain magnolia immature flower、 bigleaf magnolia bark、 Magnolia rostrata w. w. smith、 purple yulan Magnolia、 magnolia bioudii、 Mt. Huang magnolia bark、 M.szechuanica Hu 、 M.insignis(Wall.)Bl 、 Manglietia chingii Dandy、 Manglietia yuyuanensis Law、 Guangxi Manglietia、 liriodendron 、 biond magnolia flower、 shikimmi 、 Michelia maudiae、 Qinshi Manglietia、Magnolietia patungensis、 Michelia champaca L..
Euphorbiaceae	2	phyllanthi fructus、 aleurites montana
lauraceae	4	red nanmu、 thinleaf machilus 、 camphortree bark 、 Neolitsea levinei Merr.
Juglandaceae	3	Engelhardia roxburghiana Wall 、 wild walnut 、 Juglans mandshurica Maxim.
myricaceae	1	arbutus
araliaceae	1	Manglietia szechuanica Hu.
Scrophulariaceae	1	Paulownia tomentosa (Thunb.) Steud.
Theaceae	1	schima root-bark
Leguminosae	3	Albizziakal Kora(Roxb).Prain.、 Ormosia balansae 、 albiziae
Oleaceae	1	Fraxinus rhynchophylla Hance

Table 1. Families and varieties of plants identified with Magnolia officinalis

using silica gel G [21]. (5) Juglans mandshurica Maxim.,Wild walnut, Paulownia tomentosa (Thunb.) Steud.and Mountain yulanMagnolia were identified with benzene-methanol (27:1) as developer and 1% vanillin sulfuric acid solution as coloration using silica gel G [22-25]. (6) Tianmu mountain magnolia immature flower was identified with benzene-ethyl acetate-methanol (27:1) as developer using silica gel G [26]. (7)Mt. Huang magnolia bar k, Manglietia yuyuanensis Law, Michelia maudiae were identified with benzene-methanol (27:1) as developer and 5% vanillin sulfuric acid solution as coloration using silica gel G [27]. (8) Qinshi Manglietia was identified with chloroform-methanol as developer and 5% vanillin sulfuric acid solution as coloration using silica gel G [28]. (9)Engelhardia roxburghiana Wall was identified with benzene-methanol (9:1) as developer and 1% vanillin sulfuric acid solution as coloration using silica gel G [29]. High performance liquid chromatography(HPLC) detection showed the total amount of magnolol and honokiol in Magnolia wilsonii, sprenger magnolia bark, and sargent magnolia bark were corresponding with PRC codex 2005 which was on Permaphase ODS, under the condition of mobile phase of benzene:phosphate(70:30) with the flow rate of 1.0ml/min. The calibration curves showed linear regression $r > 0.9989$. The recoveries ranged from 99.04% to 105.45%. [30]. But there was no magnolol and honokiol in white yulan Magnolia, purple yulan Magnolia, magnolia bioudii and Wudang yulan magnolia on Permaphase ODS，under the condition of mobile phase of benzene:water (74.5:25.5) with the flow rate of 1.0ml/min. Most of manglietia and Mountain yulan Magnolia contain small amounts of magnolol and honokiol [31]. The randomly amplified polymorphic DNA was also used to identify the certified products and the adulterants and substitutes of Magnolia officinalis like yulan magnolia, magnolia bioudii, Wudang yulan magnolia, purple yulan Magnolia, Mountain yulan Magnolia, Manglietia chingii Dandy, M.insignis(Wal1.)Bl and liriodendron.The result showed that the DNA Fingerprinting of Magnolia officinalis was very different from that of these adulterants and substitutes [32]. 15 samples of cortex Magnolia officinalis from different origin, 1 standard sample of Magnolia officinalis and 1 Wudang yulan magnolia were identified by 1H Nuclear magnetic resonance spectroscopy. The fingerprint showed that 1H-NMR could be an accurate and feasible method for the quality control of Magnolia officinalis [33]. Powder X-ray diffraction fourier fingerprint pattern was developed to identify and analyze Magnolia officinalis. Experiments and analysis were carried out on 3 samples of cortex Magnoliae officinals, 3 samples of cortex Magnolia bilobae, 14 samples of substitute and one counterfeit of cortex Magnolia officinals. It was found that this method can be used for identification on Chinese medicinal material Cortex Magnolia officinals [34].The characteristic chromatogram for cortex Magnolia officinalis was established by using polyamide chromatography (PC) to identify the cortex Magnolia officinalis from different origin and its substitute and false products. The result showed that this method could be used for the identification and quality evaluation for cortex Magnolia officinalis [35].

4.2 Influence factors and determinative methods of quality of Magnolia officinalis

The content of magnolol and honokiol of Magnolia officinalis collected from 7 provinces, 11 counties and Jingning provenance testing forest of Zhejiang province were detected as quality standards by using HPLC. And the correlation analysis between the factors which would affect the quality of Magnolia officinalis and the content of magnolol and honokiol was applied. The result showed that many factors would affect the quality of Magnolia officinalis significantly, such as provenance, producing area, blade profile, DBH, tree height, crown width, tree age, bar thickness, powder color, oiliness, grindability, bark type and position of sampling, etc. Among them, provenance, blade profile, powder color, bark thickness, DBH and position of sampling were more significant factors, especially the variety [36]. However some other researches showed tree age and length of storage period would be two factors which affected the quality of Magnolia officinalis [37-38]. After analysis, geographical position and Climate, blade profile and variety firstly maybe would affect the quality of Magnolia officinalis, especially the provenances with a sharpened leaf tip from Hubei Province has a highest content of phenols, and that with a concave leaf tip from the Lushan Mountain has a lowest content of phenols [39-40]. Secondly, there was positive correlation between the growth factors of Magnolia officinalis including tree age, DBH, tree height, crown width and content of phenols of Magnolia officinalis, especially the DBH [41]. Thirdly, appearance characters including bark thickness, powder color, grindability and bark roughness were regarded as the main traditional basis for the quality evaluation of Magnolia officinalis, which accorded with the research [42]. Position of sampling was also a basis for the quality evaluation of Magnolia officinalis which included dry hide, root bark, shoot cortex, etc. Content of phenols of root bark from Magnolia officinalis was 3-5 times higher than that of shoot cortex from Magnolia officinalis [41].

Besides the TLC and HPLC, amplified fragment length polymorphism analysis was applied as a method for further study with molecular markers in the field of genetic diversity, for breeding new cultivars, and for genetic relationships with Magnolia officinalis [43]. First derivative of UV spectrophotometry was also used to analyze compositions of Magnolia officinalis. The result showed that this method could eliminate interference of other impurity and make all samples exhibit maximum absorbance at 300nm [44]. A gas chromatography/mass spectrography was developed to identify the compositions of Magnolia officinalis, including magnolol, honokiol, δ-selinene and β-eudeomol, etc. And the content of magnolol and honokiol were determined [45]. The second order derivative synchronous fluorescence spectra of magnolol, honokiol and their mixture in 0.08%-0.16% methanol solution were studied. The experiment results indicated that their second order derivative synchronous fluorescence spectra were separated absolutely, which eliminated the disturbance between them [46]. To detect the contents of six trace elements (Fe ,Cu ,Zn ,Mn ,Ca ,Mg) in cortex Magnolia officinalis by flame atomic absorption spectroscopy, the contents of six trace elements (Fe ,Cu ,Zn , Mn ,Ca and Mg) were determined by calibration curve method. The result showed that the Cortex Magnolia officinalis is rich in trace elements which are necessary for people [47]. Quantitative Measurement of magnolol and honokiol was tested by using excitation–emission Matrix Fluorescence coupled with second–order calibration algorithm. It showed that the second-order calibration methods could quantify the analysis of interest from overlapped chromatographic profiles and give the accurate predicted results by utilizing mathematical-separation instead of physics-separation [48]. Fluorescent determination of magnolol has been effected employing the sensitivity- and stability-enhancing action of the non-ionic surface active emulsifier OP. As a result, the accuracy of determination was raised by 2 orders of magnitude as compared to that of ultraviolet spectrophotometry [49]. A highly sensitive and selective method was developed for the determination of honokiol and magnolol by HPLC-electrochemical detection, using a microbore column. The result showed that this method could be proposed for the determination of honokiol and magnolol in traditional Chinese medicines and human plasma sample [50].

All above-mentioned researches showed there were four kinds of factors mainly affecting the quality of Magnolia officinalis. And many methods had been used to determinate the content or compositions of Magnolia officinalis for the identification or quality control. Making and following the comprehensive and well-considered plans to develop famous region drugs would benefit protecting the environment, rare Chinese Medicine and highlighting characteristic of Chinese Medicines significantly.

5. References

[1] Chinese Pharmacopoeia Commission, *Pharmacopoeia of the People's Republic of China*, vol. 1, 2005,176.

[2] Z.L.Zheng, Y.S.Zheng, *Journal of Fujian Forestry Science and Technology*, 2010, 37, 103

[3] W.B.Duan,*Chinese Journal of Misdiagnostics*, 2002, 2, 797.

[4] Q.J.Shen,*Base Journal of Chinese Materia Medica*, 1997, 11, 14.

[5] M.Xu,*Journal of Modern Applied Pharmacy*, 1995,12,22.

[6] L.Wei,*Base Journal of Chinese Materia Medica*,2000,14,32.
[7] S.L.Yu,M.R.Zhu,Z.P,Li, Shandong Journal of Traditional Chinese Medicine,1998, 17, 227.
[8] S.H.,Yang,*Strait Pharmaceutical Journal*,1994,6 ,67.
[9] H.P.Zhu,*Shandong Journal of Traditional Chinese Medicine*.2008,27,629..
[10] C.Q.Xu,L.W.Cao,F.J.Xiang, Jorunal of Chinese Medicinal Materials, 1994, 17, 16.
[11] C.Q.Xu,L.W.Cao,F.J.Xiang,China Journal of Chinese Meteria Medica,1994,19,579
[12] Q.H.Wang,*Journal of Practical Traditional Chinese Internal Medicine*,2007,21,94.
[13] S.X.Peng,Modern Journal of Integrated Traditional Chinese and Western Medicine,2008,17,5642
[14] Y.Liu,Z.L.Yang, *Nonwood Forest Research*,2002,20,45.
[15] H.L.Zhang,*Chinese Journal of Modern Applied Pharmacy*,2000,17,108.
[16] X.Yu,Y.C.Zhuang,J.X.Yi,*Lishizhen Medicine and Materia Medica Research*,2008,19,2023.
[17] H.Chen,*Yunnan Journal of Traditional Chinese Medicine and Materia Medica*,1999, 20,40.
[18] W.G.Song,Strait Pharmaceutical Journal, 2003, 15, 57.
[19] J.G.Ye,Y.L.Wang, Heilongjiang Journal of Traditional ChineseMedicine, 2000, (6), 57.
[20] Z.M.Bai,X.X.Su, Research and Practice on Chinese Medicines, 2007, 21, 28.
[21] Y.Cao,Research and Practice on Chinese Medicines, 2004,18,33.
[22] A.W.Sun,*Chinese Licensed Pharmacist*,2007,(6),30.
[23] Q.Peng,*Journal of Chinese Medicinal Materials*,1992,15,20.
[24] Q.Peng,Journal of Chinese Medicinal Materials,1993, 16, 15.
[25] S.H.Wang,B.H.Li,M.Liu,Journal of Chinese Medicinal Materials,1999, 22,397.
[26] Q.Q.Yang,*Lishizhen Medicine and Materia Medica Research*, 2005,16,42.
[27] S.F.Li,F.Zhu,J.H.Wang, Journal of Chinese Medicinal Materials,1992, 15,16.
[28] H.D.Fu,J.M.Zheng, *China Pharmaceuticals*, 2008,17,67.
[29] R.L.Lin,*Strait Pharmaceutical Journal*, 2004, 16, 79.
[30] Y.P.Zhou,X.M.Fu,*Medical Journal of the Chinese People' s Armed Police Forces*,2002,13,618.
[31] .W.Su,C.Q.Xu,C.H.Sui,R.Q.Sun,Y.J.Wang,H.L.Liu,X.H.Shen, *Journal of She-nyang Pharmaceutical University*,1992,9 ,185.
[32] B.L.Guo, M.Wu, J.P.S, J.S.Li, *Journal of pharmaceutical practice*, 2000, 18, 314
[33] Y.Nie, W.F.Yao, W.B.Shen. Jiangsu Journal of Traditional Chinese Medicine, 2008, 40, 91
[34] L.Wu, L.Ma, Q.T.Zheng, W.Z.Song, Y.Lv. *Chinese Traditio nal Patent Medicine*, 2004,26, 861
[35] H.M.Jiang, D.H.Sun, J.Q.Lu, F.Huang, Y.Cao. *China Hospital pharmacy Journal*, 2004, 24, 221
[36] J.P.Si, Z.K.Tong, Y.R.Zeng. China Journal of Chinese Materia Medica, 2000, 25, 466
[37] Y.R.Zeng, Z.K.Tong, Y.Q.Zhu, J.P.Si, X.P.Pan. Journal of Chinese Materia Medica, 1999, 22, 379
[38] X.Y.Jiang, J.P.Si, Y.R.Zeng, Y.Q.Zhu. Journal of Zhejiang University of Traditional Chinese Medicin, 2003, 27, 82
[39]] Z.Li, M.Zhang, X.Lin, Y.M.Hou. *China Journal of Chinese Materia Medica*, 1989, 14, 15
[40] J.P.Si. Journal of Chinese Materia Medica, 2000, 23, 373
[41] J.P.Si, X.P.Pan, M.Y.Pan, R.Liu, X.L.Mei. *Journal of Zhejiang Forestry Science and Technology*, 1994,14,21
[42] Y.Q.Zhu, Y.R.Zeng, X.P.Pan, J.P.Si, Z.L.Wang. *Journal of Zhejiang Forestry College*, 1999, 16, 387
[43] Y.F.Jiang, J.P.Si, H.H.Huang, L.J.Cheng. *Journal of Zhejiang Forestry College*, 2010, 27, 304

[44] X.M.Wang, T.M.Ding, C.Chen. China Journal of Chinese Materia Medica, 1992, 17, 169

[45] Y.Wang. Strait Pharmaceutical Journal, 1998, 10, 45

[46] J.Yang, D.S.Yu, S.P.Liu, G.F.Tian, B.B.M.*Chinese Journal of Analytical Chemistry*, 2009, 37, 107

[47] J.L.Li, S.Z.Wu, Y.B.Li, L.Yu, Q.S.Li. *China Pharmacy*, 2008, 19, 2843

[48] L.Q.Hu, C.L.Ying, Y.Yang, L.W.Chui. *Journa l of Pingdingshan University*, 2010, 25, 53

[49] W.J.Liu, B.Q.Wang, Z.G.Pang, H.Cheng. *China Journal of Chinese Materia Medica*, 1991, 16, 101

[50] D.L.Wang, Q.S.Wang, D.R. Jin. *Chinese Journal of Pharmaceutical Analysis*, 2007, 11, 1820

14

Phytochemicals as Antidepressants: The Involvement of Serotonin Receptor Function, Stress Resistance and Neurogenesis

Rui Wang[1] and Ying Xu[2]
[1]Program of Pharmacology, Weill Graduate School of Medical Science,
Cornell University, New York, NY,
[2]Department of Behavioral Medicine and Psychiatry,
West Virginia University Health Science Center, Morgantown, WV,
USA

1. Introduction

Mood disorders are among the most prevalent forms of mental illness and a major cause of morbidity worldwide. Depression is one of the top ten causes of morbidity and mortality worldwide based on a survey by the World Health Organization (Berton and Nestler, 2006). Depression (major depressive disorder, major depression, unipolar depression, clinical depression) is a chronic, recurring and potentially life-threatening mood disorder that has been estimated to affect 21% of the world population (Schechter et al., 2005). It is estimated that 40% of the risk for depression is genetic, though the specific genes involved in the risk is still limited understanding. The other 60% non-genetic risk remains poorly defined, with suggestions as diverse as acute or chronic stress, childhood trauma, viral infections and even random processes during brain development might be involved (Akiskal, 2000; Berton and Nestler, 2006).

Stress occurs in every day life. Among psychiatric disorders, depression is probably the most common stress-related diseases. The theoretical premise is that depression is the outcome of an eventual inability to cope with a stream of dissimilar unpleasant stimuli imposed by the environment (Ferretti et al., 1995). The link between genetic predisposition and life stressors in the etiology of depression remains unclear because the mode of transmission of mood disorders is likely to be complex. However, interactions between a genetic predisposition and some environmental stressors are probably necessary to induce depression (Caspi and Moffitt, 2006). In addition, not only the hypothalamic-pituitary-adrenal (HPA) axis, but also brain neuronal systems, including the monoaminergic systems and in particular the serotonin (5-HT) containing neuronal one, play critical roles in stress-related disorders (Lanfumey et al., 2008; Xu et al., 2006). The structural alterations of neurons in stress-induced depression, such as a progressive decrease in the volume of the frontal cortex and hippocampus, have also been found to be related to dysfunctions of HPA axis, abnormalities in 5-HT and its receptors (Drevets, 2000; Reinés et al., 2008; Tsuji et al., 2001). But, so far, no clear consensus has evolved in pathological mechanism of inter-neuronal communication and post-receptor signal transduction of depression.

Early theories of depression focused on imbalance of neurotransmitter system, especially depletion of the serotonin (5-HT), norepinephrine (NE) and/or dopamine in depression and related mood disorders, since the efficacy of tricyclic antidepressants and monoamine oxidase inhibitors (MAOIs) in the treatment of these disorders. Current theoretical and experimental developments in serotonin and noradrenaline research extend the previous studies, the robust therapeutic effects of newer antidepressants are discovered, such as selective serotonin reuptake inhibitors (SSRIs), noradrenaline reuptake inhibitors (NRIs) and serotonin and noradrenaline reuptake inhibitors (SNRIs). However, the current therapeutic options of depression are far from ideal: most of the pharmacological interventions are not effective in more than 50% cases, and are often associated with a range of serious side effects and drug-drug/drug-food interactions (Baker et al., 2003; Meijer et al., 2004).

Polyphenolic nutraceuticals (phytochemicals) present in vegetables and fruits are believed to reduce the risk of several major diseases including cardiovascular, autoimmune and neurodegenerative disorders. Six such polyphenols are curcumin, low molecular proanthocyanidin, resveratrol, fisetin, piceatannol and ferulic acid, which have been used throughout Asia as traditional herbal medicines. They show strong antioxidant and anti-inflammatory properties. The wide ranging activity of these compounds and the repeated demonstration that they can decrease the stress response, oxidative damage, inflammation, neuronal damage and act as neuroprotectants, strongly suggest these compounds might have a significant impact on stress-induced depression and other affective disorders.

In this review, we integrate our current knowledge to define the present state of depression and assessment of the position of serotoninergic function in the pathophysiology of depression. We also summarize the status of a few novel approaches and compounds that are under investigation for the treatment of major depression. We attempt to provide a progress report on the pharmacological profile of multiple polyphenolic phytochemicals as promising herbal antidepressants.

2. Biological correlates of stress-induced depression and neurogenesis: Evidence for serotoninergic function

2.1 Stress, corticosterone and depression

Glucocorticoid release is regulated by the HPA axis in physical conditions. Corticotropin-relaesing hormone (CRH) released by the paraventricular nucleus of the hypothalamus stimulates the release of corticotropin (ACTH) from the anterior pituitary, which, in turn, stimulates glucocorticoid secretion from the adrenal cortex. HPA axis is an essential component of an individual's capacity to cope with stress (Berton and Nestler, 2006). Stress may be described as any environmental change, either internal or external, that disturbs the maintenance on homeostasis (Leonard, 2005). The stress response is to maintain homeostasis, which includes a series of physiological reactions such as endocrine activation (especially of the HPA axis) and cardiovascular changes (Sapolsky, 2003). The symptomatology, such as irritability, anxiety and a feeling of being unable to cope with, may ultimately result in depression when exposure to a prolonged and sustained stress (Lanfumey et al., 2008). Chronic stress often acts as a trigger to the onset of major depression and is associated with a decreased sensitivity to HPA axis feedback inhibition by cortisol in primates or corticosterone in rodents. Excessive stimulation of the axis further increases the secretion of glucocorticoids, which affects many aspects of peripheral and neuronal function, including immune, epithelial cell growth and energy mebabolism, neuronal connections, and synaptic transmission (McEwen and Stellar, 1993).

It is a common finding that around 50% of depressed patients (80% if severely depressed) show hyperactivity of the HPA axis (Young et al., 1991). Interestingly, similar changes in the hyperactivity of the HPA axis have been reported in animals subjected to chronic stress (Leonard, 2005). Elevated corticosterone level is a hallmark of HPA axis feedback inhibition evidenced by animal studies (Centeno and Volosin, 1997). This feedback is mediated by two types of corticosteroid receptors in the brain, the mineralocorticoid receptor (MR) and the GR (McEwen, 2000). The MR is a high-affinity receptor which binds corticosterone at low concentration (Kd ~0.5nM). MR is almost completely occupied (90%) by basal corticosterone levels and this contributes to maintaining homeostasis. When normal secretion of glucocorticoids is altered during stress, leading to increased levels of corticosterone, GR becomes substantially occupied by the hormone ligand. GR has a widespread distribution in limbic regions such as the hippocampus, paraventricular nucleus (PVN), the locus coeruleus and the dorsal raphe nucleus (DRN) (Harfstrand et al., 1986; Reul and de Kloet, 1986). Glucocorticoids diffuse passively through cellular membranes and bind to intracellular glucocorticoid receptors (GR), causing their translocation into the nucleus (Gillespie and Nemeroff, 2005). In the nucleus, these ligand-activated transcription factors bind to specific DNA response elements and alter gene expression. In the brain, glucocorticoid-regulated gene changes mediate a variety of effects on neuronal excitability, neurochemistry and structural plasticity (McEwen, 2000).

2.2 Serotonin and its receptors in depression

5-HT was discovered in 1948 and is a phylogenetically conserved neurotransmitter (Rapport et al., 1948; Barnes and Sharp, 1999). It is synthesized from L-tryptophan both in the peripheral nervous system and the CNS, via tryptophan hydroxylase 1 and 2, respectively (Walther et al., 2003). In the CNS, 5-HT neurons are localized in the raphe nuclei and project, via ascending and descending pathways, to a wide range of brain regions (Dahlström and Fuxe, 1964). These receptors affect a wide range of physiological and psychopathological processes such as mood disturbances, sleep, temperature control appetite, sexual behavior, movement, pain perception, and gastrointestinal motility. It is well established that the 5-HT is a phylogenetically conserved monoaminergic neurotransmitter which is crucial for a number of physiological processes and is dysregulated in several disease states including depression, anxiety and schizophrenia. As an important neurotransmitter, serotonin exerts its functions through 14 5-HT subtypes receptors. Exposure of experimental animals to various stressors, such as restraint stress and electroshock, has been shown to increase the turnover of serotonin and its receptors in the frontal cortex, hippocampus, amygdala and other brain regions (Inoue et al., 1994).

Fourteen different 5-HT receptors have been cloned and pharmacologically characterized (Barnes and Sharp, 1999; Dahlstrom and Fuxe, 1964; Walther et al., 2003; Millan et al., 2008). The human 5-HT receptors are divided into 7 distinct families (5-HT$_{1-7}$) (Davis et al., 2002). With the exception of the 5-HT$_3$ receptor as a ligand-gated ion channel, all other serotonin receptors (5-HT$_{1A-F}$, 5-HT$_{2A-C}$, 5-HT$_4$, 5-HT$_5$, 5-HT$_6$, 5-HT$_7$) are G protein-coupled receptors that activate an intracellular second messenger cascade to produce an excitatory or inhibitory response. Activation of the specific G-protein can affect enzymes (5-HT$_1$- and 5-HT$_5$-class receptors decrease cAMP formation; 5-HT$_2$-class receptors increase inositol triphosphate and diacylglycerol formation; and 5-HT$_4$, 5-HT$_6$ and 5-HT$_7$ receptors increase cAMP formation) and the function of cation channels especially K^+ and Ca^{2+} (Kushwaha and Albert, 2005).

5-HT, as an important neurotransmitter, has long been reported to exert an important mitogenic action in the central neural system (CNS) during development (Lauder et al., 1981; Whitaker-Azmitia,1991). In the adult CNS, serotonin is involved in neuronal and synaptic plasticity, and its action on the serotonin $5-HT_{1A}$ receptor is particularly significant in this regard (Azmitia and Whitaker-Azmitia, 1997). It was also found that the powerful mitogenic effect of fenfluramine (a releaser of serotonin throughout the CNS) on the granule cell layer of the adult rat dentate gyrus (DG) could be completely blocked by pretreatment with a specific $5-HT_{1A}$ antagonist (Jacobs, 2002).

The $5-HT_{1A}$ and $5-HT_{2A}$ receptors are the most studied receptors in relation to affective disorders. It has been shown, in both human and animal studies, that $5-HT_{1A}$ (Blier et al., 1993; Nishi et al., 2009), $5-HT_{1B}$ (Benjamin et al., 1990; Clark et al., 2002; Kaiyala et al., 2003; O'Connor et al., 1994; Saudou et al.,1994; Sari, 2004), $5-HT_{2A}$ (Bhagwagar et al., 2006), and a 5-HT transporter (5-HTT) (Bhagwagar et al., 2007) play important roles in affective disorders as well as the action of antidepressants. Evidence is accumulating that dysfunction in the brain serotonergic system relates to mood and behavior disorders (Soares and Mann, 1997). The $5-HT_{1A}$ receptor is not only a presynaptic autoreceptor (as described earlier) but also a postsynaptic receptor, which is similar to the $5-HT_{2A}$ receptor and highly distributed in limbic areas and hypothalamus. In rodents, 60% of the neurons in the prefrontal cortex are expressing $5-HT_{1A}$ and/or $5-HT_{2A}$ receptors (Amargós-Bosch et al., 2004). Both of these receptors are expressed in different cell types including pyramidal cells and GABAergic inter neurons in both frontal cortex and hippocampus. The 5-HT neurons in the dorsal raphe are regulated by somatodendritic presynaptic $5-HT_{1A}$ receptors and distal feedback via postsynaptic 5-HT receptors which regulate the glutamatergic neurons in the prefrontal cortex (Celada et al., 2001; Martín-Ruiz et al., 2001; Puig et al., 2003).

The potential role of $5-HT_{1A}$ receptors in the function and structure (e.g. DG neurogenesis) of hippocampus-related depressive disorders has been reported earlier (Gould, 1999; Radley and Jacobs, 2002), and the $5-HT_{1A}$ receptor is present at a particularly high concentration in the hippocampus, especially in the DG. The consistent neuroendocrine evidence in depression has already demonstrated a reduction in $5-HT_{1A}$ receptor function and number (Porter et al., 2004; Riedel et al., 2002; Drevets et al., 1999). The clinical reports have pointed out that the low level of $5-HT_{1A}$ receptors represents a risk factor in mood disorders (O'Neill and Conway, 2001; Cryan et al., 2005). Animal studies also suggest that the increase in the neurotransmission at postsynaptic $5-HT_{1A}$ receptors may mediate the therapeutic effects of some antidepressants (Welner et al., 1989). In addition, many studies suggest that increases in adult neurogenesis after the SSRI administration require the activation of $5-HT_{1A}$ receptors (Santarelli et al., 2003), which is consistent with the results that $5-HT_{1A}$ receptor antagonists or knockout mice decrease or lack cell proliferation in the dentate gyrus, respectively (Radley and Jacobs, 2002; Santarelli et al., 2003). Furthermore, it has been reported that the antidepressant effect of SSRIs are mediated by $5-HT_{1A}$ receptors (Tatarczynska et al., 2002; Hirano et al., 2002) by changing the receptor-medicated G-protein-coupled inwardly rectifying potassium (GIRK) currents (Cornelisse et al., 2007). Therefore, $5-HT_{1A}$ is definitely involved in depression as well as the action of antidepressants.

Recent studies have also pointed out an important role for $5-HT_2$ receptors in the pathology of depression as well as the action of many antidepressants (Cryan and Leonard, 2000; Cryan and Lucki, 2000; Boothman et al., 2006). Treatment of some established antidepressants results in a reduction of $5-HT_2$ receptor density in rat frontal cortex (Klimek et al., 1994; Subhash et al., 1997). Indeed, most antidepressants can primarily down-regulate 5-HT$_{2A}$ receptors, which indicates the therapeutical potential of this receptor (Toth and Shenk, 1994). In addition, some 5-HT$_{2A/2C}$ receptor antagonists are found to enhance the antidepressant-like effects of SSRIs when given jointly (Redrobe and Bourin, 1997; Redrobe and Bourin, 1998), which suggests that the antagonism of these receptors may be implicated in the action of such antidepressants. Moreover, it has been reported that mRNA levels of 5-HT$_{1A}$ and 5-HT$_2$ remained unchanged after the treatment of imipromine or citalopram, implying that the antidepressant outcome may involve the changes of the 5-HT receptor density as well as the functional effects of 5-HT receptors (Butler et al., 1993; Burnet et al., 1994; Spurlock et al., 1994).

2.3 Neurotrophic mechanisms in depression

Animal studies have already shown that acute or chronic stress can activate HPA axis and inhibit the cell proliferation in adult hippocampus (Warner-Schmidt and Duman, 2006; Paizanis et al., 2007). It has been shown that the psychosocial and physical stressors can inhibit the neurogenesis in various animal models and thus lead to decreased cell proliferation and survival (Joëls et al., 2007). In the chronic stressed model, both neurogenesis and proliferation were reduced in all rats (Joëls et al., 2007, Li et al., 2006). Moreover, treatment with diverse antidepressants, such as lithium, will reverse these changes (Knijff et al., 2007).

It is widely accepted that both stress and corticosteroid can decrease the levels of some neurotrophic factors in hippocampus while many classes of antidepressant as well as electroconvulsive shock treatment can reverse the decrease and prevent the action of stress, which is the base of the neurotrophic mechanism of depression (Duman and Monteggia, 2006). Neurotrophic factors, such as BDNF, NGF, neurotrophin-3 (NT-3), NT-4, NT-5 and NT-6, have been shown to enhance the cell proliferation and neurogenesis in the subgranular layer of the dentate gyrus (Banasr et al., 2004). These neurotrophic factors are critical to the viability and function of the neurons. Local infusion of BDNF into the midbrain or hippocampus regions has antidepressant-like effects in behavioral animal models of depression (Siuciak et al., 1994; Duman and Monteggia, 2006). For human studies, reduced levels of BDNF were detected in postmortem brain tissues of the depressed patients while antidepressant treatment can reverse it (Chen et al., 2001). All these data suggest that the action of antidepressants might be mediated via activating BDNF signaling in the hippocampus.

Increasing evidence has shown that the neuroprotective effects of the neurotrophic factors are mainly mediated by inhibiting the cell death/apoptosis pathways (Du et al., 2003) BDNF, as a major neurotrophic factor, can initiate various signaling pathways, such as MAPK/ERK and PI-3K/Akt pathways, through binding to its tyrosine kinase TrkB receptor and thus activate the downstream molecules which can promote neurogenesis and cell survival. The phosphor-ERK and PI-3K/Akt can further phosphorylate and activate cyclic adenosine monophosphate (cAMP) response element binding (CREB) (Banasr et al., 2004; Chen and Manji, 2006). For instance, BDNF and CREB levels are decreased in cerebral cortex of depressive patients, while the treatment of antidepressants can enhance the BDNF levels in patients (Karege et al., 2002). In the CREB knockout mice, BDNF up-regulation is abolished after the antidepressant treatment (Conti et al., 2002). Moreover, a variety of antidepressants, regardless of their mechanisms, up-regulate the BDNF expression in rodent hippocampus, while the non-antidepressant drugs are not effective (Duman and Monteggia,

2006). In addition, the phosphorylation of CREB will consequently activate the transcription of many survival-promoting genes, such as B-cell lymphoma 2 (bcl-2) and BDNF.

Bcl-2, a critical anti-apoptotic protein, has been shown to be upregulated by mood stabilizers in multiple animal studies (Chen et al., 1999; Manji et al., 2000; Chang et al., 2009). Reduced level of bcl-2 was also observed after stress: bcl-2 mRNA level was decreased by 70% when exposed to aggressive social stress after ischemia. Moreover, overexpression of bcl-2 will attenuate the infracts caused by high level of corticosterone (DeVries et al., 2001). Actually, the survival-promoting effect of CREB might be attributed to its induction of bcl-2 transcription (Finkbeiner, 2000). There is accumulating evidence that CREB is a common target for different classes of antidepressants. Various kinds of antidepressants significantly increase the Phospho-CREB level as well as CREB binding activity in rat hippocampus (Nibuya et al., 1996; Koch et al., 2003). Moreover, the activation of CREB will in turn promote the transcription and synthesis of more BDNF (Riccio et al., 1999).

As discussed above, the serotonergic system is intensely involved in the pathology and treatment of depression (Mattson et al., 2004). It is also widely accepted that 5-HT receptor activation is important for the pharmacotherapeutic effects of antidepressants (Ivy et al., 2003). Actually, there exist interactions between BDNF and serotonin systems (Martinowich and Lu, 2008). A critical pathway following 5-HT stimulation is cAMP/PKA signaling transduction which results in the phosphorylation of CREB (Nestler et al., 2002). Moreover, the CREB activation can induce BDNF transcription and then increase cell proliferation (Tao et al., 1997). Indeed, there is crosstalk between the two pathways: the activation of 5-HT receptors coupled to cAMP production and CREB activation can induce transcription of BDNF gene; on the other hand, increased BDNF synthesis will promote the growth and sprouting of 5-HT neuron axons which can increase the neuronal plasticity and survival (Mamourias et al., 1995). For example, BDNF can promote the neurogenesis of 5-HT neurons (Mamounas et al., 1995) and change the 5-HT receptor expression (Lyons et al., 1999). Moreover, the activation of 5-HT receptors will lead to the phosphorylation of the transcription factor cAMP responsive element binding protein (CREB), which will start the transcription of BDNF (Mattson et al., 2004). All these observations indicate the downregulation of neurotrophic factors might mediate, at least in part, the decreased neurogenesis and structural damage in the stressed brain. Under the "neurogenesis hypothesis", neurtotrophic factors might also serve as promising targets for the treatment of depression.

3. Phytochemicals as antidepressants

3.1 Phytochemicals and serotonergic system

Health benefits associated with Mediterranean diets are due to the large intake of functional plant foods and beverages, i.e., fruits, vegetables, cereals, legumes, nuts, wine, beer, and olive oil, containing a great array of bioactive phytochemicals or nutraceutical compounds. Therefore, the low risk of chronic diseases, such as coronary hearth disease and certain cancers, observed in some population groups, results from a diverse eating style, either in term of foods or food components. The paradigm of the relationship between the chemical diversity of a particular food and the array of its biological activities may be symbolized by grape. Despite the extensive knowledge about phenylpropanoids, principally polyphenols (stilbenes and anthocyanins) and condensed tannins (proanthocyanidins), in grape and wine, little it is known about the other compounds, such as tetrahydro-b-carbolines.

Recently, it has been attached importance to the dietary indoleamines, melatonin, and serotonin, in different plant foods, including grape, thus further supporting the hypothesis that health benefits, associated with Mediterranean dietary style, are due to plant food chemical diversity. Besides, because of plant sessile status, synthesis of phytochemicals represents a major strategy for counteracting unfavorable conditions, in terms of natural selection, biological evolution, and biodiversity.

Plant natural products can be roughly ascribed to three main classes of compounds, phenylpropanoids, isoprenoids, and alkaloids, widely distributed in plant foods and medicinal herbs (Facchini, 2001; Holstein and Hohl, 2004; Iriti and Faoro, 2004). Polyphenolic phytochemicals, which are active components found in many medicinal plants and regulate a variety of enzymes as well as cell receptors, are a group of plant secondary metabolites characterized by the presence of more than one phenolic unit which is linked directly to the aromatic rings (Bravo, 1998). These compounds are categorized by the number of phenol rings as well as the structural elements linked between the rings. The major classes include phenolic acids, flavonoids, stilbenes and lignans (Manach et al., 2004). A growing number of researchers have shown interests in polyphenolic phytochemicals. The major reasons include their antioxidative effects and potentials in preventing oxidative stress-induced diseases, such as neurodegenerative diseases and cancer (Scalbert et al., 2005).

Curcuma longa, one of the most extensively studied phytochemicals, is a major constituent of many traditional Chinese medicines, such as Xiaoyao-san, and has been used widely in Asian countries to manage mental disorders effectively. Curcumin is a major active component of C. longa and its antidepressant-like effect has been previously demonstrated in animal models of depression such as the forced swimming test (Xu et al., 2005) and chronic unpredictable mild stress modle (Li et a., 2009). Moreover, the antidepressant effect of curcumin can be potentiated by various kinds of antidepressants when given jointly, such as fluoxetine, venlafaxine, and bupropion. Enhanced serotonin level has also been found in mice after curcumin administration (Kulkarni et al., 2008). The concomitant administration of curcumin and piperine, a bioavailability enhancer, showed a significantly enhanced level of serotonin (Bhutani et al., 2009). Wang et al., also demonstrated that the antidepressant effect of curcumin in the forced swimming test may involve 5-HT receptors, especially 5-HT1A/1B and 5-HT$_{2C}$ subtypes (Wang et al., 2008). The recent study also showed that curcumin attenuated the stress-induced decrease in 5-HT$_{1A}$ mRNA level in rat hippocampus (Xu et al., 2007).

Resveratrol is a key antioxidant that present in grapes and red wine. The trans-resveratrol, as the active component of Polygonum cuspidatum which is traditionally used to treat neropsychiatric disorders in Asia countries, has been studied for anti-inflammation, amelioration of learning and memory impairment, and neuroprotection (Tredici et al., 1999; Chen et al., 2007; Kumar et al., 2007; Ranney and Petro, 2009). The recent studies have already shown the inhibitory effects of resveratrol on noradrenaline and 5-HT uptake activity in rats (Yáñez et al., 2006). Moreover, significantly decreased immobility time in mouse model of despair tests as well as the enhanced levels of serotonin and noradrenaline in brain regions have been demonstrated after trans-resveratrol application (Xu et al., 2010). The reduced activity of MAO, which catalyze the oxidative deamination of dietary amines and monoamine neurotransmitters, such as 5-HT, have been shown in both in vivo and in vitro experiments (Mazzio et al., 1998; Xu et al., 2010). All these data indicate the antidepressive effect of Resveratrol.

Proanthocyanidins, known as oligonols (catechin-type monomers, dimmers and trimmers) and oligomeric proanthocyanidins (oligomers), exists commonly in plants, such as grape seeds (DalBó et al., 2006). People have shown that proanthocyanidins have a wide range of pharmacological activities, including antioxidant effect, antinociceptive and cardioprotective properties (Preuss et al., 2000; Uchida et al., 2008; Sato et al., 2001). Recently, Xu et al. have shown that proanthocyanidin can reduce the duration of immobility in both tail suspension and forced swimming test. Moreover, significantly enhanced 5-HT concentrations were found in frontal cortex, hippocampus and hypothalamus of mice after the proanthocyanidin administration (Xu et al., 2010). However, the mechanisms underlying the antidepressant effect of proanthocyanidin is still not clear.

3.2 Phytochemicals and neurotrophic mechanisms
The emerging neurotrophic hypothesis of antidepressant actions suggests that the stress-induced BDNF reduction could, at least in part, induce the structural damage as well as the reduced neurogenesis, and most antidepressant treatment share the effect of increasing BDNF and neurogenesis, which might be via downstream mechanisms (Duman et al., 1997; Duman, 2004). Through cAMP-PKA and IP3-Ca^{2+} dependent protein kinase secondary messenger systems, CREB can be regulated by 5-HT receptors (Duman, 1998; Rajkumar and Mahesh, 2008). The activation of CREB will start the BDNF transcription, which leads to the activation of downstream cascades including Ras-Raf-ERK and PI-3K/AKT via the TrkB receptor (Berton and Nestler, 2006). Accordingly, the chronic treatment of antidepressants increases cell proliferation and neurogenesis, accompanied with enhanced phosphorylated CREB (Sasaki et al. 2007; Li et al., 2009).

A number of researches have suggested that phytochemicals are neuroprotective. In the transient middle cerebral artery occlusion animal model, Cyanidin-3-O-beta-D-glucopyranoside extracted from mulberry extract showed a neuroprotective effect against the brain injury (Kang et al., 2006). Low concentration of (–)-epigallocatechin-3-gallate from green tea can reduce the neuronal cell death in serum-starved cells, and promote the neurite outgrowth (Reznichenko et al, 2005). Low dose of curcumin has been shown to activate the ERK signaling and enhance the neurogenesis in adult hippocampus, which indicates its capability to enhance neural plasticity and repair (Kim et al., 2008b). The oral administration of 10 and 20 mg/kg curcumin to mice can prevent the stress-induced decrease of BDNF level in hippampus and enhance the hippocampal neurogenesis, which suggests that curcumin might protect hippocampal neurons from further damage in response to chronic stress via up-regulating BDNF in hippocampus (Xu et al., 2007). Curcumin application also prevents the cultured rodent cortex cells against glutamate excitotoxicity (Wang et al., 2008). Recently, it has been demonstrated in the chronic unpredictable mild stress (CUMS) rats, curcumin was also able to improve the CREB activity (Li et al., 2009). More importantly, studies have also shown that curcumin exerts the neuroprotective effects via BDNF/TrkB-mediated PI-3K/Akt and MAPK/Erk cascades, and thus stimulating the transcription factor CREB (Wang et al., 2008; Wang et al., 2010).

It has been reported that resveratrol and its methylated derivertives exhibit neuroprotective effects in SH-SY5Y cells against parkinsonian mimetic 6-hydroxydopamine (6-OHDA)-induced neurotoxicity (Chao et al., 2010). Pretreatment of resveratrol has been shown to provide neuroprotection in animal models of cerebral ischemia (Della-Morte et al., 2009), which might be mediated through NMDA and estrogen receptor (Saleh et al., 2010). Moreover, Piceatannol (3,4,3',5'-tetrahydroxy-*trans*-stilbene) isolated from the seeds of

Euphorbia lagascae, is a metabolite of resveratrol existing in grapes and red wine (Ferrigni et al., 1984; Larrosa et al., 2004). Previous studies have shown that piceatannol exhibited protective effect against Aβ-induced neuronal cell death in cultured PC-12 cells (Kim et al., 2008). The following studies further demonstrated that the neuroprotective effect against oxidative stress is likely due to the inhibition on JNK (Kim et al., 2008) or c-Jun N-terminal kinase activity (Jang et al., 2009). Although the mechanisms of the neuroprotective effects of resveratrol and piceatannol are still unclear, their diverse pharmacological properties have already attracted wide attention.

Fisetin (3,3′,4′7′-tetrahydroxylflavone) is a flavonoid which exists in many plants and foods, such as strawberries (Arai et al., 2000). Recently, people have demonstrated that fisetin can protect neuronal cells from oxidative stress induced cell death, and demonstrate neurotrophic effect of improving the differentiation of PC-12 cells (Ishige et al., 2001), which might depend on the activation of ERK signaling pathway (Sagara et al., 2004). Moreover, the recent studies found that fisetin can facilitate long-term memory in rats, which is mediated via ERK signaling and the CREB phosphorylation (Maher et al., 2006). All these data indicate that fisetin has neurotrophic effect and can promote cell proliferation, and therefore it may be useful in treating mental disorders, including depression.

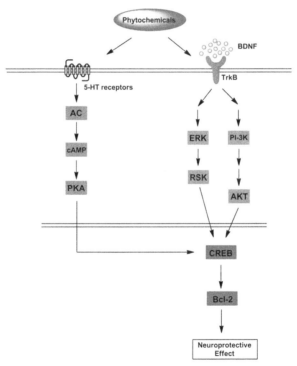

Fig. 1. Neuroprotective pathways targeted by phytochemicals. The activated BDNF receptor TrkB will initiate ERK and PI-3K signaling pathways. 5-HT receptors, which are usually coupled to G proteins, will activate the AC/PKA cascade. Phytochemicals can stimulate both 5-HT and BDNF signaling cascades which interweave and result in activation of CREB, and thus exert their neuroprotective effects.

Ferulic acid (4-hydroxy-3-methoxycinnamic acid; FA) is an ample phenolic phytochemical found in plant components (Srinivasan et al., 2007). Ferulic acid has been reported to have a number of pharmacological activities including antioxidative, anti-inflammatory, anti-cancer, anti-diabetic, anti-atherogenic and neuroprotective effects (Mukhopadhyay et al., 1982; Kawabata et al., 2000; Balasubashini et al., 2004; Kim and Kim, 2000; Yogeeta et al., 2006). Ferulic acid can prevent neurons from $A\beta$-induced cell death, which is associated with its antioxidative activity (Sultana et al., 2005; Picone et al., 2007). The recent studies found that oral administration of ferulic acid can attenuate the stress-induced behavior in the depression-like model mice. Moreover, treatment of ferulic acid can increase the CREB phophorylation. Accordingly, BDNF mRNA level in the hippocampus is also enhanced (Yabe et al., 2010). Although the molecular mechanisms of the antidepressant effect of ferulic acid still needs to be clarified, the current result indicated its therapeutic potential in the treatment of depressive disorder.

4. Future directions

It is widely accepted that phytochemicals are neuroprotective. The actions of the antidepressive effects of phytochemicals appear to involve many mechanisms, including monoamine neurotransmitters-based mechanism, HPA axis-based mechamism, and neurotrophic factors, or neurogenesis, based mechanisms. All these effects seem to be associated with the activation of the signaling cascades in brain, which can trigger a number of responses, such as promoting the neuronal survival and differentiation and inhibiting neuronal apoptosis. Despite the great advances in our understanding of depression, little is known about the antidepressant mechanisms of many phytochemicals because their antidepressant effects always involve multiple complex mechanisms. Therefore, it is very important to identify the bio-molecules and signaling network that can be specifically regulated by individual phytochemical.

There are many advantages of phytochemicals in regard to application to development of antidepressants. For instance, phytochemicals are natural products, or even isolated from some herbal medicines, so they can be readily moved to the clinical trials on humans. Moreover, chemical analogues of the druggable phytochemcals can be developed for better bioavailability and lower toxicity. However, although the consensus is developing that phytochemcals are potential antidepressant candidates, our understanding and knowledge of the active phytochemicals as well as their mechanisms of actions are limited. It is therefore of critical need to develop high-throughput assays to identify antidepressive phytochemicals. Further *in vivo* and *in vitro* studies are required to reveal in more details about the antidepressive mechanisms of phytochemcals.

5. References

Akiskal HS. Mood disorders: introduction and overview. In: Comprehensive Textbook of Psychiatry. B.J. Sadock and V.A. Sadock, (eds). Lippincott, Williams & Wilkins, 2000. 1284-1298.

Amargós-Bosch M, Bortolozzi A, Puig MV, Serrats J, Adell A, Celada P, Toth M, Mengod G, Artigas F. Co-expression and in vivo interaction of serotonin1A and serotonin2A receptors in pyramidal neurons of prefrontal cortex, Cereb. Cortex 2004; 14, 281–299.

Arai Y, Watanabe S, Kimira M, Shimoi K, Mochizuki R, Kinae N. Dietary intakes of flavonols, flavones and isoflavones by Japanese women and the inverse correlation between quercetin intake and plasma LDL cholesterol concentration. J Nutr. 2000;130(9):2243-2250.

Azmitia BC, Whitaker-Azmitia PM. Development and adult plasticity of serotoninergic nevirons and their target cells. In: Baumgarten HG, Gothert M, editors. Handbook of experimental pharmacology. Berlin: Springer; 1997; 1-39.

Baker CB., Johnsrud MT., Crismon ML, Rosenheck RA, Woods SW. Quantitative analysis of sponsorship bias in economic studies of antidepressants. Br. J. Psychiatry. 2003; 183, 498-506.

Balasubashini MS, Rukkumani R, Viswanathan P, Menon VP. Ferulic acid alleviates lipid peroxidation in diabetic rats. Phytother Res. 2004;18(4):310-314.

Bambico FR, Nguyen NT, Gobbi G. Decline in serotonergic firing activity and desensitization of 5-HT1A autoreceptors after chronic unpredictable stress. Eur Neuropsychopharmacol. 2009;19(3):215-228.

Banasr M, Hery M, Printemps R, Daszuta A. Serotonin-induced increases in adult cell proliferation and neurogenesis are mediated through different and common 5-HT receptor subtypes in the dentate gryus and the subventricular zone. Neuropsychopharmacology. 2004;29(3):450-460.

Barden N. Regulation of corticosteroid receptor gene expression in depression and antidepressant action. J. Psychiatry Neurosci. 1999; 24, 25-39.

Barnes NM, Sharp T. A review of central 5-HT receptors and their function, Neuropharmacology 1999; 38: 1083–1152.

Benjamin D, Lal H, Meyerson LR. The effects of 5-HT1B characterizing agents in the mouse elevated plus-maze. Life Sci. 1990; 47 (3), 195–203.

Berton O, Nestler EJ. New approaches to antidepressant drug discovery: beyond monoamines. Nat. Rev. Neurosci. 2006;7(2):137-151.

Bhagwagar Z, Hinz R, Taylor M, Fancy S, Cowen P, Grasby P.Increased 5-HT(2A) receptor binding in euthymic, medication-free patients recovered from depression: a positron emission study with [(11)C]MDL 100, 907. Am J Psychiatry. 2006;163(9):1580-1587.

Bhagwagar Z, Murthy N, Selvaraj S, Hinz R, Taylor M, Fancy S, Grasby P, Cowen P. 5-HTT binding in recovered depressed patients and healthy volunteers: a positron emission tomography study with [11C] DASB. Am J Psychiatry. 2007;164(12):1858-1865.

Bhutani MK, Bishnoi M, Kulkarni SK. Anti-depressant like effect of curcumin and its combination with piperine in unpredictable chronic stress-induced behavioral, biochemical and neurochemical changes. Pharmacol Biochem Behav. 2009;92(1):39-43.

Blier, P., Lista, A., De Montigny, C., Differential properties of pre- and postsynaptic 5-hydroxytryptamine1A receptors in the dorsal raphe and hippocampus: II. Effect of pertussis and cholera toxins. J. Pharmacol. Exp. Ther. 1993; 265, 16–23.

Boothman LJ, Mitchell SN, Sharp T. Investigation of the SSRI augmentation properties of 5-HT2 receptor antagonists using in vivo microdialysis. Neuropharmacology 2006; 50, 726–732.

Bravo L. Polyphenols: chemistry, dietary sources, metabolism, and nutritional significance. Nutr Rev. 1998;56(11):317-33.

Butler MO, Morinobu S, Duman RS. Chronic electroconvulsive seizures increase the expression of serotonin2 receptor mRNA in rat frontal cortex. J Neurochem 1993; 61:1270-1276.

Burnet PW, Michelson D, Smith MA, Gold PW, Sternberg EM. The effect of chronic imipramine administration on the densities of 5-HT$_{1A}$ and 5-HT$_2$ receptors and the abundances of 5-HT receptor and transporter mRNA in the cortex, hippocampus and dorsal raphe of three strains of rat. Brain Res 1994; 638: 311-324.

Caspi A, Moffitt TE. Gene-environment interactions in psychiatry: joining forces with neuroscience. Nat. Rev. Neurosci. 2006; 7, 583-590.

Celada P, Puig MV, Casanovas JM, Guillazo G, Artigas F. Control of dorsal raphe serotonergic neurons by the medial prefrontal cortex: Involvement of serotonin-1A, GABA(A), and glutamate receptors. J Neurosci. 2001;21(24):9917-9929.

Centeno VA, Volosin M. Chronic treatment with desipramine: effect on endocrine and behavioral responses induced by inescapable stress. Physiol. Behav. 1997; 62, 939-944.

Chang YC, Rapoport SI, Rao JS. Chronic administration of mood stabilizers upregulates BDNF and bcl-2 expression levels in rat frontal cortex. Neurochem Res. 2009;34(3):536-541

Chao J, Li H, Cheng KW, Yu MS, Chang RC, Wang M. Protective effects of pinostilbene, a resveratrol methylated derivative, against 6-hydroxydopamine-induced neurotoxicity in SH-SY5Y cells. J Nutr Biochem.2010;21(6):482-489.

Chen B, Dowlatshahi D, MacQueen GM, Wang JF, Young LT. Increased hippocampal BDNF immunoreactivity in subjects treated with antidepressant medication. Biol Psychiatry. 2001;50(4):260-265.

Chen G, Huang LD, Jiang YM, Manji HK. The mood-stabilizing agent valproate inhibits the activity of glycogen synthase kinase-3. J Neurochem. 1999;72(3):1327-1330.

Chen G, Manji HK. The extracellular signal-regulated kinase pathway: an emerging promising target for mood stabilizers. Curr Opin Psychiatry. 2006;19(3):313-323.

Chen LW, Wang YQ, Wei LC, Shi M, Chan YS. Chinese herbs and herbal extracts for neuroprotection of dopaminergic neurons and potential therapeutic treatment of Parkinson's disease. CNS Neurol Disord Drug Targets. 2007;6(4):273-281.

Chen MJ, Nguyen TV, Pike CJ, Russo-Neustadt AA. Norepinephrine induces BDNF and activates the PI-3K and MAPK cascades in embryonic hippocampal neurons. Cell Signal. 2007;19(1):114-128.

Clark MS, Sexton TJ, McClain M, Root D, Kohen R, Neumaier JF. Overexpression of 5-HT1B receptor in dorsal raphe nucleus using Herpes Simplex Virus gene transfer increases anxiety. J Neurosci. 2002; 22(11):4550-4562.

Cornelisse LN, Van der Harst JE, Lodder JC, Baarendse PJ, Timmerman AJ, Mansvelder HD, Spruijt BM, Brussaard AB. Reduced 5-HT1A and GABAB receptor function in dorsal raphe neurons upon chronic fluoxetine treatment of socially stressed rats. J. Neurophysiol., 2007; 98, 196-204.

Conti AC, Cryan JF, Dalvi A, Lucki I, Blendy JA. cAMP response element-binding protein is essential for the upregulation of brain-derived neurotrophic factor transcription, but not the behavioral or endocrine responses to antidepressant drugs. J Neurosci. 2002;22(8):3262-3268.

Cryan JF, Leonard BE. 5-HT1A and beyond: the role of serotonin and its receptors in depression and the antidepressant response. Hum. Psychopharmacol. 2000; 15, 113-135.

Cryan JF, Lucki I. Antidepressant-like behavior effects mediated by 5-hydroxytryptamine (2C) receptors. J. Pharmacol. Exp. Ther. 2000; 295, 1120-1126.

Cryan JF, Valentino RJ, Lucki I. Assessing substrates underlying the behavioral effects of antidepressants using the modified rat forced swimming test. Neurosci. Biobehav. Rev. 2005; 29, 547-569.

Dahlström A, Fuxe K, Localization of monoamines in the lower brain stem, Experientia. 1964; 20: 398-399.

DalBó S, Jürgensen S, Horst H, Soethe DN, Santos AR, Pizzolatti MG, Ribeiro-do-Valle RM. Analysis of the antinociceptive effect of the proanthocyanidin-rich fraction obtained from Croton celtidifolius barks: evidence for a role of the dopaminergic system. Pharmacol Biochem Behav 2006;85:317-323.

Davis KL, Charney D, Coyle JT, Nemeroff CB. (Eds.), Neuropsychopharmacology: The Fifth Generation of Progress, 5th ed., Lippinkott Williams & Wilkins, Nashville, 2002.

Della-Morte D, Dave KR, DeFazio RA, Bao YC, Raval AP, Perez-Pinzon MA. Resveratrol pretreatment protects rat brain from cerebral ischemic damage via a sirtuin 1-uncoupling protein 2 pathway. Neuroscience. 2009;159(3):993-1002.

DeVries AC, Joh HD, Bernard O, Hattori K, Hurn PD, Traystman RJ, Alkayed NJ. Social stress exacerbates stroke outcome by suppressing Bcl-2 expression. Proc Natl Acad Sci. 2001; 98(20):11824-11828.

Drevets WC, Frank E, Price JC, Kupfer DJ, Holt D, Greer PJ, Huang Y, Gautier C, Mathis C. PET imaging of serotonin 1A receptor binding in depression. Biol. Psychiatry 1999; 54, 597-606.

Drevets WC. Neuroimaging studies of mood disorders. Biol. Psychiatry 2000; 48, 813-829.

Du J, Gould TD, Manji HK: Neurotrophic signaling in mood disorders; in Finkel T, Gutkind JS (eds): Signal Transduction and Human Disease. Hoboken, Wiley, 2003: 411-446.

Duman RS, Heninger GR & Nestler EJ. A molecular and cellular hypothesis of depression. Arch. Gen. Psychiatry 1997; 54, 597-606.

Duman RS. Novel therapeutic approaches beyond the serotonin receptor. Biol. Psychiary 1998; 44, 324-335.

Duman RS. Structural alterations in depression: cellular mechanism underlying pathology and treatment of mood disorders. CNS Spectr. 2002, 7, 140-142, 144-147.

Duman RS. Role of neurotrophic factors in the etiology and treatment of mood disorders. Neuromolecular Med. 2004; 5, 11-25.

Duman RS, Monteggia LM. A neurotrophic model for stress-related mood disorders. Biol. Psychiatry 2006, 59, 1116-1127.

Facchini PJ. Alkaloid biosynthesis in plants: biochemistry, cell biology, molecular regulation and metabolic engineering. Annu Rev Plant Physiol Plant Mol Biol. 2001; 52:29-66.

Ferretti C, Marinella B, Gamalero SR, Ghi, P. Biochemical and behaviour changes induced by acute stress in a chronic variate stress model of depression: the effect of amitripltyline. Eur. J. Pharmacol. 1995; 280, 19-26.

Ferrigni NR, McLaughlin JL, Powell RG, Smith CR. Use of potato disc and brine shrimp bioassays to detect activity and isolate piceatannol as the antileukemic principle from the seeds of Euphorbia lagascae. J Nat Prod 1984;47:347–352.

Finkbeiner S. CREB couples neurotrophin signals to survival messages. Neuron. 2000; 25(1):11-14.

Gillespie CR, Nemeroff CB. Hypercortisolemia and depression. Psychosom. Med. 2005; 67, S26-S28.

Gould E. Serotonin and hippocampal neurogenesis. Neuropsychopharmacology 1999; 21:46S–51S.

Harfstrand A, Fuxe K, Cintra A, Agnati LF, Zini I, Wikstrom AC, Okret S, Yu ZY, Goldstein M, Steinbusch H, Verhofstad A, Gustafsson JA. Glucocorticoid receptor immunoreactivity in monoaminergic neurons of rat brain. Proc. Natl. Acad. Sci. 1986; 83, 9779-9783.

Hirano K, Yamada S, Kimura R. Effects of fluvoxamine and fluoxetine on 5-HT$_{1A}$ and 5-HT$_{2A}$ receptors in mouse brain. Pharmacol. Rev. Commun. 2002; 12, 215-221.

Holstein SA, Hohl RJ. Isoprenoids: remarkable diversity of form and function. Lipids 2004; 34:293–309.

Inoue T, Tsuchiya K, Koyama T. Regional changes in dopamine and 5-hydroxytryptamine activation with various intensity of physical and psychological stress in rat brain. Pharmacol. Biochem. Behav. 1994, 49, 911-920.

Iriti M, Faoro F. Plant defense and human nutrition: the phenylpropanoids on the menu. Curr. Top. Nutr. Res. 2004; 2:47–65.

Ishige K, Schubert D, Sagara Y. Flavonoids protect neuronal cells from oxidative stress by three distinct mechanisms. Free Radic Biol Med. 2001;30(4):433-446.

Ivy AS, Rodriguez FG, Garcia C, Chen MJ, Russo-Neustadt AA. Noradrenergic and serotonergic blockade inhibits BDNF mRNA activation following exercise and antidepressant. Pharmacol. Biochem. Behav. 2003; 75: 81-88.

Jacobs BL. Adult brain neurogenesis and depression. Brain Behav. Immun. 2002;16:602–609.

Jang YJ, Kim JE, Kang NJ, Lee KW, Lee HJ. Piceatannol attenuates 4-hydroxynonenal-induced apoptosis of PC12 cells by blocking activation of c-Jun N-terminal kinase. Ann N Y Acad Sci. 2009;1171:176-182.

Joëls M, Karst H, Krugers HJ, Lucassen PJ. Chronic stress: implications for neuronal morphology, function and neurogenesis. Front Neuroendocrinol. 2007;28(2-3):72-96.

Kaiyala KJ, Vincow ES, Sexton TJ, Neumaier JF. 5-HT$_{1B}$ receptor mRNA levels in dorsal raphe nucleus: inverse association with anxiety behavior in the elevated plus maze. Pharmacol. Biochem. Behav. 2003, 75 (4), 769–776.

Kang TH, Hur JY, Kim HB, Ryu JH, Kim SY. Neuroprotective effects of the cyanidin-3-O-beta-Dglucopyranoside isolated from mulberry fruit against cerebral ischemia. Neurosci Lett. 2006;391(3):122-126.

Karege F, Perret G, Bondolfi G, Schwald M, Bertschy G, Aubry JM. Decreased serum brain-derived neurotrophic factor levels in major depressed patients. Psychiatry Res. 2002; 109(2):143-148.

Kawabata K, Yamamoto T, Hara A, Shimizu M, Yamada Y, Matsunaga K, Tanaka T, Mori H. Modifying effects of ferulic acid on azoxymethane-induced colon carcinogenesis in F344 rats. Cancer Lett. 2000;157(1):15-21.

Kim HJ, Lee KW, Lee HJ. Protective effects of piceatannol against beta-amyloid-induced neuronal cell death. Ann N Y Acad Sci. 2007;1095:473-82.

Kim HJ, Lee KW, Kim MS, Lee HJ. Piceatannol attenuates hydrogen-peroxide- and peroxynitrite-induced apoptosis of PC12 cells by blocking down-regulation of Bcl-XL and activation of JNK. J Nutr Biochem. 2008a;19(7):459-466.

Kim SJ, Son TG, Park HR, Park M, Kim MS, Kim HS, Chung HY, Mattson MP, Lee J. Curcumin stimulates proliferation of embryonic neural progenitor cells and neurogenesis in the adult hippocampus. J. Biol. Chem. 2008b;283(21):14497-14505.

Kim SR, Kim YC. Neuroprotective phenylpropanoid esters of rhamnose isolated from roots of Scrophularia buergeriana. Phytochemistry. 2000;54(5):503-509.

Klimek V, Zak-Knapik J, Mackowiak M. Effects of repeated treatment with fluoxetine and citalopram, 5-HT uptake inhibitors, on 5-HT1A and 5-HT2 receptors in the rat brain. J. Psychiatry Neurosci. 1994; 19, 63-67.

Knijff EM, Breunis MN, Kupka RW, de Wit HJ, Ruwhof C, Akkerhuis GW, Nolen WA, Drexhage HA. An imbalance in the production of IL-1beta and IL-6 by monocytes of bipolar patients: restoration by lithium treatment. Bipolar Disord. 2007;9(7):743-753.

Koch JM, Kell S, Aldenhoff JB. Differential effects of fluoxetine and imipramine on the phosphorylation of the transcription factor CREB and cell-viability. J. Psychiatr. Res. 2003; 37: 53-59.

Kushwaha N, Albert PR. Coupling of 5-HT1A autoreceptors to inhibition of mitogen-activated protein kinase activation via G beta gamma subunit signaling. Eur. J. Neurosci. 2005; 21, 721-732.

Kulkarni SK, Bhutani MK, Bishnoi M. Antidepressant activity of curcumin: involvement of serotonin and dopamine system. Psychopharmacology (Berl) 2008;201:435-442

Kumar A, Naidu PS, Seghal N, Padi SS. Neuroprotective effects of resveratrol against intracerebroventricular colchicine-induced cognitive impairment and oxidative stress in rats. Pharmacology. 2007;79(1):17-26.

Ishige K, Schubert D, Sagara Y. Flavonoids protect neuronal cells from oxidative stress by three distinct mechanisms. Free Radic Biol Med. 2001;30(4):433-446.

Lanfumey L, Mongeau R, Cohen-Salmon C, Hamon M. Corticosteroid-serotonin interactions in the neurobiological mechanisms of stress-related disorders. Neurosci Biobehav Rev. 2008;32(6):1174-1184.

Larrosa M, Tomas-Barberan FA, Espin JC. The grape and wine polyphenol piceatannol is a potent inducer of apoptosis in human SKMel-28 melanoma cells. Eur J Nutr 2004;43:275-84.

Lauder JM, Wallace JA, Krebs H. Roles for serotonin in neuroembryogenesis. Adv. Exp. Med. Biol. 1981;133:477-506.

Leonard BE, 2005. The HPA and immune axes in stress: the involvement of the serotonergic system. Eur. Psychiatry. 20, S302-306.

Lesch KP, Mayer S, Disselkamp-Tietze J., Hon A., Wiesmann M., Osterheider M., Schulte H.M., 1990. 5-HT1A receptor responsivity in unipolar depression. Evaluation of ipsapirone-induced ACTH and cortisol secretion in patients and controls. Biol. Psychiatry. 1990; 28, 620-628.

Li YC, Wang FM, Pan Y, Qiang LQ, Cheng G, Zhang WY, Kong LD. Antidepressant-like effects of curcumin on serotonergic receptor-coupled AC-cAMP pathway in chronic unpredictable mild stress of rats. Prog Neuropsychopharmacol Biol Psychiatry. 2009;33(3):435-449.

Li YF, Chen HX, Liu Y, Zhang YZ, Liu YQ, Li J. Agmatine increases proliferation of cultured hippocampal progenitor cells and hippocampal neurogenesis in chronically stressed mice. Acta Pharmacol Sin. 2006;27(11):1395-1400

Li YF, Huang Y, Amsdell SL, Xiao L, O'Donnell JM, Zhang HT. Antidepressant- and anxiolytic-like effects of the phosphodiesterase-4 inhibitor rolipram on behavior depend on cyclic AMP response element binding protein-mediated neurogenesis in the hippocampus. Neuropsychopharmacology. 2009;34(11):2404-19.

Lyons WE, Mamounas LA, Ricaurte GA, Coppola V, Reid SW, Bora SH, Wihler C, Koliatsos VE, Tessarollo L. Brain-derived neurotrophic factor-deficient mice develop aggressiveness and hyperphagia in conjunction with brain serotonergic abnormalities. Proc. Natl. Acad. Sci. 1999; 96, 15239-15244.

Maher P, Akaishi T, Abe K. Flavonoid fisetin promotes ERK-dependent longterm potentiation and enhances memory. Proc Natl Acad Sci. 2006;103(44):16568-73.

Mamounas LA, Altar CA, Blue ME, Kaplan DR, Tessarollo L, Lyons WE. BDNF promotes the survival and sprouting of serotonergic axons in the rat brain. J. Neurosci., 1995; 15, 7929-7939.

Manji HK, Lenox RH. The nature of bipolar disorder. J Clin Psychiatry. 2000;61 Supp 13:42-57.

Manach C, Scalbert A, Morand C, Rémésy C, Jiménez L. Polyphenols: food sources and bioavailability. Am J Clin Nutr.2004; 79(5):727-47.

Martín-Ruiz R, Puig MV, Celada P, Shapiro DA, Roth BL, Mengod G, Artigas F. Control of serotonergic function in medial prefrontal cortex by serotonin-2A receptors through a glutamate-dependent mechanism. J Neurosci. 2001; 21(24):9856-9866.

Martinowich K, Lu B. Interaction between BDNF and serotonin: role in mood disorders. Neuropsychopharmacology 2008; 33: 73-83.

Mattson MP, Maudsley S, Martin B. BDNF and 5-HT: a dynamic duo in age-related neuronal plasticity and neurodegenerative disorders. Trends Neurosci. 2004; 27(10):589-594.

Mazzio EA, Harris N, Soliman KF. Food constituents attenuate monoamine oxidase activity and peroxide levels in C6 astrocyte cells. Planta Med. 1998;64(7):603-606.

McEwen BS, Stellar E. Stress and the individual. Mechanisms leading to disease. Arch. Intern. Med. 1993; 153, 2093-2101.

McEwen BS. The neurobiology of stress: from serendipity to clinical relevance. Brain Res. 2000; 886, 172–189.

Meijer WE, Heerdink ER, Nolen WA, Herings RM, Leufkens HG, Egberts AC. Association of risk of abnormal bleeding with degree of serotonin reuptake inhibition by antidepressants. Arch. Intern. Med. 2004; 164, 2367-2370.

Millan MJ, Marin P, Bockaert J, Mannoury la Cour C. Signaling at G-protein-coupled serotonin receptors: recent advances and future research directions. Trends Pharmacol Sci. 2008;29(9):454-464.

Mukhopadhyay A, Basu N, Ghatak N, Gujral PK. Anti-inflammatory and irritant activities of curcumin analogues in rats. Agents Actions. 1982;12(4):508-515.

Nestler EJ, Barrot M, DiLeone RJ, Eisch AJ, Gold SJ, Monteggia LM. Neurobiology of depression. Neuron 2002; 34, 13-15.

Nishi K, Kanemaru K, Diksic M. A genetic rat model of depression, Flinders sensitive line has a lower density of 5-HT$_{1A}$ receptors, but a higher density of 5-HT1B receptors, compared to control rats. Neurochem. Int. 2009; 54 (5–6), 299–307.

Nibuya M, Nestler EJ, Duman RS. Chronic antidepressant administration increases the expression of cAMP response element binding protein (CREB) in rat hippocampus. J Neurosci. 1996;16(7):2365-72.

Nibuya M, Morinobu S, Duman RS. Regulation of BDNF and trkB mRNA in rat brain by chronic electroconvulsive seizure and antidepressant drug treatments. J Neurosci 1995; 15: 7539 –7547.

O'Connor JJ, Rowan MJ, Anwyl R. Long-lasting enhancement of NMDA receptor-mediated synaptic transmission by metabotropic glutamate receptor activation. Nature 1994; 367 (6463): 557–559.

O'Neill MF, Conway MW. Role of 5-HT1A and 5-HT1B receptors in the mediation of behavior in the forced swim test in mice. Neuropsy- chopharmacology 2001; 24, 391–398.

Paizanis E, Kelaï S, Renoir T, Hamon M, Lanfumey L. Life-long hippocampal neurogenesis: environmental, pharmacological and neurochemical modulations. Neurochem. Res. 2007; 32, 1762–1771.

Picone P, Bondi ML, Montana G, Bruno A, Pitarresi G, Giammona G, Di Carlo M. Ferulic acid inhibits oxidative stress and cell death induced by Ab oligomers: improved delivery by solid lipid nanoparticles. Free Radic Res. 2009; 43(11):1133-1145.

Preuss HG, Wallerstedt D, Talpur N, Tutuncuoglu SO, Echard B, Myers A, et al. Effects of niacin-bound chromium and grape seed proanthocyanidin extract on the lipid profile of hypercholesterolemic subjects: a pilot study. J Med 2000; 31:227–246.

Porter RJ, Gallagher P, Watson S, Young AH. 2004. Corticosteroid-serotonin interactions in depression: a review of the human evidence. Psychopharmacology (Berl). 2004;173(1-2):1-17

Puig MV, Celada P, Díaz-Mataix L, Artigas F. In vivo modulation of the activity of pyramidal neurons in the rat medial prefrontal cortex by 5-HT2A receptors: relationship to thalamocortical afferents. Cereb Cortex. 2003;13(8):870-882.

Radley JJ, Jacobs BL. 5-HT1A receptor antagonist administration decreases cell proliferation in the dentate gyrus. Brain Res 2002;955:264–267.

Rajkumar R, Mahesh R. Assessing the neuronal serotonergic target-based antidepressant stratagem: impact of in vivo interaction studies and knockout models. Curr Neuropharmacol. 2008;6(3):215-234.

Ranney A, Petro MS. Petro, Resveratrol protects spatial learning in middle-aged C57BL/6 mice from effects of ethanol. Behav Pharmacol. 2009;20(4):330-336.

Rapport MM, Green AA, Page IH., Crystalline Serotonin. Science. 1948; 108(2804):329-330.

Reznichenko, L., Amit, T., Youdim, M. B. and Mandel, S. Green tea polyphenol (–)-epigallocatechin-3-gallate induces neurorescue of long-term serum-deprived PC12 cells and promotes neurite outgrowth. J. Neurochem. 2005; 93, 1157–1167.

Redrobe JP, Bourin M. Partial role of 5-HT2 and 5-HT3 receptors in the activity of antidepressants in the mouse forced swimming test. Eur. J. Pharmacol. 1997; 325, 129–135.

Redrobe JP, Bourin M. Clonidine potentiates the effects of 5-HT1A, 5-HT1B and 5-HT2A/2C receptor antagonists and 8-OH-DPAT in the mouse forced swimming test. Eur. Neuropsychopharm. 1998; 8, 169–173.

Reul JM, de Kloet ER. Anatomical resolution of two types of corticosterone receptor sites in rat brain with in vitro autoradiography and computerized image analysis. J. Steroid Biochem. 1986; 24, 269-272.

Riedel W, Klaassen T, Griez E, Honig A, Menheere P, Van Praag HM, 2002. Dissociable hormonal, cognitive and mood responses to neuroendocrine challenge: evidence for receptor-specific serotonergic dysregulation in depressed mood. Neuropsychopharmacology. 26, 358-367.

Reinés A, Cereseto M, Ferrero A, Sifonios L, Podestá MF, Wikinski S. Maintenance treatment with fluoxetine is necessary to sustain normal levels of synaptic markers in an experimental model of depression: correlation with behavioral response. Neuropsychopharmacology 2008; 33, 1896-1908.

Riccio A, Ahn S, Davenport CM, Blendy JA, Ginty DD (1999). Mediation by a CREB family transcription factor of NGF-dependent survival of sympathetic neurons. Science 286: 2358–2361.

Sagara Y, Vanhnasy J, Maher P. Maher, Induction of PC12 cell differentiation by flavonoids is dependent upon extracellular signal-regulated kinase activation. J Neurochem. 2004;90(5):1144-1155.

Saleh MC, Connell BJ, Saleh TM. Resveratrol preconditioning induces cellular stress proteins and is mediated via NMDA and estrogen receptors. Neuroscience. 2010; 166(2):445-454.

Santarelli L, Saxe M, Gross C, Surget A, Battaglia C, Dulawa S, et al. Requirement of hippocampal neurogenesis for the behavioral effects of antidepressants. Eur J Pharmacol 2003; 301:805–809.

Sari Y. Serotonin1B receptors: from protein to physiological function and behavior. Neurosci. Biobehav. Rev. 2004; 28 (6), 565–582.

Sapolsky RM. Taming stress. Sci. Am. 2003; 289: 86-95.

Sasaki T, Kitagawa K, Omura-Matsuoka E, Todo K, Terasaki Y, Sugiura S, Hatazawa J, Yagita Y, Hori M. The phosphodiesterase inhibitor rolipram promotes survival of newborn hippocampal neurons after ischemia. Stroke 2007; 38:1597–1605.

Sato M, Bagchi D, Tosaki A, Das DK. Grape seed proanthocyanidin reduces cardiomyocyte apoptosis by inhibiting ischemia/reperfusion-induced activation of JNK-1 and C-JUN. Free Radic Biol Med 2001;31:729–737.

Saudou F, Amara DA, Dierich A, LeMeur M, Ramboz S, Segu L, Buhot MC, Hen R. Enhanced aggressive behavior in mice lacking 5-HT1B receptor. Science 1994; 265 (5180), 1875–1878.

Scalbert A, Manach C, Morand C, Rémésy C, Jiménez L. Dietary polyphenols and the prevention of diseases. Crit Rev Food Sci Nutr. 2005;45(4):287-306.

Schechter LE, Ring RH, Beyer CE, Hughes ZA, Khawaja X, Malberg JE, Rosenzweig-Lipson S. Innovative approaches for the development of antidepressant drugs: current and future strategies. J. Am. Soc. Exp. Neurother. 2005; 2, 590-611.

Siuciak JA, Altar CA, Wiegand SJ, Lindsay RM. Antinociceptive effect of brain-derived neurotrophic factor and neurotrophin-3. Brain Res. 1994;633(1-2):326-30.

Spurlock G, Buckland P, O'Donovan M, McGuffin P. Lack of the effect of antidepressant drugs on the levels of mRNAs encoding serotonergic receptors, synthetic enzymes and 5-HT transporter. Neuropharmacology 1994; 33:433-440.

Srinivasan M, Sudheer AR, Menon VP. Ferulic Acid: therapeutic potential through its antioxidant property. J Clin Biochem Nutr. 2007;40(2):92-100.

Soares JC, Mann JJ. The functional neuroanatomy of mood disorders. J. Psychiatr. Res. 1997; 31, 393–432.

Subhash MN, Jagadeesh S. Imipramine-induced changes in 5-HT2 receptor sites and inositoltrisphosphate levels in rat brain., 1997. Neurochem Res. 22, 1095-1099.

Sultana R, Ravagna A, Mohmmad-Abdul H, Calabrese V, Butterfield DA. Ferulic acid ethyl ester protects neurons against amyloid beta- peptide(1-42)-induced oxidative stress and neurotoxicity: relationship to antioxidant activity. J Neurochem. 2005 Feb;92(4):749-758.

Tao X, Finkbeiner S, Arnold DB, Shaywitz AJ, Greenberg ME. Calcium influx regulates BDNF transcription by a CREB family transcription factor-dependent mechanism. Neuron 1997; 20: 709–726.

Tatarczynska, E., Klodzinska, A., Chojnacka-Wojcik, E. Effects of combined administration of 5-HT1A and/or 5-HT1B receptor antagonists and paroxetine or fluoxetine in the forced swimming test in rats. Pol. J. Pharmacol. 2002; 54, 615-623.

Toth M, Shenk T. Antagonist-mediated down-regulation of 5-hydroxytryptamine type 2 receptor gene expression: modulation of transcription. Mol. Pharmacol., 1994; 45, 1095-1100.

Tredici G, Miloso M, Nicolini G, Galbiati S, Cavaletti G, Bertelli A. Resveratrol, map kinases and neuronal cells: might wine be a neuroprotectant? Drugs Exp Clin Res. 1999; 25(2-3):99-103.

Tsuji M, Takeda H, Matsumiya T. Protective effects of 5-HT1A receptor agonists against emotional changes produced by stress stimuli are related to their neuroendocrine effects. Br. J. Pharmacol. 2001; 134, 585-595.

Uchida S, Hirai K, Hatanaka J, Hanato J, Umegaki K, Yamada S. Antinociceptive effects of St. John's wort, Harpagophytum procumbens extract and grape seed proanthocyanidins extract in mice. Biol Pharm Bull 2008;31:240–245.

Walther DJ, Peter JU, Bashammakh S, Hörtnagl H, Voits M, Fink H, Bader M. Synthesis of serotonin by a second tryptophan hydroxylase isoform. Science. 2003;299(5603):76

Warner-Schmidt JL, Duman RS. Hippocampal neurogenesis: opposing effects of stress and antidepressant treatment. Hippocampus 2006; 16, 239–249.

Wang R, Xu Y, Wu HL, Li YB, Li YH, Guo JB, Li XJ. The antidepressant effects of curcumin in the forced swimming test involve 5-HT1 and 5-HT2 receptors. Eur J Pharmacol. 2008; 578(1):43-50

Wang R, Li YB, Li YH, Xu Y, Wu HL, Li XJ. Curcumin protects against glutamate excitotoxicity in rat cerebral cortical neurons by increasing brain-derived neurotrophic factor level and activating TrkB. Brain Res. 2008;1210:84-91.

Wang R, Li YH, Xu Y, Li YB, Wu HL, Guo H, Zhang JZ, Zhang JJ, Pan XY, Li XJ. Curcumin produces neuroprotective effects via activating brain-derived neurotrophic factor/TrkB-dependent MAPK and PI-3K cascades in rodent cortical neurons. Prog Neuropsychopharmacol Biol Psychiatry. 2010;34(1):147-153.

Welner SA, De Montigny C, Desroches J, Desjardins P, Suranyi-Cadotte BE. Autoradiographic quantification of serotonin 1A receptors in rat brain following antidepressant drug treatment. Synapse 1989; 4:347–352.

Whitaker-Azmitia PM. Role of serotonin and other neurotransmitter receptors in brain development: basis for developmental pharmacology. Pharmacol Rev. 1991; 43(4):553-561.

Xu Y, Ku BS, Yao HY, Lin YH, Ma X, Zhang YH, Li XJ. Antidepressant effects of curcumin in the forced swim test and olfactory bulbectomy models of depression in rats. Pharmacol Biochem Behav. 2005;82(1):200-206.

Xu Y, Ku B, Cui L, Li X, Barish PA, Foster TC, Ogle WO. Curcumin reverses impaired hippocampal neurogenesis and increases serotonin receptor 1A mRNA and brain-derived neurotrophic factor expression in chronically stressed rats. Brain Res. 2007;1162:9-18.

Xu Y, Ku B, Tie L, Yao H, Jiang W, Ma X, Li X. Curcumin reverses the effects of chronic stress on behavior, the HPA axis, BDNF expression and phospphorylation of CREB. Brain Res. 2006; 1122: 56-64.

Xu Y, Li S, Chen R, Li G, Barish PA, You W, Chen L, Lin M, Ku B, Pan J, Ogle WO. Antidepressant-like effect of low molecular proanthocyanidin in mice: involvement of monoaminergic system. Pharmacol Biochem Behav. 2010; 94(3):447-53.

Xu Y, Wang Z, You W, Zhang X, Li S, Barish PA, Vernon MM, Du X, Li G, Pan J, Ogle WO. Antidepressant-like effect of trans-resveratrol: Involvement of serotonin and noradrenaline system. Eur Neuropsychopharmacol. 2010; 20(6):405-13.

Yabe T, Hirahara H, Harada N, Ito N, Nagai T, Sanagi T, Yamada H. Ferulic acid induces neural progenitor cell proliferation in vitro and in vivo. Neuroscience. 2010; 165(2):515-24.

Yáñez M, Fraiz N, Cano E, Orallo F. Inhibitory effects of cis- and trans-resveratrol on noradrenaline and 5-hydroxytryptamine uptake and on monoamine oxidase activity. Biochem Biophys Res Commun. 2006; 344(2):688-95.

Yogeeta SK, Gnanapragasam A, Kumar SS, Subhashini R, Sathivel A, Devaki T. Synergistic interactions of ferulic acid with ascorbic acid: its cardioprotective role during isoproterenol induced myocardial infarction in rats. Mol Cell Biochem. 2006;283(1-2):139-146.

Young EA, Haskett RF, Murphy-Weihberg V, Watson SJ, Akil H. Loss of glucocorticoid fast feed back in depression. Arch. Gen. Psychiatry. 1991; 48, 693-699.

15

Separation and Quantification of Component Monosaccharides of Cold Water-Soluble Polysaccharides from *Ephedra sinica* by MECC with Photodiode Array Detector

Haixue Kuang, Yong-Gang Xia and Bing-You Yang
Key Laboratory of Chinese Materia Medica,
(Heilongjiang University of Chinese Medicine), Ministry of Education, Harbin,
China

1. Introduction

The *Ephedra* plant, or "Mahuang" of traditional Chinese medicine, is one of the oldest medicinal plants known to mankind. More than 45 species of *Ephedra* plants exist and are indigenous to regions of Asia, North, Central and South America and Europe. Mahuang contains ephedrine alkaloids as their principal components, which are primarily localized in the aerial parts of the plant [1]. In recent years, many herbs used in popular medicine have been reported to contain polysaccharides with a great variety of biological activities and the polysaccharides are also demonstrated to be one of the main bioactive constituents of *Ephedra* plant except for a series of ephedrine alkaloids [2-4]. For these reasons, great interest arose on the reliable analytical methods of the Mahuang polysaccharides, which can be used for exploring the new functional products with polysaccharides due to its pharmacological importance and application in the pharmaceutical industry. Immunosuppressive effects of acidic polysaccharides from the stems of *E. sinica* have been demonstrated by carbon clearance test, delayed type hypersensitivity reaction and humoral immune response *in vivo* [2].

The commonly used separation techniques for carbohydrate analysis are gas chromatography (GC), high-performance liquid chromatography (HPLC), and capillary electrophoresis (CE) [5-7]. GC is a very classical method to analyze monosaccharide compositions of polysaccharides. Neutral monosaccharides are derivatized by silylation or acetylation before analysis, whereas acidic monosaccharides such as glucuronic acid and galacturonic acid can not be derivatized at all [8]. The uronic acid contents can be calculated by the difference between before and after carboxyl reduction of polysaccharides [9, 10]. So it is very laborious to calculate the uronic acid contents by GC method. Most of the HPLC and CE techniques are often used labeling with either fluorescence or UV tags for enhanced detection because these native carbohydrates are lack of chromophores or fluorophores in the structure. The reagent 1-phenyl-3-methyl-5-pyrazolone (PMP) is one of the popular labels that react with the reducing carbohydrate under mild conditions, requiring no acid catalyst and causing no desialylation and isomerization [11-16]. CE seems to possess several advantages over HPLC by offering higher separation efficiencies, yielding shorter analysis time, requiring small sample amounts, and consuming lower amounts of expensive reagents and solvents. It has the potential to become an important analytical separation tool for carbohydrate determination. Capillary zone electrophoresis (CZE) has been developed and successfully applied to analyze and quantify the aldoses and uronic acids [11-16]. However, few reports were proposed using MECC for the separation of the aldoses and uronic acids. The present paper is specifically concerned with the simultaneous separation of the 8 monosaccharides (aldoses and uronic acids) possibly found in natural herbs using pre-column PMP derivatization MECC and UV detection at 254 nm. Furthermore, the developed MECC method was applied to the quantitative analysis of component monosaccharides in the cold water-soluble polysaccharides from E. sinica.

2. Materials and methods

2.1 Rragents and standards
D-mannose (Man), L-rhamnose (Rha), D-glucose (Glc), D-galactose (Gal), L-arabinose (Ara), D-xylose (Xyl), D-glucuronic acid (GlcUA), D-galacturonic acid (GalUA) and sulfuric acid (H_2SO_4) were purchased from Sigma (St. Louis, USA). Trifluoroacetic acid (TFA) was obtained from Merck (Darmstadt, Germany). 1-Phenyl-3-methyl-5-pyrazolone (PMP), purchased from Beijing Reagent Plant (Beijing, China), was recrystallized twice from chromatographic grade methanol before use. Throughout the study deionised water was used, prepared by a Milli-Q water system (Millipore, MA, USA). The pH value of the electrolyte solution was measured with a Sartorius PB-20 pH meter with Sartorius pH/ATC electrode (Sartorius, CO, Germany) calibrated with commercial buffers of pH 7.00, 10.00, and 12.0 (Titrisol, Merck kGaA, Germany). All other chemicals were of the highest grade available.

2.2 Plant material
The dry stems of E. sinica were collected in March 2007 from Datong of Shanxi Province, China and identified by Prof. Zhenyue Wang of Heilongjiang University of Chinese Medicine. The voucher specimen (20070016) was deposited at Herbarium of Heilongjiang University of Chinese Medicine, Harbin, P. R. China.

2.3 Extraction of polysaccharides from E. sinica
The dry stems of E. sinica were ground to powders, and submitted to extractions as follows: dry powders (1.0 kg) were extracted 3 times with 10 vol of 95% EtOH under reflux for 3 h each time to remove lipids. The residue was dried in air and then extracted 3 times with 10 vol of distilled water for 24 h (each time) at 4 °C. The combined aqueous extracts were filtered, concentrated 10-fold, and 95% EtOH added to final concentration of 80%. The precipitate was dissolved in 600 mL of water and deproteinated 15 times with 200 mL of 5:1 chloroform -n-butanol as described by Staub (1965). The resulting aqueous fraction was extensively dialyzed (cut-off M_w 3500 Da) against tap water for 48 h and distilled water for 48 h and precipitated again by adding a 5 fold volume of ethanol. After centrifugation, the precipitate was washed with anhydrous ethanol and then dissolved in water and lyophilised to yield the cold water soluble polysaccharide (8.5 g) was collected by centrifugation (3000 rpm, 10 min, 20 °C).

2.4 MECC equipment and conditions

The analysis of PMP-labeled monosaccharides was carried out on a P/ACE MDQ capillary electrophoresis instrument (Beckman Coulter, Fullerton, CA, USA). An integrated P/ACE 32 Karat Station (software version 4.0) was used to perform the data collection and to control the operational variables of the system. Separation was carried out in an unmodified fused silica capillary (48.5 cm × 50 µm i.d., effective length 40 cm). Both the capillary and samples were thermostatted to 25 °C. The samples were injected with a pressure of 0.5 psi for 5 s. The separation voltage was raised linearly within 0.2 min from 0 to 20 kV. Detection was done with direct UV monitoring using a photodiode array detector at wavelength 254 nm.

A new capillary from Yongnian Optical Fiber Factory (Hebei Province, China) was activated by washing consecutively with each of 0.1 M phosphoric acid (15 min), water (10 min), 0.1M sodium hydroxide (15 min), and water (10 min). At the beginning of each working day, the capillary was prewashed with 0.1 M phosphoric acid (2 min), water (2 min), 0.1 M sodium hydroxide (2 min), water (2 min) and running buffer (2 min), respectively. Between analyses the capillaries were consecutively rinsed with 0.1 M sodium hydroxide (1 min), water (1 min) and running buffer (1 min).

2.5 Complete acid hydrolysis

20 mg of polysaccharide sample was dissolved in 2 ml of 2 M TFA in an ampoule (5 ml). The ampoule was sealed under a nitrogen atmosphere and kept in boiling water bath to hydrolyze the polysaccharide into component monosaccharides for 10 h. After being cooled to room temperature, the reaction mixture was centrifuged at 1000 rpm for 5 min. The supernatant was collected and dried under a reduced pressure. The hydrolyzed and dried sample solutions are added with 1 ml distilled water and then ready for the following experiments.

2.6 Derivatization procedure

PMP derivatization of monosaccharides was carried out as described previously with proper modification [11-17]. 200 µl of individual standard monosaccharide, or mix standard monosaccharide solutions, or the hydrolyzed polysaccharide samples were placed in the 2.0 ml centrifuge tubes, respectively, then 0.5 M methanol solution (100 µl) of PMP and 0.3 M aqueous NaOH (100 µl) were added to each. Each mixture was allowed to react for 30 min at 70 °C water bath, then cooled to room temperature and neutralized with 100 µl of 0.3 M HCl. The resulting solution was performed on liquid-liquid extraction with same volume of isoamyl acetate (two times) and chloroform (one time), respectively. After being shaken vigorously and centrifuged, the organic phase was carefully discarded to remove the excess reagents. Then the aqueous layer was filtered through a 0.45 µm membrane and diluted with water before MECC analysis.

2.7 Method validation

The regression equations were calculated in the form of $y = a\,x + b$, where y was the peak areas and x was the concentration of analytes. The signal-to-noise of 3:1 and 10:1 were used to establish LOD and LOQ, respectively. The measurement of intra- and inter-day variability was utilized to determine the precision of this newly developed method. The intraday variation was determined by analyzing the same mixed standard water solution for five times within 1 day. While for inter-day variability test, the solution was examined in triplicate for consecutive 3 days. Stability of sample solution was tested at 0, 4, 8, 12, 24 and 48 h within 2 days. All solutions were kept at 4 °C before analysis. The analytes showed stable in water solution (RSD < 3.45%) at 4 °C during the tested period.

3. Results and discussion

3.1 Method development

We can only label carbohydrates according to Fig. 1 [16], usually yields neutral sugar derivatives which become negatively charged in aqueous basic solutions due to the partial dissociation of the enolic hydroxyl group of the PMP tag. In this study, the method development was achieved by optimizing background electrolyte pH, SDS and borax concentration of the buffer, applied voltage and capillary temperature.

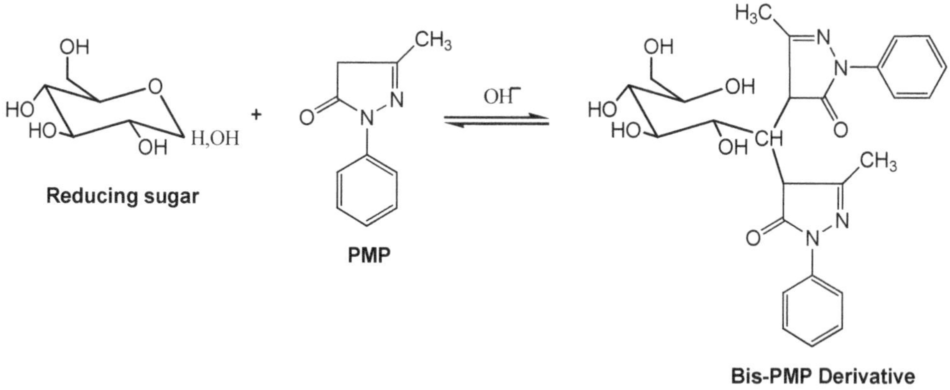

Fig. 1. Illustration of condensation reaction with PMP

3.1.1 Effect of pH

The effect of pH on the separation was also investigated in the pH range from 9.7 to 10.75 using borate buffer solutions as background electrolytes. Fig. 2 is comparison of four pH electrolytes in the analysis of 8 carbohydrates, from which the separation conditions are revealed more clearly. The result reveals that the pH of buffer had great influence on the resolutions and the migration time. Supposing an appropriate pH (9.70) chosen, ara and glc have been co-eluted as one peak. Only man, gal, glcUA and galUA have the high resolutions. If a higher pH (10.0 or 10.23) is adopted, there are poor resolutions between ara and glc. And if we use pH 10.75, good symmetry and the resolution for each analyte was achieved. Thus pH 10.75 was chosen as the optimal running buffer condition.

3.1.2 Effect of buffer and SDS concentration

The separation of PMP-labeled carbohydrates was very sensitive to borate buffer concentrations and SDS concentration in MECC. In this study, borate concentration in the range of 20–33 mM was evaluated (Fig. 3). The results indicated that the migration time of PMP-labeled carbohydrates generally increased with a gradual increasing of buffer

concentrations. Taking the shorter run-time and good resolution into consideration, 25 mM
borate buffer solution was selected and the maximum resolution was obtained.

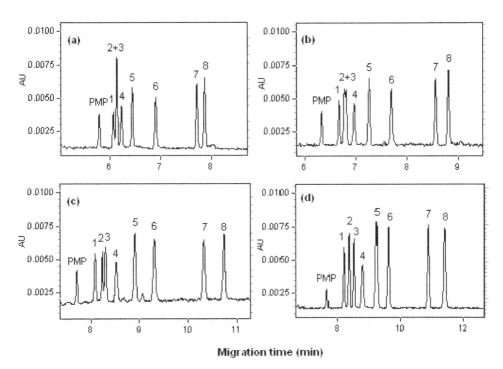

Migration time (min)

Fig. 2. Comparison of electropherograms of PMP derivatives of 8 standard
monosaccharides with 25 mM borate buffer and 30 mM SDS at four pH electrolytes, 1 mM
each. Peak identities: 1, xyl; 2, ara; 3 glc; 4 rha; 5, man; 6, gal; 7, glcUA; 8, galUA. Separation
conditions: applied voltage, +20 kV; Separation conditions: +25 kV; detection, 254 nm direct
mode; injection pressure, 0.5 psi for 5 s; capillary, fused-silica 40.0/48.5 cm (Ldet/Ltot);
separation temperature, 25 °C. The pH of borate buffer: (a) pH 9.70; (b) pH 10.00; (c) pH
10.23; (d) pH 10.75

Different concentrations of SDS (25, 30 and 35 mM) at pH 10.75 and 25 mM borate buffer on
the separation of analytes were studied (Fig. 4). It was found that Xyl and Ara were not well
separated at 20 mM SDS with poor resolution, but best resolution and highest theory plates
were achieved at 30 mM SDS. Increasing SDS concentration, however, remarkably increased
the migration time of all analytes. Therefore, 30 mM SDS was chosen as the optimal SDS
concentration thus it was chosen for the further experiments.

3.1.3 Effect of capillary temperature and voltage
The temperature of the analysis may sometimes be important in MECC, as fluctuations in
the temperature may affect the viscosity of the running buffer, leading to higher analyte
electrophoretic mobilities and shorter analysis time. The temperature changes can also affect

the pH of the buffer. In this case, 25 °C is most optimal. In addition, the effects of three voltage values (10-28 kV) on separation of the analytes also were studied. The results showed that the good resolution and acceptable migration time were achieved at 25 kV.

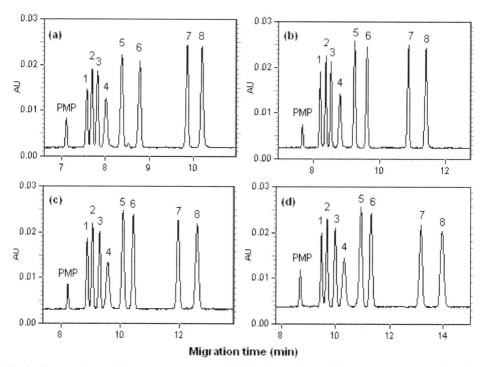

Fig. 3. Comparison of electropherograms of PMP derivatives of 8 standard monosaccharides at four buffer concentration electrolytes, 1 mM each. Borate concentration: (a) 20 mM; (b) 25 mM; (c) 27 mM; (c) 30 mM. Peak identities and other analytical conditions were in Fig. 2.

To achieve optimal separation, the operation at 20 mM of borax and 30 mM SDS at pH 10.75, capillary temperature 25 °C and applied voltage 20 kV, a complete baseline resolution for carbohydrate derivatives can be achieved within the shortest time. Under the proposed conditions, the separation of nine PMP-labeled carbohydrates is achieved within 12 min. The separation of standard mixture consisting of 8 PMP-labeled carbohydrates is shown in Fig. 5A.

3.2 Validation of the method developed

The MECC method was validated in terms of linearity, reproducibility, limit of detection (LOD) and precision. The linearity was verified by the analysis of six points in the range of 37.5 - 600.00 μM, and the linear regression parameters of the calibration curves were shown in Table 1. As a consequence, the good linearity (correlation coefficient $R^2 > 0.9993$) between y (peak area ratio of the analytes with internal standard) and x (concentration of the standards) was achieved in the tested range. Furthermore, LOD of each tested analyte was obtained by injecting 0.5 psi for 5 s of gradational dilutions of a standard mixture

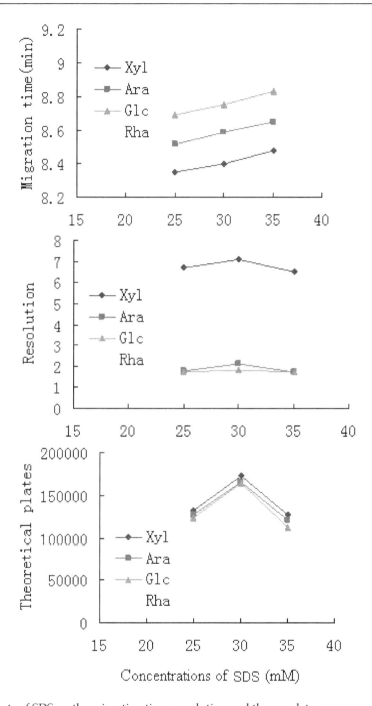

Fig. 4. Effects of SDS on the migration time, resolution and theory plates.

derivatized as mentioned above in the derivatization procedure, followed by the comparison of peak height with baseline noise level and a signal-to-noise ratio (S/N) of 3 assigned the detection limit. The results showed that the LOD of the monosaccharides was in the range from 10.5 to 11.7 µM (Table 1), indicating that the sensitivity of the method was satisfactory.

Carbohydrats[a]	Regression equation $(y = a + b\,x)$[b]		correlation coefficient	LOD[c] (µM)	LOQ[d] (µM)
	a	b			
Xyl	-0.2106	0.0134	0.9998	10.5	33.6
Ara	-0.2681	0.0172	0.9994	11.2	35.8
Glc	-0.1576	0.0078	0.9993	11.4	36.4
Rha	-0.1196	0.0086	0.9997	11.7	37.5
Man	-0.1049	0.0203	0.9995	10.9	34.8
Gal	-0.26	0.0225	0.9995	11.3	36.0
GalUA	-0.4612	0.0232	0.9992	10.8	34.6

[a] Quantitated with a calibration curve at = 254 nm
[b] The y and x are peak area ratio of the analytes to internal standard (GlcUA) and concentration of the analytes (37.5-600µM), respectively
[c] LOD corresponds to concentrations giving a signal-to-noise ratio of 3.
[d] LOQ corresponds to concentrations giving a signal-to-noise ratio of 10.

Table 1. Linearity of CE method of different carbohydrate

Carbohydrats	Intra-day precision (RSD%, n = 5)		Inter-day precision (RSD%, n = 3)	
	Retention time	Peak area	Retention time	Peak area
Xyl	1.25	2.38	1.36	3.21
Ara	2.03	2.97	1.58	3.56
Glc	1.69	1.97	2.21	4.03
Rha	2.31	2.46	1.99	3.69
Man	2.09	2.36	2.16	2.79
Gal	1.95	2.57	1.94	2.88
GlcUA	1.85	2.77	2.37	4.35
GalUA	1.38	2.89	1.96	4.27

Table 2. Precision of the retention time and peak area of analytes in the present method

Moreover, method precision was also determined by measuring repeatability (intra-day variability) and intermediate precision (inter-day variability) of retention time and peak area for each tested monosaccharide. The precision of method was calculated as the coefficient of variation (RSD) for five successive injections of each tested monosaccharide at the concentration of 1 mM and the results were summarized in Table 3. The results showed that the intra-day reproducibility (RSD values) were less than 2.31% for the migration time and 2.97% for the peak areas, and the interday RSD values were less than 2.37% for the migration time and 4.35% for the peak areas, indicating that the method precision was satisfactory.

Component	added amount (µM)	found amount (µM)	recovery(%)[a] means ± SD	RSD (%)[b]
Ara	270	270.2	100.15 ± 4.03	4.02
Glc	62	61.7	99.51 ± 3.63	3.65
Rha	35	35.4	105.13 ± 2.79	2.76
Man	25	24.6	98.45 ± 2.86	2.91
Gal	53	53.5	103.97 ± 3.51	3.48
GalUA	30	29.7	97.28 ± 3.73	3.83

a Recovery (%) = [(mean of measured concentration−spiked concentration)/spiked concentration]×100.
b RSD (%) = (SD/mean)×100

Table 3. Recoveries of six monosaccharides in sample analysis (n= 6)

3.3 Analysis of the cold water-soluble polysaccharide extract from E. sinica

This experiment was designed to develop a rapid, repeatable and accurate MECC method for the quantification of the component carbohydrates in the cold water-soluble polysaccharide extract from E. sinica. In order to evaluate the applicability of the proposed method, the polysaccharide was hydrolyzed with 2M TFA, and PMP-labeled as described in the experimental section and finally, the released monosaccharide derivatives were analyzed by the described MECC method under the optimized conditions using GlcUA as internal standard. Fig. 5B shows a typical chromatogram of the cold water-soluble polysaccharide sample. As can be seen, the PMP derivatives of the component monosaccharides released from the Mahuang polysaccharide sample could be still baseline separated and the component monosaccharides could be identified by comparing with the chromatogram of the mixture of standard monosaccharides (Fig. 5A). The results showed that the cold water-soluble polysaccharide extract from E. sinica was a typical heteropolysaccharide and was composed of arabinose, glucose, rhamnose, mannose, galactose and galacturonic acid in the molar rate of 4.36:1.43:1.00:0.55:0.41:0.85:0.45, and their corresponding mole percentages were 57.24%, 13.12%, 7.16%, 5.40%, 11.17%, and 5.87% (mol%), respectively. It was clear that the predominantly composition monosaccharides in the cold water-soluble polysaccharide extract from E. sinica were arabinose up to 57.24% (mol%) of total carbohydrates, and only 5.87% of total carbohydrates was galacturonic acid.

Furthermore, recovery experiments were performed in order to investigate the accuracy of the method. Known amounts of each monosaccharide solute were added to the sample detected, and the resulting spiked sample was subjected to the entire analytical sequence. Each solute was spiked at a close concentration with the sample and recoveries were calculated based on the difference between the total amount determined in the spiked samples and the amount observed in the non-spiked samples. All analyses were carried out in triplicate. The results showed that the recoveries of all the monosaccharides ranged between 97.28% and 105.13% and the RSD values were within 2.76–4.02% (Table 3). Such results further demonstrated that this method is precise and practical for the analysis of polysaccharide samples from E. sinica.

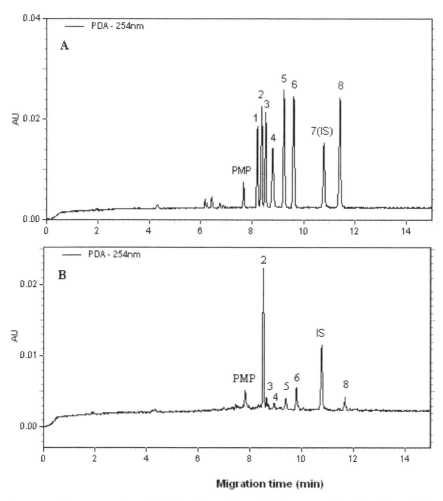

Fig. 5. Electropherograms of PMP derivatives of standard monosaccharides (A) and the sample (B). Peak identities and other analytical conditions were in Fig. 2.

4. Conclusions

In recent years, the monosaccharides PMP derivatives mentioned above were successfully separated by CZE and HPLC although the analysis was accomplished for a long time [11-16]. However, in this study, as shown in Fig. 5A, various PMP derivatives of monosaccharides were shown to separate quite nicely in MECC within 12 min and seven composition monosaccharides were successfully identified and the assay results were satisfactory. The separation is based on the differential distribution of the PMP derivatives between the aqueous mobile phase and the micellar phase. The applicability of the SDS micellar system was extended to the identification and quantitation of monosaccharides obtained from carbohydrate hydrolyzates from polysaccharide. The shape of the peaks was

very sharp and it was clear that a substantial improvement in the separation of neutral sugar
and uronic acid derivatives was obtained by MECC method, and thus, the analytical cost is
lower and is also eco-friendly for its non-consumption of organic solvents as compared with
other analytical techniques.

5. Acknowledgements

The authors wish to thank financial support for this study by the Major State Basic Research
Development Program of China (973 Program 2006CB504708), State Key Creative New Drug
Project of 12th Five-year Plan of China (2011ZX09102-006-01), National Natural Science
Foundation of China (30973870), China Postdoctoral Science Foundation project
(20110490111), Heilongjiang Postdoctoral Science Foundation project (LBH-Z10019) and
Heilongjiang University of Chinese Medicine Doctor Innovative Foundation project
(B201002).

6. References

[1] Jiangsu New Medical College (1986). *Dictionary of Chinese Materia Medica*. Shanghai:
    Shanghai people's press; p. 2221-2224.
[2] Kuang, H. X., Xia, Y. G., Yang, B.Y., Wang, Q. H., and Wang, Y. H. Screening and
    comparison of the immunosuppressive activities of polysaccharides from the stems
    of *Ephedra sinica* Stapf. *Carbohydrate Polymers*, 2010, 83 (2), 787-795.
[3] Cheng, R. M., Zhu, G. X., and Xu, Z. Y. (2001). Effect of different extracts from Ephedra
    on cell immunity. *Journal of Nanjing TCM University*, 17, 234–236.
[4] Meng, D. L., Yan, S. H., and Xu, Z. Y. (2007). Effect of ephedran on erythrocytolysin
    formation of mouse caused by sheep erythrocyte. *Journal of Jiangsu University*, 17,
    379–381.
[5] Guo, L., Xie, M. Y., Yan, A. P., and Wan, Y. Q. (2006). Simultaneous determination of five
    synthetic antioxidants in edible vegetable oil by GC-MS. *Analytical and Bioanalytical
    Chemistry*, 386, 1881-1887.
[6] Daotian, F., and Roger, A. (1995). Monosaccharide composition analysis of
    oligosaccharides and glycoproteins by high-performance liquid chromatography.
    Analytical Biochemistry, 227, 377-384.
[7] Lv, Y., Yang, X. B., Zhao, Y., Ruan, Y., Yang, Y., and Wang, Z. Z. (2009). Separation and
    quantification of component monosaccharides of the tea polysaccharides from
    Gynostemma pentaphyllum by HPLC with indirect UV detection. *Food Chemestry*, 112,
    742-746.
[8] Chen, Y., Xie, M. Y., Wang, Y. X., Nie, S. P., and Chang, L. (2009). Analysis of the
    monosaccharide composition of purified polysaccharides in *Ganoderma atrum* by
    capillary gas chromatography. *Phytochemical Analysis*, 20, 503-510.
[9] Perry, M. B., MacLean, L. L., Patrauchan, M. A., and Vinogradov, E. (2007). The structure
    of the exocellular polysaccharide produced by *Rhodococcus sp*. RHA1. *Carbohydrate
    Research*, 342, 2223-2229.
[10] Xia, Y. G., Liang, J., Yang, B. Y., Wang, Q. H., and Kuang, H. X. A new method for
    quantitative determination of two uronic acids by CZE with direct UV detection.
    Biomedical chromagraphy, doi:10.1002/bmc.1564.

[11] Andersen, K. E., Bjergegaard, C., Mller, P., Srensen, J. C., and Srensen, H. (2003). High performance capillary electrophoresis with indirect UV detection for determination of α-galactosides in leguminose and brassicaceae. *Journal of Agricultural and Food Chemistry, 51,* 6391-6397.

[12] Daotian, F. and Roger, A. (1995). Monosaccharide composition analysis of oligosaccharides and glycoproteins by high-performance liquid chromatography. *Analytical Biochemistry, 227,* 377-384.

[13] Honda, S., Akao, E., Suzuki, S., Okuda, M., Kakehi, K., and Nakamura, J. (1989). High performance liquid chromatography of reducing carbohydrates as strongly ultraviolet-absorbing and electrochemically sensitive 1-phenyl-3-methyl-5-pyrazolone derivatives. *Analytical Chemistry, 180,* 351-357.

[14] Honda, S., Suzuki, S., and Taga, A. (2003). Analysis of carbohydrates as 1-phenyl-3-methyl-5 -pyrazolone derivatives by capillary/microchip electrophoresis and capillary electrochro -matography. *Journal of Pharmaceutical and Biomedical Analysis, 30,* 1689-1714.

[15] Wang, Q. J. and Fang, Y. Z. (2004). Analysis of sugars in traditional Chinese drugs. *Journal of Chromatography B, 812,* 309-324.

[16] Xia, Y. G., Wang, Q. H., Liang, J., Yang, B. Y., Li, G. Y., and Kuang, H. X. Development and application of a rapid and efficient CZE method coupled with correction factors for determination of monosaccharide composition of acidic hetero-polysaccharides from *Ephedra sinica. Phytochemical Analysis,* 2011, 22, 103-111.

[17] Zhang, L. Y., Xu, J., Zhang, L. H., Zhang, W. B., and Zhang, Y. K. (2003). Determination of 1-phenyl-3-methyl-5-pyrazolone-labeled carbohydrates by liquid chromatography and micellar electrokinetic chromatography. *Journal of Chromatography B, 793,* 159-165.

Permissions

The contributors of this book come from diverse backgrounds, making this book a truly international effort. This book will bring forth new frontiers with its revolutionizing research information and detailed analysis of the nascent developments around the world.

We would like to thank Haixue Kuang, for lending his expertise to make the book truly unique. He has played a crucial role in the development of this book. Without his invaluable contribution this book wouldn't have been possible. He has made vital efforts to compile up to date information on the varied aspects of this subject to make this book a valuable addition to the collection of many professionals and students.

This book was conceptualized with the vision of imparting up-to-date information and advanced data in this field. To ensure the same, a matchless editorial board was set up. Every individual on the board went through rigorous rounds of assessment to prove their worth. After which they invested a large part of their time researching and compiling the most relevant data for our readers. Conferences and sessions were held from time to time between the editorial board and the contributing authors to present the data in the most comprehensible form. The editorial team has worked tirelessly to provide valuable and valid information to help people across the globe.

Every chapter published in this book has been scrutinized by our experts. Their significance has been extensively debated. The topics covered herein carry significant findings which will fuel the growth of the discipline. They may even be implemented as practical applications or may be referred to as a beginning point for another development. Chapters in this book were first published by InTech; hereby published with permission under the Creative Commons Attribution License or equivalent.

The editorial board has been involved in producing this book since its inception. They have spent rigorous hours researching and exploring the diverse topics which have resulted in the successful publishing of this book. They have passed on their knowledge of decades through this book. To expedite this challenging task, the publisher supported the team at every step. A small team of assistant editors was also appointed to further simplify the editing procedure and attain best results for the readers.

Our editorial team has been hand-picked from every corner of the world. Their multi-ethnicity adds dynamic inputs to the discussions which result in innovative outcomes. These outcomes are then further discussed with the researchers and contributors who give their valuable feedback and opinion regarding the same. The feedback is then collaborated with the researches and they are edited in a comprehensive manner to aid the understanding of the subject.

Apart from the editorial board, the designing team has also invested a significant amount of their time in understanding the subject and creating the most relevant covers. They scrutinized every image to scout for the most suitable representation of the subject and create an appropriate cover for the book.

The publishing team has been involved in this book since its early stages. They were actively engaged in every process, be it collecting the data, connecting with the contributors or procuring relevant information. The team has been an ardent support to the editorial, designing and production team. Their endless efforts to recruit the best for this project, has resulted in the accomplishment of this book. They are a veteran in the field of academics and their pool of knowledge is as vast as their experience in printing. Their expertise and guidance has proved useful at every step. Their uncompromising quality standards have made this book an exceptional effort. Their encouragement from time to time has been an inspiration for everyone.

The publisher and the editorial board hope that this book will prove to be a valuable piece of knowledge for researchers, students, practitioners and scholars across the globe.

List of Contributors

John W.M. Yuen, Sonny H.M. Tse and Jolene Y.K. Yung
School of Nursing, The Hong Kong Polytechnic University, Hong Kong SAR, China

Yuhui Zhou
Nanjing University of Chinese Medicine, China
Tianjing Medical University General Hospital, China
Hongkong Baptist University, Hongkong, China

Fei Xiong, Zhenzhou Huang, Luyu Zheng, Miao Jiang, Yuping Tang, Jian Ma, Zhen Zhan, Jinao Duan and Xu Zhang
Nanjing University of Chinese Medicine, China

Ming Jiang
Hongkong Baptist University, Hongkong, China

Ying Xu and Chong Zhang
Department of Behavioral Medicine and Psychiatry, West Virginia University, WV, USA

William O. Ogle
Crayton Pruitt Family Department of Biomedical Engineering and Evelyn F. & William L. Mcknight Brain Institute, University of Florida, Gainesville, FL, USA

Huige Li
Department of Pharmacology, University Medical Center, Johannes Gutenberg University, Mainz, Germany

Rui-Zhi Zhao
Second Affiliated Clinical College, Guangzhou University of Chinese Medicine, Nei Huan XiLu, Guangzhou Daxue Cheng, Guangzhou, China

Qihe Xu, Yuen Fei Wong, Shanshan Qu, Qingyang Kong, Qin Hu, Mazhar Noor and Bruce M. Hendry
King's College London, Department of Renal Medicine, The Rayne Institute, London, United Kingdom

Xiu-Li Zhang and Xin-Miao Liang
Multi-Component TCM Group, Dalian Institute of Chemical Physics, Chinese Academy of Sciences, Dalian PR China

Adrián Angel Inchauspe
La Plata National University, Argentina

Lulu Fu and Hong Xu
Victoria University, Endeavour College of Natural Health, Australia

Yong Wang and Chunhui Luo
College of Bioscience, Shenzhen University, Shenzhen, China

Chenggang Huang, Bin Wu, Zhixiong Li, Yihong Tang and Zhaolin Sun
Shanghai Institute of Materia Medica, Chinese Academy of Sciences, Shanghai, China

Shuang Liu
Haerbin University of Commerce, Haerbin, China

Ke Wang and Longhai Jian
Shanghai Institute for Food and Drug Control, Shanghai, China

Shuyun Liu
Shanghai Institute of Materia Medica, Chinese Academy of Sciences, Shanghai, China
Shuguang Hospital, Shanghai University of Traditional Chinese Medicine, Shanghai, China

Dae Youn Hwang
Pusan National University, Republic of Korea

Zhen-Feng Chen, Hong Liang and Yan-Cheng Liu
Guangxi Normal University, China

Guo Li
Jiangxi University of Traditional Chinese Medicine, Nanchang, Jiangxi, PRC

Rui Wang
Program of Pharmacology, Weill Graduate School of Medical Science, Cornell University, New York, NY, USA

Ying Xu
Department of Behavioral Medicine and Psychiatry, West Virginia University Health Science Center, Morgantown, WV, USA

Haixue Kuang, Yong-Gang Xia and Bing-You Yang
Key Laboratory of Chinese Materia Medica, (Heilongjiang University of Chinese Medicine), Ministry of Education, Harbin, China

Printed in the USA
CPSIA information can be obtained
at www.ICGtesting.com
JSHW011443221024
72173JS00004B/920